Bladder Tumors and Other Topics in Urological Oncology

ETTORE MAJORANA INTERNATIONAL SCIENCE SERIES

Series Editor:

Antonino Zichichi

European Physical Society

Geneva, Switzerland

(LIFE SCIENCES)

Volume 1   **BLADDER TUMORS AND OTHER TOPICS IN UROLOGICAL ONCOLOGY**

Edited by M. Pavone-Macaluso, P. H. Smith, and F. Edsmyr

Bladder Tumors and Other Topics in Urological Oncology

Edited by

M. Pavone-Macaluso
University Polyclinic Hospital
Palermo, Italy

P. H. Smith
St. James University Hospital
Leeds, England

and

F. Edsmyr
Radiumhemmet
Stockholm, Sweden

Associate Editors:
M. R. G. Robinson and M. A. Aske

Plenum Press · New York and London

Library of Congress Cataloging in Publication Data

International Urological Oncology Course, 2d, Erice, Italy, 1978.
  Bladder tumors and other topics in urological oncology.

  (Ettore Majorana international science series: Life sciences; v. 1)
  "Proceedings of the Second International Urological Oncology Course, held in
Erice, Sicily, November 4—8, 1978."
  Sponsored by the Urological Group of the European Organisation for Research in
the Treatment of Cancer and others.
  Includes index.
  1. Bladder—Cancer—Congresses. 2. Genito-urinary organs—Cancer—Congresses.
I. Pavone-Macaluso, M. II. Smith, Philip Henry. III. Edsmyr, Folke, 1926—
IV. Title. V. Series.
RC280.B5I53 1978   616.9'94'6   79-20614
ISBN 0-306-40308-0

Proceedings of the Second International Urological Oncology Course,
held in Erice, Sicily, November 4—8, 1978

© 1980 Plenum Press, New York
A Division of Plenum Publishing Corporation
227 West 17th Street, New York, N.Y. 10011

Preface

This volume is a report of the proceedings of the Second International Urological Course held in the Ettore Majorana Centre in Erice, Sicily from the 4-8 November 1978. The meeting was sponsored by the Urological Group of the EORTC (European Organisation for Research in the Treatment of Cancer), the WHO Collaborating Centre for Bladder Cancer, the European Urological Association, the Italian Research Council (CNR), Italian League against Tumours, Italian Government and Regional Sicilian Government.

Contributions were accepted on the understanding that the editors could make certain changes leading towards a uniformity of style but accepting as a priority the importance of early publication, if necessary at the expense of stylistic perfection.

Editorial notes have been inserted at infrequent intervals, sometimes to summarise discussions and at others in an attempt to clarify certain issues or to highlight conflicting opinions. Although the work has been divided amongst the editors and co-editors it is only proper to acknowledge that the major role in collating and in correcting much of the material has fallen on Mrs M Aske who has also typed the manuscript. We should also like to acknowledge the kindness of the Yorkshire Regional Cancer Organisation who allowed Mrs Aske to devote much of her time to this work, Miss S Barrowby who has also given considerable secretarial assistance and the Department of Medical Photography, St James's University Hospital, Leeds whose staff are responsible for many of the illustrations.

Although the majority of contributions in this volume are concerned with carcinoma of the bladder a few papers of special interest dealing with other urological tumours have been included.

The next International Course on Urological Oncology will deal especially with tumours of the kidney and prostate and will be held in Erice in June 1981.

Contents

PART 2

BLADDER CANCER

AETIOLOGY, CYTOLOGY AND CARCINOMA IN SITU

DIAGNOSIS, PROGNOSIS AND CLINICAL ASPECTS

IMMUNOLOGY AND IMMUNOTHERAPY

SURGICAL TREATMENT

NEW TREATMENTS OF MULTIPLE SUPERFICIAL TUMORS

CHEMOTHERAPY

PART 3

PROSTATIC CANCER

PART 4

TUMORS OF THE MALE GENITALIA

Part 1
General Aspects of Urological Oncology

TNM CLASSIFICATION OF UROLOGICAL TUMOURS - 1978 EDITION

B VAN DER WERF-MESSING

Rotterdam Radiotherapy Institute, Groene Hilledijk 297

Rotterdam, The Netherlands

INTRODUCTION

The TNM classification of the UICC primarily aimed to describe the clinical extent of the malignancy without using surgical procedures except for the diagnostic biopsy. The purpose of the classification is to allow a comparison of various types of treatment (surgical, chemotherapeutic, radiotherapeutic, immunological etc.). It also helps in selecting the most appropriate type of treatment for the patient and in predicting prognosis.

The first TNM classification was developed under the leadership of Pierre Denoix of the Institut Gustave Roussy in Villejuif. The third edition of the TNM classification appeared at the Buenos Aires Cancer Congress in 1978.

The classification describes T, which is the extent of the primary growth; N, which means the involvement of lymph nodes, regional and in certain sites the juxta-regional nodes, and M, which denotes the presence or absence of distant metastases.

The third edition has been built up by joint cooperation of the German, American, Canadian TNM-Committee and the American Joint Committee. Various international organisations also contributed to this classification.

The third edition introduced some fundamental new aspects:-

1. Pathological TNM classification; ie. a postsurgical pathological classification has been added, based on the findings

3

during surgery and the pathological examination of the operative
specimen (p TNM).

2.   In cases of combined modality treatment (preoperative
radiotherapy or preoperative chemotherapy or a combination of both)
the symbol y precedes the P-classification (yP TNM).

3.   The third edition also offers the possibility of
classifying recurrences: the symbol r identifies this situation
(r TNM).

Apart from the above mentioned new general policies, the
urological classification has not changed essentially as compared
with the classification edited in 1972-1974, though there are minor
changes:

1.   The M-classification has been simplified and reduced to
MO and M1. To M1 optionally the involved organ can be added.

2.   As in the second edition, it is optional to add the
histological degree of differentiation of the growth, but in this
third edition, for prostate, bladder and kidney the grade GO has
been omitted, as it refers to benign disease, which is not
classified in the UICC TNM classification.

3.   The absence or presence of lymphatic invasion (l) and of
venous invasion (v) is optionally included in the classification.

                    CARCINOMA OF THE BLADDER

The T categories underwent a slight alteration:

Tis   applies to preinvasive carcinoma, carcinoma in situ or flat
      tumour.
Ta   indicates non-invasive papillary carcinoma.
T1   applies to tumours infiltrating the lamina propria.

The N categories have not been changed.

M categories. Biochemical tests to indicate the existence of
distant metastases are considered unreliable and have been deleted.

The p TNM corresponds to the clinical TNM classification.

According to various reports in the literature the T classification is very relevant and corresponds well with prognosis, but
the N classification appears so far to be unreliable. Apparently
more experience with regard to assessing lymphography in cases of
bladder cancer is required. The M classification is satisfactory.

PROSTATIC CANCER

There are no changes of the TNM classification in the third edition as compared with the previous edition. The postsurgical pathological classification corresponds roughly to the clinical classification with two minor exceptions.

T1 indicates an intracapsular tumour, surrounded by palpable normal gland. pT1 is a focal (single or multiple) carcinoma. T2 is a tumour confined to the gland, a nodule deforming contour but with lateral sulci and seminal vesicles not involved; pT2 is a diffuse carcinoma with or without extension to the capsule.

The N and M categories (both clinical and pathological) have not been changed.

Data from the literature shows that the clinical T categories and the pathological T categories correspond well with prognosis, but that the clinical N categories appear to be unreliable. Again more experience of radiographic assessment of lymph nodes is probably required. The pathological N categories have a good relationship with prognosis.

The M categories are reliable prognostic factors.

MALIGNANT TESTICULAR TUMOURS

There is no substantial change in the clinical TNM classification and in the pathological TNM classification.

In practice the T classifications are hardly ever used as prognosticators. The N categories appear to be of great prognostic importance: Lymph node involvement based on radiography appears to be reliable in about 70% of the cases. Both clinical and pathological involvement of lymph nodes worsen prognosis significantly.

CARCINOMA OF THE KIDNEY

The third edition classification is similar to the 1972-1974 classification. Biochemical tests to indicate the presence or absence of distant metastases have been abolished. Data from the literature (1,2) show that the clinical T classification based on angiography is unreliable. The P classification also appears to be unsatisfactory. The most reliable prognostic factor so far is renal vein involvement. Perhaps future CT-scan evaluation of renal vein involvement might contribute to a better classification.

REFERENCES

1.   Das, G., Chisholm, G. D. and Sherwood, T., Can Angiography
     stage Renal Carcinoma? Brit. J. Urol. 49, 611-614 (1977).

2.   van der Werf-Messing, B., van der Heul, R. O. and
     Ledeboer, R. Ch., Renal cell carcinoma trial. Cancer Clin.
     Trials, 1, 13-21 (1978).

T CATEGORY IN RENAL CARCINOMA

G D CHISHOLM

Department of Urology, Western General Hospital, Edinburgh
and Department of Surgery, University of Edinburgh,
Scotland

In the 1974 recommendations for the TNM classification of
urological tumours, the difficulty in achieving an accurate T
category for renal tumours was emphasised (Wallace et al, 1975).
In order to improve the accuracy of this T category it was recommended that an arteriogram was necessary and if this could not be done
then the minimum requirements could not be met ie. Tx.

Because the usefulness of arteriography has not always been
apparent in clinical practice, a comparison was made of the arteriogram findings (T category) and histopathological findings (P
category) in 36 patients with renal carcinoma (Das et al, 1977).

Using the standard abdominal aortogram and selective renal
arteriogram there was a 40% error rate in the T category. The main
error was overstaging: eight T3/P2 tumours appeared to be invading
the renal capsule or hilum on x-ray but this was not confirmed when
the specimen was examined. This error seemed to be due to the gross
deformity that occurred with some of these tumours - producing a
vascular pattern well beyond the renal outline. Histopathologically,
the capsule can be greatly stretched over the mass, but intact ie.
P2. Even tumours with vessels that are extra renal in origin can
also be wholly intrarenal ie. P2. Such angiograms cannot be taken
as evidence of tumour extension.

This study has shown that the inclusion of angiography to
improve the accuracy of the T category in renal tumours was not
justified. Since it is unlikely that any of the current investigative methods can reliably distinguish T2 from T3 tumours, the use
of a T category should either be abandoned or left as Tx until a
more accurate technique becomes available. It is concluded that the

only reliable method of describing the local extension of these
tumours consists of histopathological category (P) and invasion of
veins (V).

REFERENCES

1.   Wallace, D. M., Chisholm, G. D. and Hendry, W. F.   TNM
     classification for urological tumours (UICC) - 1974.   Brit. J.
     Urol. 47, 1-12 (1975).

2.   Das, G., Chisholm, G. D. and Sherwood, T.   Can angiography
     stage renal carcinoma?   Brit. J. Urol. 49, 611-614 (1977).

TNM CLASSIFICATION OF URINARY BLADDER TUMOURS: VALUE OF Ta CATEGORY

FOR NON INFILTRATING EXOPHYTIC TUMOURS

H RUBBEN, H H DAHM, J BUBENZER AND W LUTZEYER

Departments of Urology and Pathology, Rhineland-

Westfalian Technical Highschool, Aachen, Germany

ABSTRACT

The 1974 TNM classification of the UICC was tested. These data show that the differentiation between non infiltrating tumour and those invading the lamina propria is important to establish adequate treatment. Ta G1 tumours are treated effectively by transurethral resection (TUR) whereas T1 tumours often need more extensive operation if recurrence occurs.

The classification reestablished in 1974 by the UICC for urinary bladder tumours does not differentiate between exophytic tumours not infiltrating the lamina propria and those extending beyond the urothelial basement membrane. This study evaluated the clinical importance of the sub-division of the T1 category into Ta and T1 (Figure 1).

We examined a total of 179 bladder tumours, which were followed for three years or longer and met the following criteria:

1. histologically diagnosed bladder tumours
2. assessment of stage and grade
3. original tumour category T1 (UICC 1974)
4. patients treated by TUR
5. sub-division into: Ta exophytic, non infiltrating and T1 invading the lamina propria

Ninety-seven percent of patients with Ta G1 tumours and 90% with Ta G2 tumours survived more than three years, but only 92% with

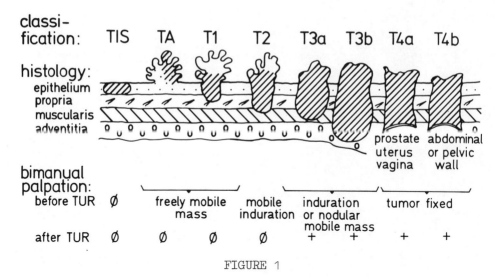

FIGURE 1

T1 G1 and 74% with T1 G2 tumours survived. Patients with poorly
differentiated and undifferentiated tumours showed a bad clinical
course, if treated by TUR (Table I).

The sub-division into Ta and T1 categories is of special
interest when planning the therapy of recurrent transitional cell
carcinoma. Whereas the percentage of primary tumours having a bad
clinical course (increase of grade or stage or death due to the
tumour) was not significantly different in Ta and T1 carcinomas,
recurrent T1 tumours showed a worse prognosis than recurrent Ta
tumours. This is shown by the fact that none of 14 patients with
even more than 10 Ta G1 recurrences died from their tumour within
three years following the last TUR.

TABLE I

% 3 YEAR SURVIVAL RATE

1960-77

T/G	1	2	3
Ta	97	90	–
	(96/99)	(26/29)	(1/3)
T1	90	72	–
	(9/10)	(23/32)	(3/6)

TABLE II

PRIMARY OR RECURRENT TUMOURS, WHICH ARE FOLLOWED BY A TUMOUR
WITH AN INCREASE OF GRADE OR STAGE OR WHICH CAUSED THE DEATH OF
THE PATIENT WITHIN THREE YEARS

	Primary Tumour	Recurrence
Ta	7/50 (14%)	5/81 (6%)
T1	8/34 (24%)	7/14 (50%)

These data show that the differentiation between non infiltrating exophytic tumours and tumours invading the lamina propria is important to establish the appropriate treatment. Ta G1 tumours are effectively treated by TUR, whereas T1 tumours need more extensive operation if recurrence occurs (Table II).

Editorial note (MP-M)   These presentations on TNM were followed by a long and stimulating discussion. Most participants objected to the amendments inflicted upon the 1974 TNM classification. It was said among other things that:- a) the five year interval for testing the value of the 1974 classification had not yet elapsed; b) that this seemed like a sort of premature revolution made without a large consensus of opinion. In particular it was noted that large representative groups, which are particularly active in the clinical field of urological oncology, such as the WHO and EORTC urological groups, were excluded from a preliminary discussion on a very important topic such as this; c) the splitting of the former T1 category into Ta and T1 is misleading and is likely to cause confusion in the future, as many people will still refer to T1 to indicate both O and A stages of the Jewett-Marshall's classification, whereas others will use it only for tumours invading the lamina propria. As Rübben's papers indicate, it is likely that the last group of tumours do have a worse prognosis. Their subdivision is therefore right, but the new terminology did not please everybody. Some aggressive discussants said that the symbol Ta, unheard of previously in TNM terminology, was an abortion rather than a premature delivery. A more logical subdivision should have been established into T1a and T1b, resembling the analogous subdivision into T3a and T3b, T4a and T4b.

Professor van der Werf-Messing replied to the various questions and objections with her usual politeness and charm. She was not, of course, personally responsible for such alterations and she also felt that some questions put by the audience were justified. The

UICC committee had felt, however, that the symbol "Ta" instead of
T1a was a better choice, because of the fact that T1 means an
invasive carcinoma in other organ sites, whereas a papillary bladder
tumour limited to the mucosal layer is obviously not an infiltrating
carcinoma. This new terminology was strongly supported by an
American group of pathologists and its acceptance appeared to be a
fair price to pay for a wider acceptance of the TNM classification among urologists and oncologists in the USA.

In conclusion, in spite of a few controversial points, the new
TNM classification adds a greater precision to a simplified, short-
hand like, description of the tumour. If my understanding of the new
terminology is correct, pT1 and pT2 will be employed instead of P1
and P2, etc. Furthermore, I also understood that a distinction is
proposed depending on whether the classification is based upon
clinical examination, biopsy or pathology from the surgical specimen
(respectively cTNM, bTNM, pTNM).

In addition, the new symbols yTNM and rTNM should be employed
respectively following adjuvant therapy and in the case of recurrent
tumours.

Hopefully we will soon become accustomed to this new jargon.

PREDNIMUSTINE

I KÖNYVES

AB LEO, Research Laboratories

Helsingborg, Sweden

ABSTRACT

Prednimustine is a chlorambucil ester of prednisolone, effective in various experimental tumours. Clinically, Prednimustine is effective in haematological disorders and in breast, prostate and ovarian cancer. Controlled clinical trials of Prednimustine have been started in various malignant diseases.

————

The adverse effects on rapidly proliferating cell tissues, above all on the bone marrow, have limited the dosage of various drugs with cytostatic properties. For this reason, during the last 20 years, a large number of research centres have tried to find new drugs with improved selectivity.

The synthesis of antineoplastic agents with hormones as biological carriers of various cytostatic groups appeared to us a useful approach. Our working hypothesis was to utilise the cellular specificity of various steroids, because of the presence of steroid receptors in some malignant cells. Furthermore, it was anticipated that the passage of the cytostatic agents across the cell membranes might be facilitated for these more lipophilic compounds (9).

Whitmore reported as early as 1956 that treatment with a high dose of corticosteroids can be effective as palliative therapy in patients with advanced prostatic cancer (13). Today it is generally accepted that temporary subjective improvement can be noted after adrenocorticoid treatment and this type of steroid can be the last step of the therapeutic programme in patients with prostatic cancer.

13

It is suggested that the action of corticosteroids may have a different mechanism from that due to antiandrogenic therapy.

Corticosteroids are used also in combination with various cytostatic agents as an integral part of some regimens for the treatment of leukemias, lymphomas and also in some solid tumours, as disseminated mammary cancer.

There are two main ways of synthesising corticosteroid cyto-static compounds: one being the attachment of cytostatic agents directly to one of the carbon atoms of the steroidal skeleton, the other by linking these agents by means of a connecting group to the steroids. We selected the second way because of the possibility of preparing drugs of low reactivity in these types of compounds, producing low toxicity also.

On the basis of this consideration, we have synthesised different series of glucocorticosteroids, where these hormones are substituted in the 21-position. From the glucocorticosteroids prednisolone was chosen on the basis of several advantageous pharmacological and clinical properties.

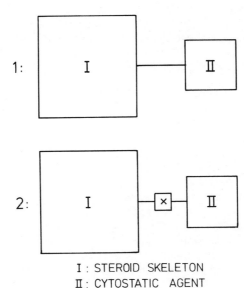

I : STEROID SKELETON
II : CYTOSTATIC AGENT
X : CONNECTING GROUP

FIGURE 1

POSSIBLE WAYS TO CONNECT
CYTOSTATIC AGENTS TO STEROID HORMONES

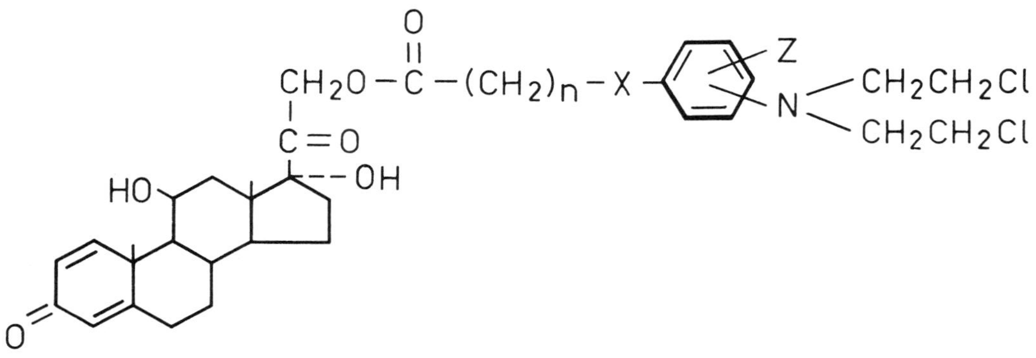

n = 0, 1, 2 or 3

X = Oxygen, sulphur or a carbon-carbon bond

Z = Hydrogen or lower alkyl group

The position of the group $-N\begin{smallmatrix} CH_2CH_2Cl \\ CH_2CH_2Cl \end{smallmatrix}$ is meta or para to X

FIGURE 2

THE GENERAL FORMULA OF PREDNISOLONE -
21-(N-BIS(2-CHLOROETHYL)-AMINO)-PHENYL-CARBOXYLIC ACID ESTERS

We found the highest activity against experimental tumours when we linked these steroids with various nitrogen mustard substituted aromatic carboxylic acids.

As can be seen in Figure 2, we have varied the length of the acid components by making n equal to 0, 1, 2 or 3. Further variations have been attained by incorporating an oxygen or a sulphur atom into the side chain. As is evident from the general formula, the cytostatic group can be in meta or para positions to the acid part. The antitumour properties of these compounds depended on the number of $-CH_2$ groups in the chain, as well as on the position of the alkylating group. Further variations have been attained by building an oxygen or a sulphur atom into the side chain (8).

After preliminary screening, we selected Prednimustine, Leo 1031 the chlorambucil ester of prednisolone, for further experimental evaluation.

In experimental tumour systems, a favourable therapeutic index for Prednimustine was reported when compared to chlorambucil and the equivalent mixture of prednisolone plus chlorambucil. This was due mainly to a low toxicity, which is in good agreement with the report by van Putten and co-workers who studied the cell killing effectiveness of Prednimustine on L1210 cells in comparison to resting and rapidly proliferating normal stem cells. The ratio of effectiveness against L1210 cells compared to resting cells was 23, which is higher than those observed for any other alkylating agent tested in the same system (5).

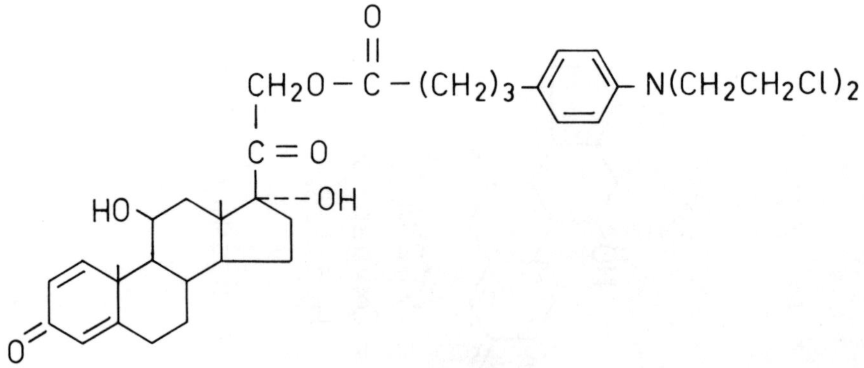

FIGURE 3

THE STRUCTURAL FORMULA OF PREDNIMUSTINE (INN)
(LEO 1031, NSC 134087, EORTC 1502, R.B. 1539)

The pharmacokinetics of Prednimustine have been investigated by the Institute of Cancer Research, Sutton, UK, The Roswell Park Memorial Institute, Buffalo, USA as well as by our Research Laboratories in Helsingborg, Sweden. The enzymes involved in the hydrolysis showed a species specificity and the extent of hydrolysis was greater in the human and animal tumours studied than in plasma or bone marrow. The differences in hydrolytic activity may contribute to the low myelotoxicity of Prednimustine (14).

Against this background, Prednimustine was introduced into clinical use about five years ago. Since the components of Prednimustine, prednisolone and chlorambucil, have been used mostly in haematological disorders, it was originally tried in chronic lymphocytic leukemia and in non-Hodgkin's lymphomas, and later in patients with acute non-lymphocytic leukemia (1,7,2).

The results of various Phase II trials were reported from European and American clinics in more than 300 patients with haematological disorders. After the preliminary trials, the intermittent regimen looks superior to continuous therapy (6). The following controlled comparative studies are in progress on Prednimustine in haematological disorders:

1.   The Central Swedish Haematology Cooperative Group has started a study on patients with chronic lymphocytic leukemia and well differentiated lymphoma, where Prednimustine in continuous and intermittent schedule is being compared with the effect of the combination of Chlorambucil and Prednisolone.

2.   The EORTC Leukemia and Haematosarcoma Group recently started a randomised trial where Prednimustine is compared with Chlorambucil in patients with chronic lymphocytic leukemia.

3.   The intermittent schedule of Prednimustine will be compared with the Cyclophosphamide + Vincristine + Prednisone regimen in patients with non-Hodgkin's lymphomas of favourable histology in a multicenter trial in Sweden.

The Central Swedish Haematology Cooperative Group started in 1977 a randomised study comparing the effect of Prednimustine + Vincristine combination to that of the combination of Thioguanine + Cytosine Arabinoside in elderly patients with acute non-lymphocytic leukemia.

In clinical screening against solid tumours, Prednimustine as a single drug appears effective in the treatment of breast and ovarian cancer (11,12).

The experience with Prednimustine in the treatment of prostatic carcinoma is limited. Catane and co-workers, Roswell Park Memorial

Institute, Buffalo, found in a pilot study 13% objective and 35% subjective response in 23 patients. All the patients had prior oestrogen therapy or orchidectomy or both, six of the patients had previous radiation therapy and eight previous chemotherapy (Table I). The criteria for objective and subjective response in this and in the following trial were those defined by the National Prostatic Cancer Project (3).

This Cooperative Group started the protocol 400 in March 1976 and the evaluation was made in January 1978. The patients in this study were randomised between Estracyt and Prednimustine and Prednimustine alone. All patients were in very advanced stages of the disease, they had failed on adequate hormone therapy and had prior extensive irradiation, at least 2,000 rad to the pelvis. The members from the nine hospitals in these cooperative trials found about the same percentage of objective and subjective response, 13 and 32 respectively, as reported in the first study (14).

Prednimustine was responsible for discontinuation of the treatment in 8% of the patients because of nausea and vomiting. Reversible thrombocytopenia or leucopenia was noted in about 20%.

In our opinion, the results obtained in the United States in this indication can improve when we switch over to intermittent therapy instead of continuous therapy. In this way, we can obtain a reduction of myelosuppression which is the dose-limiting toxic effect of the drug (4).

We are interested now in finding cytostatic agents of the non-alkylating type, which are useful to combine with Prednimustine in

TABLE I

CLINICAL RESULTS OF PREDNIMUSTINE THERAPY IN PATIENTS

WITH PROSTATIC CANCER

STUDY	AUTHOR	NO. OF PATIENTS EVALUATED	RESPONSE[1]	
			OBJECTIVE	SUBJECTIVE
I	Catane et al[2]	23	13%	35%
II	Murphy et al[3]	62	13%	32%

[1] According to NPCP-criteria, J. Urol. 114, 909 (1975).

[2] Brit. J. Urol. 50, 29 (1978).

[3] J. Urol. In Press, with permission of Dr G P Murphy, Roswell Park Memorial Institute.

a combination schedule for the treatment of patients resistant to antiandrogenic and Estracyt therapy.

REFERENCES

1. Brandt, L., Könyves, I. and Möller, T. R.   Acta Med. Scand. 197, 317-322 (1975).

2. Brandt, L. and Könyves, I.   Eur. J. Cancer, 13, 393-398 (1977).

3. Catane, R., Kaufman, J. H., Madajewicz, S., Mittelman, A. and Murphy, G. P.   Brit. J. Urol., 50, 29-32 (1978).

4. Clinical Screening Cooperative Group of EORTC.   Biomed., 27, 158-161 (1977).

5. Evenaar, A. H., Wins, E. H. R. and van Putten, L. M.   Eur. J. Cancer, 9, 773-774 (1974).

6. Hayat, M.   Lecture published in compilation on Working Conference at Leo, March 1976.

7. Håkansson, L., Könyves, I., Lindberg, L. G. and Möller, T. Oncology, 35, 103-106 (1978).

8. Könyves, I., Fex, H. and Högberg, B.   Proc. 8th Int. Congress Chemotherapy, Ed. G. K. Daikos, Vol. III, Antineoplastic Chemotherapy, 791-795 (1974).

9. Könyves, I. and Liljekvist, J.   Excerpta Medica International Congress Series No. 375, 98-105 (1976).

10. Könyves, I., Nordenskjöld, B., Plym Forshell, G., de Schryver, A. and Westerberg-Larsson, H.   Eur. J. Cancer, 11, 841-844 (1975).

11. Murphy, G. P., Gibbons, R. P., Johnson, D. E., Prout, G. R. Jr., Schmidt, J. D., Soloway, M. S., Loening, S. A., Chu, T. M., Gaeta, J. F., Saroff, J., Wajsman, Z., Slack, N. H. and Scott, W. W.   J. Urol. In Press (1979).

12. Lele, S. B., Piver, M. S., Barlow, J. and Murphy, G. P. Oncology, 35, 101-102 (1978).

13. Whitmore, W. F. Jr.   Amer. J. Med. 21/5, 697-713 (1965).

14. Wilkinson, R., Gunnarsson, P. O., Plym-Forshell, G., Renshaw, J. and Harrap, K. R.   Excerpta Medica International Congress Series No. 420, 260-273 (1978).

ORGOTEIN EFFICACY IN AMELIORATING SIDE EFFECTS DUE TO RADIATION

THERAPY

F EDSMYR, K B MENANDER-HUBER and W HUBER

The Radiumhemmet, The Karolinska Hospital, Stockholm and

Diagnostic Data Inc., Mountain View, CA 94043, USA

INTRODUCTION

Orgotein, the generic name for drug versions of Cu-Zn superoxide dismutases (SOD), is a new anti-inflammatory drug (1) which has been shown to be very safe in man and animals (2). In veterinary medicine orgotein has been used for some years in the treatment of arthritis and cataracts. Cu-Zn SODs are stable, soluble metalloproteins whose MW is approximately 32,000. They are found intracellularly in liver, kidney, red cells and other tissues in varying amounts (3). Both the amino acid sequence and the structural features of the protein have been determined and the essential features of the molecule are well understood (4,5).

In nature, Cu-Zn SODs occur in all cells of oxygen-consuming organisms where they dismutate superoxide anions (O_2^-) formed by a host of intracellular autooxidations (6). As a very active radical, O_2^- occurring extracellularly can be a threat to the integrity of living systems, since the concentration of SODs in mammalian plasma is very low (approx. 10 ng/ml). It has been shown that exogenous SOD in vitro inhibites the cytotoxic effects of the superoxide anion generated by phagocytosing neutrophils and macrophages (7). It has long been established that irradiation results in cell death with subsequent invasion of phagocytosing cells (8). The undesirable side effects of radiation therapy are at least partly due to such phenomena.

We initiated our studies based upon the belief that orgotein could reduce inflammatory side effects in patients receiving high-dose irradiation for pelvic tumours. As destruction of malignant cells by high-energy radiation is largely a direct-hit nuclear event

that occurs in the presence of a relatively high concentration of
superoxide dismutases in the cytosol, we felt that interference with
the tumourolytic events by extra-cellular orgotein would not occur.
That this is so is supported by in vitro as well as by in vivo
animal experiments, which document the absence of any orgotein effect
on tumour tissue for various radiation regimens, for intratumour
injections, and for systemic injections up to 400 mg/kg (9,10).

CLINICAL TRIALS

In our clinical trials we have used the following protocol.
Four or eight mg orgotein or placebo dissolved in about 1 ml Saline
injection USP was injected subcutaneously 15-30 minutes after
completion of each daily radiation session. The poorly differentiated tumours were classified according to UICC and covered
categories T2-T4. Histological grading included malignancy grades
2-4. All patients received high-energy radiation with 6MV x-rays
delivered by linear accelerator, using three-field simultaneous
irradiation with CRE factors totally similar (11). Patients were
assigned randomly, received antibacterial therapy throughout the
trial, and were permitted to use one specified anti-diarrhoeal as
needed. No other anti-inflammatory agents than orgotein were
permitted.

The effects of the experimental medication were assessed, using
parameters such as pain and dysuria, maximum voided volume, interval
between voidings during day and night, severity of diarrhoea, and
amount of medication needed to control diarrhoea. The patients were
evaluated at regular intervals after entry into the trial. One visit
always coincided with the termination of therapy. Follow-up
evaluations were done at least at about four months and two years
thereafter. Haematology and urinalysis were performed at each visit
and clinical chemistry at the beginning and end of the treatment.

In a previous double-blind, placebo-controlled study it was
demonstrated that orgotein injected after each daily irradiation
session can be used safely and effectively to ameliorate or prevent
the side effects due to high-energy radiation therapy (8,400 or
6,400 rads) of bladder tumours (10). The efficacy of orgotein over
placebo was shown by a marked reduction of bladder and bowel
disturbance in the group receiving orgotein. This was statistically
significant.

Follow-up evaluations, after completion of radiation therapy,
at four months and two years, respectively, have now been completed
for the patients in this trial. All 35 patients meeting the
selection criteria of the protocol (20 orgotein, 15 placebo) were
alive at the four months follow-up. At that time the beneficial
effects of orgotein over placebo on bladder and bowel had become,

if anything, more marked than at termination of therapy. For
instance, four of 15 patients in the placebo group still had
symptoms of proctitis, while all patients in the orgotein group
were free of it. At the two year follow-up only nine of the 35
patients were still alive (five orgotein, four placebo), a number
too small to draw any conclusion of statistical significance, but
indicating that orgotein treatment concurrent with radiation therapy
does not influence survival time. In view of the high death rate
due to tumour recurrence, no analyses of late radiation induced
side effects on bladder or bowel could be done in either group.

In a second double-blind, placebo-controlled trial 8 mg orgotein
or placebo per injection was administered to 50 patients receiving
radiation therapy (5,400 rads/seven weeks for poorly differentiated
prostatic carcinoma (Table I). Administration of medication and
evaluation of patients were performed as described above. In this
study, radiation-induced side effects were seen in considerably
fewer patients than expected from prior clinical experience. In
the patients experiencing radiation-induced side effects, parameters
lending themselves to analysis included change in overall signs

TABLE I

PROTOCOL PARAMETERS OF DOUBLE-BLIND PLACEBO-CONTROLLED STUDY
ON THE ORGOTEIN EFFICACY IN AMELIORATING SIDE-EFFECTS
DUE TO RADIATION THERAPY OF PROSTATE TUMOURS

	PROTOCOL PARAMETERS
Patient Selection	Patients with Prostate Tumours T2-T4
No. of Patients	50
Orgotein or Placebo Dosage	8 mg Subcutaneously after Completion of Daily Radiation Therapy
Radiation Dosage	5,400 rads/7 weeks
Parameters Evaluated	Maximal Voiding Volume, Frequency (Bowel and Bladder), Pain, Anti-diarrhoeal Medication used

and symptoms in bowel and bladder, and change in voiding frequency of bowel and bladder, both day and night. Again orgotein therapy relieved these side effects more effectively than placebo. In addition, the one case that had to go to surgery occurred in the placebo group. In view of the low overall frequency of serious, radiation-induced side effects, the differences between orgotein and placebo reached statistical significance only occasionally.

The two trials concluded so far show that with orgotein a single-drug therapeutic treatment of radiation-induced side effects is possible and can replace the presently used symptomatic treatment with anticholinergics, analgesics and opiates. An additional and more challenging aspect is the potential of using concomitant orgotein treatment to permit the use of higher radiation doses, and with it the possibility of a better therapeutic result. As a first attempt to explore this, we are now conducting a double-blind, placebo-controlled trial in patients suffering from poorly differentiated prostatic carcinoma, using the protocol shown in Table II. The patients will receive a radiation regimen of 5,000 rads during seven weeks directed at the prostatic gland as well as

TABLE II

PROTOCOL PARAMETERS OF DOUBLE BLIND PLACEBO-CONTROLLED STUDY ON THE ORGOTEIN EFFICACY IN AMELIORATING SIDE EFFECTS DUE TO LARGE FIELD RADIATION THERAPY OF PROSTATE TUMOURS AND ADJACENT LYMPH NODES

	PROTOCOL PARAMETERS
Patient Selection	Patients with Prostate Tumours T2-T4
No. of Patients	50
Orgotein or Placebo Dosage	16 mg Subcutaneously after completion of daily Radiation Therapy and during rest period
Radiation	6 MV x-rays, three field technique; 5,000 rads/7weeks, Prostate and Lymph Nodes; 2 weeks rest; then, 1,500 rads/2 weeks booster to Prostate alone
Parameters Evaluated	Maximal voiding volume, frequency (Bowel and Bladder), pain, anti-diarrhoeal medication used

the surrounding lymph nodes. After a two week rest interval this
is followed by a booster dose of 1,500 rads given during two weeks
and directed at the prostate only. Sixteen milligram doses of
orgotein or placebo are injected after each individual irradiation
session, and also daily during the two week rest period. In this
trial a total dose of 6,500 rads will be directed at the prostate
while a larger area, including the lymph nodes adjacent to the
prostate, will be exposed to a total dose of 5,000 rads.

CONCLUSIONS

Orgotein is an anti-inflammatory agent which minimises the
side effects of radiotherapy in patients with carcinoma of bladder
and prostate without reducing the effect of radiation therapy. In
these patients, orgotein administration concomitant with radiation
therapy did not influence the effectiveness of the irradiation
regimen either immediately or up to the final assessment at two
years.

The two double-blind, placebo-controlled trials in patients
with cancer of the bladder and prostate now completed show that
with orgotein a therapeutic, single-drug treatment of radiation-
induced side effects is possible which can replace the presently
used symptomatic treatment with anticholinergics, analgesics and
opiates.

The results obtained to date indicate that concomitant
administration of orgotein could permit the patient to tolerate
higher radiation doses and with it have the promise of a better
therapeutic result. The validity of this premise is presently being
explored in another double-blind, placebo controlled trial in
prostatic carcinoma patients exposed to an irradiation regimen where
a total dose of 6,500 rads is directed at the prostate while a larger
area, including the lymph nodes adjacent to the prostate, are exposed
to a total dose of 5,000 rads.

REFERENCES

1.   Huber, W., Menander-Huber, K. B., Saifer, M. G. P. and
      Dang, P. H-C., Studies on the clinical and laboratory
      pharmacology of drug formulations of bovine Cu-Zn superoxide
      dismutases (orgotein), in perspectives in inflammation. Eds.
      Willoughby, D. A., Giroud, J. P., Velo, G. P., Baltimore,
      University Park Press, 527 (1977).

2.   Carson, S., Vogin, E. E., Huber, W., and Schulte, T. L., Safety
      tests of orgotein, an anti-inflammatory protein. Toxicol. Appl.
      Pharmacol., 26, 184 (1973).

3.   Fridovich, I., Superoxide dismutases. Ann. Rev. Biochem. 44, 147 (1975).

4.   Steinman, H., Naik, V., Abernethy, J. and Hill, R., Bovine erythrocyte superoxide dismutase. Complete amino acid sequence. J. Biol. Chem., 249, 22, 7326 (1974).

5.   Richardson, J., Thomas, K., Rubin, B. and Richardson, D., Crystal structure of bovine Cu-Zn Superoxide dismutase at 3A resolution: chain tracing and metal ligands. Proc. Natl. Acad. Sci. USA, 72, 1349 (1975).

6.   Fridovich, I., A free radical pathology: superoxide radical and superoxide dismutases. Ann. Rep. Med. Chem., 10, 257 (1975).

7.   Salin, M. L. and McCord, J. M., Free radicals and inflammation. Protection of phagocytosing leukocytes by superoxide dismutase. J. Clin. Inv. 56, 1319 (1975).

8.   Moss, W. T., Ackermann, L. V., Therapeutic Radiology. 2nd Ed. St Louis: Mosby (1965).

9.   Hill, R. P., Personal Communication.

10. Overgaard, J., Personal Communication.

11. Littbrand, B., Edsmyr, F. and Revesz, W., A low dose fractionation scheme for the radiotherapy of carcinoma of the bladder. Bull. du Cancer, 62, 241 (1975).

12. Edsmyr, F., Huber, W.,and Menander-Huber, K. B., Orgotein efficacy in ameliorating side effects due to radiation therapy. I. Double-blind, placebo-controlled trial in patients with bladder tumours. Curr. Therap. Res. 19, 198 (1976).

METRONIDAZOLE: A RADIOSENSITISER OF THE HYPOXIC CELLS

C RIMONDI

Department of Radiation Therapy, Malpighi Hospital

Bologna, Italy

The main reasons for the low radiosensitivity of bladder cancer especially in its advanced stages are the problems of necrosis, thrombosis and fibrosis producing large areas of hypoxic cells which are radioresistant. The employment of a drug which radio-sensitise such cells offers great promise. Metronidazole (Flagyl) is a 5 nitroimidazole compound. It has shown a radiosensitising effect on hypoxic cells both in vitro and in vivo. This drug acts on the tumour, whereas it does not act on the normal tissues surrounding the growth. There is, therefore, no increased radiation damage on the normal tissues which are well vascularised and normally oxygen-ated. It acts particularly on the hypoxic cells of the tumour, which constitute its radioresistant cell subpopulation.

The radiosensitisation depends on the serum concentration of the drug. The enhancement ratio (ER) in many tests in mouse experimental tumours varies from 1.5 to 2.1 at a dose of 1 mg of drug/1 g tumour with high dose irradiation in a single fraction (Adams, 1979). In man doses of 4-6 g/m^2 produce a serum con-centration of 150-220 µg/ml two to four hours after oral administration. Similar levels are found in the tumour, even in hypoxic areas. These levels remain high for a long time halving after 10-12 hours. The ER for such drug doses used with fractionated radiotherapy (RT) is of the order of 10-20%.

At such a dose the drug is not always well tolerated by the stomach and may cause vomiting.

Due to this poor gastric tolerance the common scheme of fractionated RT was changed (Urtasun et al, 1975). The number of

fractions was reduced and each radiation dose increased to give
3,000 rads in nine fractions, three times a week.

Our experiment with Metronidazole started one year ago. In a
Phase I study in 20 patients with locally advanced cancer of many
sites. Twelve patients experienced vomiting after drug
administration and many developed anorexia; both side effects
stopped at the end of the treatment. There was no evidence of bone
marrow, hepatic or renal toxicity (Rimondi, 1978).

A randomised clinical trial has now been started in patients
with bladder cancer (T3 Nx Mo) using Metronidazole. In order to
exploit the long metabolic half life of this drug a scheme of
fractionation is used with a dose of 100 rads repeated three times
a day (Littbrand and Edsmyr, 1976), 3-7-11 hours after 4 g/m^2 drug
administration.

Because of poor gastric tolerance Metronidazole is administered
to patients every other day, radiation treatment is performed each
day following the same scheme for three weeks, five days a week up
to a total radiation dose of 4,500 rads tumour dose (TD).

Three weeks after the end of the treatment the patients are
examined both clinically and cystoscopically. If the tumour
reduction is greater than 50% radiation treatment is completed
giving another 2,000-3,000 rads in two to three weeks to the bladder
only using a pendular technique. If tumour reduction is less than
50% the patients are operated upon, when possible, usually by total
cystectomy.

Dische (1978) has proposed the use of Misonidazole, a 2
nitroimidazole compound. This drug is more efficient but is
neurotoxic at high doses. A total dose of drug of 12 g/m^2 is
divided into 20 doses administered four hours before each radiation
treatment of 20 fractions over a period of five weeks, four times
a week. The first 16 fractions are given to a large volume,
including bladder and pelvic nodes, the last four fractions only to
a small volume restricted to the known site of the tumour. The
single dose is 260 rads minimum TD up to a total dose of 5,200 rads.

The results of both these studies are awaited with great
interest.

REFERENCES

1.   Adams, G. E., Hypoxic cell radiosensitizers for radiotherapy.
      (1979) In Press.

2. Dische, S., Hypoxic cell sensitisers in radiotherapy. Int. J.
    Rad. Oncol. Biol. Phys. 4, 157-160 (1978).

3. Dische, S., Trial of Misonidazole in the radiotherapy of the
    carcinoma of the bladder. Personal Communication (1978).

4. Littbrand, B., Edsmyr, F., Preliminary results of bladder
    carcinoma irradiated with low individual dose and high total
    dose. Int. J. Rad. Oncol. Biol. Phys. 1, 1059-1062 (1976).

5. Rimondi, C., Problems and prospectives of Metronidazole in
    radiotherapy in "Radiosensitiser of hypoxic cells". Eds.
    Breccia, A., Rimondi, C. and Adams, G. E. Elsevier, Amsterdam,
    (1978).

CIS-DIAMMINE-DICHLORO-PLATINUM SINGLE DRUG AND COMBINATION CHEMOTHERAPY IN THE TREATMENT OF GENITOURINARY CANCER

G STOTER AND H M PINEDO

Division of Oncology,

University Hospital, Utrecht, The Netherlands

INTRODUCTION

Cis-diammine-dichloro-platinum is the first drug of a new class of cytotoxic agents. It has an alkylating effect and also inhibits DNA-synthesis.

———

In phase I and phase II studies cis-platinum has been shown to produce an overall response rate of 66% in testicular cancer (1-4). Except for renal cell cancer, cis-platinum is also effective in the other genitourinary tumours. Using cis-platinum as a single drug in prostatic cancer, Merrin (5) achieved partial remissions in 17 of 54 oestrogen pretreated patients (31%). This response lasted from two to 18 months. Using cis-platinum in 51 patients with advanced bladder cancer, he achieved a response in 19 (36%). The duration of the response varied from two to 13 months. The combination of cis-platinum and cyclophosphamide resulted in 47% partial remissions (6), whereas the combination of cis-platinum, adriamycin and 5-Fluoro-uracil is not very myelosuppressive.

CLINICAL EXPERIENCE

In disseminated testicular cancer the combination of cis-platinum, vinblastine and bleomycin produces about 70% complete remissions (8). Using this combination chemotherapy, according to Einhorn's regimen, we have accumulated experience in disseminated testicular non-seminomas from 1976. The main toxicity of this combination comprises the risk of renal failure due to cis-platinum,

myelosuppression and the hazard of agranulocytic sepsis due to
vinblastine, whereas bleomycin may produce pneumonitis and lung
fibrosis. Table I shows the results of chemotherapy in 40 patients
with disseminated testicular non-seminomas. The patients are
divided by histology into; intermediate, undifferentiated and
trophoblastic teratoma. Twenty-four of 40 patients (60%) achieved
a complete remission and 22 of them are still in complete remission
with a present follow-up of three to 28 months. After four cycles
of this combination chemotherapy we give maintenance chemotherapy
for two years with cis-platinum and vinblastine and stop all therapy
thereafter. Three of the complete responders are off treatment since
they have exceeded a complete remission period of two years and they
are probably cured (9). Eleven patients (28%) achieved a partial
remission. Three patients died of toxicity: one of renal failure,
one of agranulocytic sepsis, and one patient died of bleomycin lung
fibrosis. Two patients showed progression of the disease after
initial response and went off study. Our series of patients is
highly compromised for two reasons. In the first place 50% of the
patients had been pretreated with radiation and/or chemotherapy; and
in the second 90% of the patients had extensive abdominal and/or
pulmonary metastases according to Samuels' criteria (10).

Table II demonstrates the relationship between severe toxicity
and previous treatment in our patients. Twenty patients had received
therapy, 12 of whom had received radiotherapy with or without
chemotherapy. Eight patients had been pretreated with chemotherapy
alone. The remaining 20 patients had had no previous treatment
except for surgery. There is a striking preponderance of severe
bone marrow toxicity and sepsis in the radiation pretreated group
compared with the chemotherapy pretreated group and the non pretreated group. The prevalence of renal function impairment in the

TABLE I

RESULTS OF THE CHEMOTHERAPY ACCORDING TO THE HISTOLOGY

Histology	Patients	CR	PR	TD	Progression
MTI	9	6(76%)	3	-	-
MTU	24	15(63%)	5	3	1
MTT	7	3(42%)	3	-	1
Total	40	24(60%)	11(28%)	3	2

CR = complete remission; PR = partial remission; TD = toxic death
MTI = malignant teratoma intermediate; MTU = malignant teratoma
undifferentiated; MTT = malignant teratoma trophoblastic.

TABLE II

SIDE EFFECTS OF THE CHEMOTHERAPY IN RELATION TO PREVIOUS THERAPY

Side effects	Patients	Pretreatment Radio+Chemo 12	Chemo 8	No Pretreatment 20
Granulocytopenia $<500/mm^3$, >5 days	15	10	2	3
Thrombocytopenia $<50,00/mm^3$, >5 days	9	9	-	-
Sepsis	11	8	2	1
Renal Failure*	13	7	3	3

Radio = radiotherapy; Chemo = chemotherapy
Renal Failure includes all patients with serum creatinine above
1.2 mg/100 ml.

radiation pretreated group is due to septic shock and the treatment
of sepsis with potentially nephrotoxic antibiotics such as gentamicin
and cephalothin (11), in addition to the nephrotoxic effects of
cis-platinum.

CONCLUSION

In conclusion we may say that cis-platinum used as a single
agent or in combination chemotherapy, although toxic, appears to be
promising in genitourinary tumours, especially in testicular cancer.
Cis-platinum has been shown to be ineffective in renal cell cancer
(5,12).

REFERENCES

1. Hayes, D., et al. Proc. Am. Assoc. Cancer Res./Proc. Am. Soc.
    Clin. Oncol. 17, 169 (1976).

2. Merrin, C. Proc. Am. Assoc. Cancer Res./Proc. Am. Soc. Clin.
    Oncol. 17, 243 (1976).

3. Higby, D. J., et al. J. Urol. 112, 100-104 (1974).

4.   Osieka, R., et al. Dtsch. Med. Wschr. 101, 191-195 (1976).

5.   Merrin, C. Treatment of genitourinary tumours with cis-
     diammine-dichloro-platinum. Experience in 250 patients.
     (In Press).

6.   Yagoda, A., et al. Cancer 41, 2121-2130 (1978).

7.   Williams, D. 3., Rohm, R. J., Donohue, J. F. and Einhorn, L. H.
     Proc. Am. Assoc. Cancer Res./Proc. Am. Soc. Clin. Oncol. C37,
     316 (1978).

8.   Einhorn, L. H. and Donohue, J. Annals of Internal Medicine, 87,
     293-298 (1977).

9.   MacKay, E. N. and Sellers, A. H. Canad. Med. Ass. J. 94, 889-
     899 (1966).

10. Samuels, M. L., et al. Cancer Treatment Reviews, 3, 185-204
     (1976).

11. Gonzalez-Vitale, J. C., et al. Cancer Treat. Rep. 62, 693-
     698 (1978).

12. Rodrigues, L. H. and Johnson, D. E. Urology 11, 4, 344-346
     (1978).

THE AIMS AND ACTIVITIES OF THE EORTC UROLOGICAL GROUP

P H SMITH

Department of Urology, St James's University Hospital
Leeds, England
Chairman, EORTC Urological Group

AIMS

The EORTC Urological Group was formed in 1976 of two previously existing groups and its aim was to bring together those European Urologists interested in research into the problems presented by patients with neoplasms of the genito-urinary tract. It was recognised that the group's main interest would lie in clinical research and that the presence of the Data Centre was essential if clinical studies were to be implemented, monitored and analysed satisfactorily.

To encourage active and committed Urologists to join the group and to contribute cases as rapidly as possible it was decided to appoint National Coordinators responsible for recruitment within their own country, for the organisation of national meetings and for the translation of protocols. Study Coordinators were also appointed to deal with the implementation and analysis of each protocol.

We also formed Chemotherapy and Pathology Panels to obtain competent advice in these fields, and are now considering the formation of a Panel in Radiotherapy.

It was. hoped that doctors interested in basic science and other scientists would gradually come to work together with the clinicians on a local, national or international basis but no attempt has yet been made to set up a formal scientific advisory committee.

This arrangement has worked satisfactorily and has allowed the group to undertake studies in patients with cancer of the bladder

and prostate. Proposals for investigation and treatment of patients
with tumours of the kidney and testis have not as yet been
implemented.

ACTIVITIES

Bladder Cancer

In patients with non invasive bladder cancer there has been
increasing interest in intravesical chemotherapy since Jones and
Swinney (1961) showed that Thiotepa could control certain papillary
tumours within the bladder. Pavone-Macaluso (1971) reviewed the
available literature and showed that intravesical chemotherapy would
reduce the recurrence rate in such tumours from 60% without treatment
to 23% with prophylactic therapy and recommended that "a trial of
topical chemotherapy should be attempted before performing a total
cystectomy for papillomatosis". The agents suggested for intravesical use include Thiotepa, Epodyl, Mitomycin C, Bleomycin,
Adriamycin and Peptichemio.

At the time the group considered this problem none of these
agents had been subjected to randomised clinical trial. The group
decided to evaluate the use of Thiotepa in comparison with VM 26,
which had shown some effect in invasive bladder cancer (Pavone-
Macaluso and EORTC, 1976) and with a control arm, in patients with
category T1, Nx, Mx bladder cancer (Figure 1). This study has now
been closed as 340 patients have been entered and the preliminary
evaluation will be reported later during the course of this meeting.
This study is to be replaced by a second study comparing Thiotepa,
Adriamycin and Cis-Platinum used intravesically and by a further
study comparing oral Pyridoxine against Placebo to investigate the
observation of Byar and Blackard (1977) that Pyridoxine, which
prevents the excretion of abnormal Tryptophan metabolites - not
infrequently found in patients with bladder cancer is associated
with a reduction in recurrence rate of non invasive bladder cancer.

For patients with invasive bladder cancer the group regards the
results of surgery and radiotherapy alone or in combination as unacceptable and has decided to evaluate the potential of cytotoxic
agents with surgery and radiotherapy.

Before introducing such adjuvant regimes it is necessary to find
agents which exert some effect on tumours without producing unacceptable toxicity (Phase I studies) and to determine for a given
tumour the incidence of remission produced by the agent or agents,
usually in patients with advanced disease (Phase II studies).

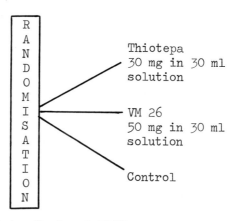

Male and
female patients
with T1, Nx, Mx
transitional cell
tumours of the
bladder.

Thiotepa
30 mg in 30 ml
solution

VM 26
50 mg in 30 ml
solution

Control

FIGURE 1 - Protocol 30751

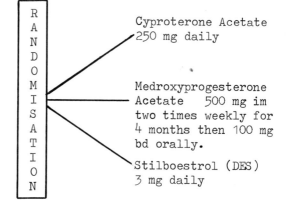

Patients with T3
or T4 carcinoma
of the prostate.

Cyproterone Acetate
250 mg daily

Medroxyprogesterone
Acetate   500 mg im
two times weekly for
4 months then 100 mg
bd orally.

Stilboestrol (DES)
3 mg daily

FIGURE 2 - Protocol 30761

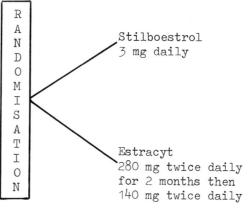

Patients with T3
or T4 carcinoma
of the prostate.

Stilboestrol
3 mg daily

Estracyt
280 mg twice daily
for 2 months then
140 mg twice daily

FIGURE 3 - Protocol 30762

A recent computer search reveals that as yet there is only a limited amount of information from Phase II studies: this is summarised on page 388 of this book and the drugs which have not yet been tested in patients with bladder cancer on page 389.

The EORTC Urological Group has already published a Phase II study using Adriamycin and 5-Fluorouracil in 43 evaluable patients with advanced disease, demonstrating a 42% remission rate (EORTC Urological Group D, 1977). Since that time it has implemented a Phase II study to compare Adriamycin, Adriamycin and 5-FU and Cyclophosphamide and is currently developing a further Phase II study to evaluate Vincristine as a single agent.

The results of the work with 5-FU and Adriamycin have been promising enough to allow the development of a trial of adjuvant chemotherapy in patients with category P3, N_0-N_2, MO bladder cancer following the use of flash radiotherapy and radical cystectomy. It is expected that this trial will become active in January 1979.

Cancer of the Prostate

The Veterans Administration Cooperative Research Group (VACURG) have shown that Stilboestrol (DES) 1 mg or 5 mg/day decreases the death rate from prostatic cancer, that DES 5 mg/day predisposed to death from cardiovascular disease and is associated with longer survival than is early treatment with DES 5 mg/day (VACURG, 1967; Byar, 1973). However, many questions remain unanswered and few randomised trials have been carried out to evaluate the many treatments which have been shown to have some effect. Treatments alternative to DES include Cyproterone Acetate, Medroxyprogesterone Acetate (MPA) and Estracyt amongst others. The group felt that it was important to obtain further information and has implemented two studies to evaluate these agents (Figure 2 and 3) both in patients with advanced prostatic cancer (category T3, T4). At the moment 202 patients have been entered in protocol 30762 and 155 in protocol 30761. These studies require approximately one hundred evaluable patients in each arm and it is hoped that both will be closed to entry within the next six to twelve months. Although these results will be of great interest it is always important to remember that cost has an influence on the choice of drugs. Cost is likely to be of particular importance in the treatment of prostatic cancer since the alternatives to Stilboestrol are from 10 - 450 x as expensive! (Smith, 1979).

There has been increasing interest in the last five years in the use of cytotoxic chemotherapy for cancer of the prostate but the incidence of objective remission so far reported is low (Smith, 1979). At this time the group is just completing a study comparing Adriamycin and Procarbazine in patients who have failed on conventional therapy. Preliminary evaluation suggests that Procarbazine in the dose used (200 mg/m^2 days 1-14 of 28 day cycle) is both toxic and ineffective.

THE FUTURE

The EORTC Urological Group is now a viable enterprise entering large numbers of patients into randomised clinical trials. I should like to take this opportunity of thanking most sincerely all those who have entered patients to the different studies. It is important that we build upon this promising start and activate further studies as soon as possible. The potential of the group is unlimited and I see no reason why two or three different studies in patients with cancer of the bladder or prostate cannot be implemented at the same time, allowing a centre or national group to join one protocol for each tumour type. In my view this would provide an element of healthy competition between centres and between countries leading to even more rapid progress.

REFERENCES

1. Jones, H. C. and Swinney, J., Thiotepa in the Treatment of Tumours of the Bladder. Lancet, 2, 615 (1961).

2. Pavone-Macaluso, M., Chemotherapy of Vesical and Prostatic Tumours. Brit. J. Urol. 43, 701-708 (1971).

3. Pavone-Macaluso, M. and EORTC Genitourinary Tract Cooperative Group A, Single Drug Chemotherapy of Bladder Cancer with Adriamycin, VM 26 or Bleomycin. Eur. Urol. 2, 138-141 (1976).

4. Byar, D. and Blackard, C., Comparisons of Placebo, Pyridoxine and topical Thiotepa in preventing recurrence of Stage I Bladder Cancer. Urology, 10, 556-561 (1977).

5. EORTC Urological Group B, The Treatment of Advanced Carcinoma of the Bladder with a combination of Adriamycin and 5-Fluorouracil. Eur. Urol. 3, 276-278 (1977).

6. Veterans Administration Cooperative Urological Research Group, Treatment and Survival of Patients with Cancer of the Prostate. Surg. Gynec. Obstet. 124, 1011-1017 (1967).

7. Byar, D., The Veterans Administration Cooperative Urological Research Group B Studies of Cancer of the Prostate. Cancer, 32, 1126-1130 (1973).

8. Smith, P. H. Eur. Urol. (1979). In Press.

WHO COLLABORATING CENTRE FOR RESEARCH AND TREATMENT OF URINARY

BLADDER AND PROSTATIC CARCINOMA

F EDSMYR

Radiumhemmet, Karolinska sjukhuset, Stockholm, Sweden
Chief, WHO Collaborating Centre for Research and
Treatment of Urinary Bladder and Prostatic Cancer

In the spring of 1974, the World Health Organisation Cancer
Unit organised a conference concerning malignant tumour diseases
throughout the world, and representatives from Vienna, Stockholm
and Moscow, in cooperation with the Cancer Unit, decided on a plan
for organising Collaborating Centres to investigate some of the ten
commonest and most serious cancer diseases. Later on, Collaborating
Centres were set up for various tumour diseases - including Tokyo
for stomach cancer, Paris for breast cancer, Leningrad for cancer
of the ovaries, Sophia for cervical cancer and Miami for lung cancer.

In March 1976 following preparatory negotiations between the
World Health Organisation and the Swedish Government, the WHO set up
a Collaborating Centre for Research and Treatment of Urinary Bladder
Cancer in Radiumhemmet and Karolinska Hospital in Stockholm. This
was the fifth in the series of WHO centres. Professor Folke Edsmyr,
Senior Physician at Radiumhemmet, became chief of the Centre.

After a number of smaller preparatory conferences, a relatively
large conference was held in Stockholm in April 1977, with 150
participants from all over the world. Topical aspects of bladder
cancer were discussed by specialists from leading centres. The
relevant papers will be published in Urological Research(1). On the
basis of these papers, collaborative work is established on certain
points where international cooperation is required to achieve quicker
research results and avoid duplication of work.

As an example of such multinational projects may be mentioned
the analysis of various radiation treatment techniques, particularly
in the external radiation treatment of bladder cancer. Different

techniques used in Stockholm, London and Rotterdam are compared with regard to radiation doses and the scope of treatment.

To discuss diagnosis and treatment (especially cytostatic) treatment) of superficial bladder cancer, a WHO Centre conference was held in Stockholm on 15 September, 1978, with participants from different urological and oncological centres in the Nordic countries as well as in Europe and Japan(2).

WHO will hold a conference at the Cancer Institute in Cairo in December 1978, with the participation of representatives from the WHO Collaborating Centre in Stockholm and specialists of the Middle East countries, discussing bilharzia and urinary bladder cancer.

Instead of organising a new Collaborative Centre, the World Health Organisation proposes that the Urinary Bladder Cancer Centre in Stockholm shall extend its activities to include cancer of the prostate. In the preliminary discussions it has become apparent that a centre in Stockholm would need increased resources to achieve its expansion. By agreement between WHO, the Swedish National Board of Health and Welfare and the Swedish Government, the Stockholm Centre has been expanded to include cancer of the prostate for an experimental period until March 1979.

On the initiative of WHO in Geneva, an international conference on prostatic cancer will be held in Stockholm on 12-15 March, 1979. To provide a basis for international cooperation this conference will deal broadly with the present status of research on cancer of the prostate. One important objective for such cooperation is to standardise morphological methods in diagnosis. Throughout the world histological examination is generally employed. There is less agreement regarding the value and reproducibility of fine needle aspiration biopsy which is far more comfortable for the patient and is possible to use on a large scale, since it can be performed in out-patient clinics. Therefore, it is necessary that fine needle aspiration biopsy be tried out on a large scale at several different centres so its value can be further analysed and in the hope that the method will gain acceptance.

While prostate cancer in the western world has a very high and steadily increasing frequency, its frequency is extremely low in the Far East. The possible reasons for this large discrepancy in incidence will be discussed at the WHO Collaborative meeting in March 1979.

During recent years, radiation treatment has become increasingly used in treatment of cancer of the prostate. In addition, American centres in the past few years have tried implantation of radioactive isotopes. At European centres, such as Stockholm and Rotterdam, external radiation treatment with different techniques has been more commonly used.

With regard to the serious cardiovascular complications of oestrogen treatment it is important to analyse the value of different cytostatic drugs in the treatment of prostate cancer. Studies are established in EORTC and a collaborative programme will begin between EORTC and the WHO Collaborating Centre in Stockholm.

REFERENCES

1.   Special Issue : Bladder Cancer Research. Urological Research 6, 4 (1978).

2.   WHO Collaborating Centre for Research and Treatment of Urinary Bladder Cancer. Diagnostics and Treatment of superficial urinary bladder tumours. Radiumhemmet, Karolinska Hospital, Stockholm, September 15, 1978. Published by Montedison Läkemed AB, Stockholm, Sweden (1979).

Editorial Note (PHS). One of the chief features of the last decade has been the emergence of many cooperative research groups, especially in the field of cancer treatment. The contributions of the two groups represented at this conference demonstrate some of the advantages to be gained from such an approach. Less clearly demonstrated but of equal value is the way in which such groups, by the regular meetings of their members, allow the rapid dissemination of knowledge, focus attention upon issues of current importance and raise the standard of patient care as successive protocols are implemented.

Part 2
Bladder Cancer

CHEMICAL CARCINOGENESIS - A REVIEW AND PERSONAL OBSERVATIONS WITH
SPECIAL REFERENCE TO THE ROLE OF TOBACCO AND PHENACETIN IN THE
PRODUCTION OF UROTHELIAL TUMOURS

L WAHLQVIST

Department of Urology
University of Umeå
Umeå, Sweden

ABSTRACT

A review of the oncogens associated with urothelial tumours but
excluding occupational chemical carcinogens has been undertaken
together with an evaluation of the role of consumption of phenacetin
and tobacco in patients with carcinoma of the renal pelvis and
bladder. The importance of infection and stone formation is
discussed.

INTRODUCTION

The incidence of urothelial tumours, renal carcinoma and
prostatic carcinoma has increased more than 100% in 12 years in
Sweden. To some extent this increase can be explained by the
increase in the numbers in the older age groups. During the same
period the incidence of gastric carcinoma has decreased. The
difference in behaviour between the two tumour types might be
explained by variable exposure to carcinogens.

From a chemical point of view the carcinogens can be divided
into three groups, including direct-acting carcinogens, pre-
carcinogens ie. agents requiring biochemical activation and
promoting agents or co-carcinogens.

From a clinical point of view Melicow's scheme of oncogens (7)
must be considered as being of importance. This includes irritants
which produce necrosis and healing eg. cyclophosphamide; initiators
in which necrosis and healing is followed by residual hyperplasia
eg. MNU (N-methyl-nitrosurea) in a single dose; and promotors, co-

carcinogens and potentiators eg. saccharine or cyclamate, when given in combination with a single dose of MNU.

The induction and/or promotion in man of urothelial neoplasia from chemicals has been studied for many years. About twenty substances have been positively identified as carcinogenic in man and several of them have been shown to produce urothelial tumours. Asbestos, nickel compounds and nitrogen mustard have been shown to be oncogenic not to the urothelium but to other tissues. Chlornafazin is a nitrogen mustard compound releasing 2-naphthylamine, which is a strong carcinogen to the urothelium.

The genesis of urothelial tumours might be due to a disturbance of tryptophan metabolism in certain cases. High levels of metabolites represent endogenous chemical carcinogens in contrast to exogenous carcinogens such as 2-naphthylamine.

NON CHEMICAL CARCINOGENESIS

Some experimental studies and some clinical observations during recent years have also drawn attention to factors other than chemical oncogens including trauma, immunosuppression, irradiation and infection.

Trauma. In animals some carcinogens are only effective if introduced into the bladder in a pellet. Pricking of the bladder wall with a needle reduced the induction time from years to one to two weeks for phenacetin fed rats (2). The effect of other types of trauma to the bladder wall seems not to have been studied experimentally. On the other hand it is well known that after treatment of a solitary bladder tumour explosive growth with many tumour satellites is often seen. The effect of electric heating knife and scissors seem not to have been evaluated. It is not yet known whether we are dealing with cells which implant or whether carcinogens in combination with trauma are responsible for the rapid recurrences. Calculi have been suspected of being involved in the genesis of carcinoma of both bladder and renal pelvis. The atypical urothelial cells found in the urine from stone patients are well known. How often such findings really indicate the genesis of a malignant neoplasia is however not known.

Immunosuppression. Attention has been drawn to transplanted patients, who have a higher frequency of malignant diseases than controls. It has been shown that patients with uremia of long duration have a higher frequency of malignant disease even before transplantation. Immunosuppressive drugs seem to be of importance in those transplanted.

Irradiation. The deposition of radioactive contrast medium (Thorotrast) in the kidney produced malignant tumours after 20-30 years. External irradiation may be of some importance in the genesis of ureteral tumours.

Infection. Infection is a common finding in paraplegic patients with long term in-dwelling catheters. After about 15 years the appearance of pathological bladder epithelium has been found and later on bladder tumours may develop. E.coli and Proteus Mirabilis have been said to form nitrosamine in urine containing nitrate. The importance of infection in the genesis of urothelial tumours seems not to have been satisfactorily investigated in clinical studies. Schistosoma haematobium is a heavy burden to man giving inflammatory reactions in the bladder wall and, in a high percentage, bladder carcinoma. The agent acting as the carcinogen is not yet identified.

CHEMICAL CARCINOGENESIS

Endogenous

Metabolites of tryptophan seem to be the only probable endogenous carcinogens. These metabolites increase after the administration of antagonists of pyridoxine and after smoking or chewing tobacco. Tobacco smoking also releases 2-naphthylamine. In England L-Tryptophan has been used as a drug for the treatment of depression and in Sweden is available in the Chemists shops to counteract spring depression.

Exogenous

1. Beverages. Epidemiological studies have shown that coffee and sweeteners (cyclamate, saccharine) are involved in the genesis of bladder tumours. The bracken pteridium aquilium is carcinogenic to the urothelium in man, water buffalo and cow. Whether the carcinogenic substance can be transmitted with milk is not known.

In the Balkans water from wells of certain depths in certain valleys causes the Balkan nephropathy as well as urothelial tumours. Silicates in the water have been suspected as the causative agent. The drinking of well water might indicate a high intake of nitrate; urinary tract infection might in such people lead to an increased risk of bladder tumours from nitrosamine.

2. Drugs. In experimental studies some analgesic drugs cause serious destruction of the kidney parenchyma. Phenacetin has been shown experimentally and clinically to have a carcinogenic effect on the urothelium (3,4,5,6). Caffeine is mutagenic to Drosophila but

seems not to have produced experimental tumours. Phenacetin--
containing analgesics are in all probability carcinogenic to the
urothelium in man. Chloroform is carcinogenic to the renal
epithelium in rat but is probably of no importance in man.
Antagonists of pyridoxine increase the excretion of tryptophan
metabolites. Chlornafazin used against erythremia was an extremely
carcinogenic drug giving a high frequency of bladder carcinomas.
Cyclophosphamide has been shown to produce bladder carcinomas after
treatment of myeloma or Hodgkin's disease and followed haemorrhagic
cystitis during the treatment. The induction time was between $3\frac{1}{2}$
and 13 years. Other cytotoxic drugs seem not yet to have been
evaluated from this point of view.

    3. Environmental Factors. Cadmium is a carcinogen in animals
and a competitive inhibitor of zinc, which is found in significant
quantities in the kidney. An association of cadmium with renal
carcinoma has been found with a synergistic effect with occupational
exposure and smoking. Cadmium may also be ingested from cigarette
tobacco but the synergistic effect can not be explained by the
cadmium in the cigarette smoke. Lead has been shown to cause renal
carcinoma in experimental studies, an association between lead and
tumours in man seems not to have been established.

    1- and 2-naphthylamine as well as 4-nitrobiphenyl and
4,4-biaminobiphenyl have caused most of the known cases of
occupational bladder carcinomas. Benzidine used in dyes and in
medical laboratories is another known occupational carcinogen.

    Epidemiological studies outside Sweden have shown either a weak
or no association between the consumption of tobacco and the
consumption of alcohol or drugs. In a Swedish study of patients with
gastric ulcer a significant association was found between a high
consumption of alcohol, sleeping pills, coffee, analgesics and
sedatives. A given correlation between smoking and the genesis of a
tumour might thus, at least in some countries, depend on factors
other than smoking. This highlights the difficulties in the
investigation of oncogenesis. The effect of alcohol on tryptophan
metabolism and thus on the genesis of bladder tumours seems not to
be known.

PERSONAL INVESTIGATIONS

    The consumption of phenacetin and tobacco has been investigated
in four groups of urological patients (Table I). The criteria for
significant consumption of phenacetin was 1 kg phenacetin and an
induction time of eight years qualified as a significant consumption
of tobacco. There was a high phenacetin consumption in 1-5% of
patients without tumour. These patients usually had a story of renal
symptoms with or without haematuria. There was, however, an

TABLE I

FREQUENCY OF HEAVY CONSUMTPION OF PHENACETIN AND TOBACCO

IN PATIENTS AT A UROLOGICAL CLINIC

	Phenacetin		Tobacco	
	M	F	M	F
Renal Carcinoma	0/10	1/7	9/10	0/7
Carcinoma of Renal Pelvis	5/10	6/11	10/10	0/11
Bladder Carcinoma	6/116	6/32	89/116	5/32
Patients without Tumours	3/150	3/59	70/150	15/59

association between phenacetin consumption and renal pelvis carcinoma as well as bladder carcinoma in women. Tobacco consumption in males was associated with these tumours. The mean induction time in 42 patients with bladder carcinoma and a high consumption of phenacetin was 30 years. The corresponding mean time for patients with renal pelvis carcinoma was 22 years. Recurrent urinary tract infection was found in 65% of the patients with renal pelvis carcinoma and in 80% of those with bladder carcinoma and high phenacetin consumption. Previous radiotherapy had been given because of gynaecological tumours in three to four patients with ureteral tumours. The high frequency of recurrent urinary tract infection in patients with bladder tumours is remarkable.

The serum creatinine values in patients with phenacetin consumption and renal pelvis carcinoma or bladder carcinoma respectively are given in Table II. There was a similar distribution in the two groups of patients. The serum creatinine value gives no information of the level of the primary urothelial tumour in patients with a high consumption of phenacetin. In 60 patients with renal pelvis carcinoma all serum creatinine values over 1.4 mg% were associated with a heavy consumption of phenacetin containing analgesics. Some of the patients had severe damage to both kidneys. Conservative parenchymal kidney surgery was performed in 21 patients. Of these 14 had a high consumption of phenacetin. In 17 of the 21 a curative operation was possible. Bladder carcinoma patients with a high serum creatinine value but without bilateral stenosis of the ureters might have bilaterally damaged kidneys because of phenacetin - containing analgesics. Also patients with normal serum creatinine values and even normal clearance values can have had a consumption of phenacetin.

TABLE II

SERUM CREATININE VALUES IN PATIENTS WITH HIGH CONSUMPTION OF
PHENACETIN CONTAINING ANALGESICS AND WITH CARCINOMA OF THE
RENAL PELVIS OR BLADDER

	Serum Creatinine (mg%)				
	1.2	1.3-2.0	2.1-4.0	4	Total
Carcinoma of Renal Pelvis	15%	42%	24%	19%	100%
Bladder Carcinoma	26%	44%	17%	13%	100%

Upper urinary tract infection was found in 65% of the patients
with renal pelvis carcinoma and only in 5% with renal carcinoma
(Table III). This difference is statistically significant and it is
not possible to exclude an association between infection of the upper
urinary tract and the development of urothelial tumours. The
incidence of stone formation in each group before or at the time of
diagnosis is the same as that for 50 year old Swedish men and it
seems that stone formation is not of importance for the genesis of
these tumours. In patients with bladder stones bladder tumours have
been found in 16% which is remarkable.

Table IV shows the localisation of the primary tumour for 81
consecutive patients. There were as many males as females. Nearly
all had a urothelial tumour, only six had renal carcinoma and pure
squamous cell carcinoma was rare. The primary tumours associated
with phenacetin consumption seem to occur as often in the upper as

TABLE III

% INCIDENCE OF UPPER URINARY TRACT INFECTION, CALCULI AND DIABETES

IN PATIENTS WITH RENAL CARCINOMA AND CARCINOMA OF THE RENAL PELVIS

	Upper Tract Infection	Lithiasis	Diabetes
Renal Carcinoma n = 155	5	13	4
Carcinoma of Renal Pelvis n = 60	65	17	7

TABLE IV

SEX DISTRIBUTION AND LOCALISATION OF THE PRIMARY TUMOUR IN 81

TUMOUR PATIENTS WITH A HEAVY CONSUMPTION OF PHENACETIN

	Males	Females
Renal Carcinoma	3	3
Carcinoma of Renal Pelvis	16	21
Ureteral Carcinoma with or without Bladder Carcinoma	6	3
Bladder Carcinoma	16	13
Total	41	40

in the lower urinary tract. The reputation of phenacetin-containing
analgesics for causing pelvic carcinomas is somewhat misleading as
bladder carcinomas are found with equal frequency.

CONCLUSIONS

Chemical and non chemical carcinogens play an important part in
the formation of bladder tumours. It is important that these bladder
carcinomas are diagnosed early and treated adequately according to
their grade and stage. The prognosis for high grade tumours is
however bad whatever the treatment. The known urothelial carcinogens
are associated with the common distribution of malignancy grades.
The elimination of carcinogens in food, drugs, tobacco, drinking
water and of occupational carcinogens can reduce the increasing
incidence of bladder tumours of all grades. In Sweden occupational
carcinogens have not been found to be of importance. Although heavy
use of tobacco and/or phenacetin-containing analgesics in Sweden has
given rise in part to the increase of urological tumours the main
part of the increase is still unexplained. Investigation for the
detection of as yet unrecognised chemical carcinogens is complicated
by oncogens acting as described by Melicow and possibly by other
factors such as trauma, calculi and infection. It seems, however,
that it is as important to find these carcinogens as it is to refine
methods for diagnosis and treatment.

REFERENCES

1.   Bergman, B., Nygaard, E. and Tomic, R., To be published 1978.

2.   Johansson, S., Urothelial hyperplasia of the urinary bladder of
      the rat induced by mechanical perforation and phenacetin
      treatment. Acta Path. Microbiol. Scand., Section A, 86, 333-
      335 (1978).

3.   Johansson, S. and Wahlqvist, L., Tumours of urinary bladder and
      ureter associated with abuse of phenacetine containing
      analgesics. Acta Path. Microbiol. Scand., Section A, 85, 768-
      774 (1977).

4.   Johansson, S. and Wahlqvist, L., A prognostic study of uro-
      thelial renal pelvic tumour. Comparison between the prognosis
      of patients treated with intrafascial nephrectomy and peri-
      fascial nephroureterectomy. Cancer. In Press (1978).

5.   Johansson, S., Angervall, L., Bengtsson, U. and Wahlqvist, L.,
      Uroepithelial tumours of the renal pelvis associated with abuse
      of phenacetin containing analgesics. Cancer, 33, 743-753
      (1974).

6.   Johansson, S., Angervall, L., Bengtsson, U. and Wahlqvist, L.,
      A clinicopathologic and prognostic study of epithelial tumours
      of the renal pelvis. Cancer, 37, 1376-1383 (1976).

7.   Melicow, M. M., The urothelium : A battleground for oncogenesis.
      J. Urol. 120, 43-47 (1978).

PATHOLOGY OF BLADDER TUMOURS. THE UROLOGIST'S POINT OF VIEW

G GRECHI and G P MINCIONE

Institute of Urology and Institute of Pathology

University of Florence, Italy

ABSTRACT

Many aspects of the pathology of bladder tumours need to be clarified, particularly:-

1.   the nature of the disease: are bladder tumours of a common origin or are they heterogeneous?

2.   are clinical "recurrences" real or merely new lesions related to the multicentricity of the disease?

3.   tumours with a clearly defined benign histologic pattern may have an unpredictable evolution; also recurrent tumours may change in grade;

4.   the dubious accuracy of clinical staging often makes the choice of therapy and prognosis difficult.

INTRODUCTION

The knowledge of the pathology of bladder tumours must influence the Urologist's activity if we are to improve the possibilities of diagnosis and treatment and reduce unsatisfactory results.

It must be emphasised at once, that some pathological features need to be clarified. The first problem concerns the nature of the disease, particularly the unanswered question as to whether bladder tumours are to be considered as uniform or heterogeneous: as for this point, polymorphism of bladder tumours and, essentially, the difference between papillary and solid growths is well known. The problem is:- are we dealing with a single oncogen and, consequently,

with the same tumour, the difference resulting from various responses
of cells with different potentials or, on the contrary, are we
dealing with more than one carcinogen each stimulating urothelial
cells in a different way and so, ab initio, the tumours must be
considered to be dissimilar? The question is important from the
practical point of view as it is known that papillary tumours
include those forms that are easier to treat and have a better
prognosis; but if the first hypothesis is the true one, in every
cases of grade O or I papillary tumour the possibility of co
existence of a solid tumour or of a carcinoma in situ ought to be
considered.

The second problem concerns the multicentricity of urothelial
neoplasms and underlines three different points of great importance
from the clinical point of view:

1.   bladder neoplasms are often multiple;

2.   a bladder neoplasm can be concomitant with or secondary
to a urothelial tumour of the upper urinary tract or of the
urethra;

3.   the difficulty of distinguishing recurrences of a bladder
tumour from new lesions.

HISTOLOGY

The histology of bladder neoplasms is well defined, but
classification criteria are various. The difficulty arises in
determining the correlation between the clinical and the histological
pattern of these tumours for which, chiefly, criteria of benignancy
need to be defined. In fact tumours with a clearly defined benign
histologic pattern may have unpredictable evolution including
recurrence and change in grade and stage. As a result some workers
consider all bladder tumours as potentially malignant and the term
"carcinoma" has been applied to all of them. We cannot agree with
such an opinion as, in our judgement, the term "carcinoma" should
be applied only to actually histologically malignant growths and not
to potentially cancerous or even to precancerous lesions. The term
"papilloma", with the meaning of a defined benign lesion, must be
maintained. The problem is to differentiate, in the pathological
study, between papillomas that will recur and become malignant and
those that will have a benign course. If it is once established
that classical histology cannot help in this field, additional help
may be found, according to recent studies, in cytogenetic evaluation
of cells in the pathological specimen, and in immunological studies.

CYTOGENETIC AND IMMUNOLOGICAL EVALUATION

In cytogenetic evaluation, the study of chromosome number does not seem to have a practical clinical value. High chromosome numbers are usually seen in high degrees of anaplasia and low chromosome numbers are related to well differentiated tumours: evidently, the findings are concomitant with histology.

A greater clinical value is to be attributed to chromosome constitution, i.e. karyotype. The finding of abnormal chromosomes, called "marker chromosomes" (Falor and Ward, 1978) in the cells of the pathological specimen seems to demonstrate a potentiality for recurrence that is not present in cases in which marker chromosomes are absent.

In our opinion these studies could represent a great aid in the diagnosis and management of bladder neoplasms dictating, in selected cases, more intensive therapy.

Another field of study that may help in predicting the natural history of an initial tumour is offered by immunology. The major blood group antigens are present on the surface of normal bladder epithelial cells and in those low grade tumours that seem to have a minor potentiality for recurrence. The loss of surface antigens in tumour cells seems to predict a malignant behaviour (Bergman and Javadpour, 1978).

CONCLUSIONS

What then are the questions of clinical value the urologist must ask the pathologist dealing with a bladder tumour specimen?

1. The grading of the tumour, with the related problems we have talked about;

2. Staging of the tumour, assessing the depth of infiltration in the muscle layers and the vascular and lymphatic invasion. It must be emphasised that pathological staging after cystectomy requires good fixation and that this is obtained by filling the bladder with 10% formalin soon after operation, in order to eliminate folding of the wall. Specimens removed by TUR may be difficult to stage;

3. Assessment of the pattern of regional lymph-nodes, to establish neoplastic invasion and also, eventually, the activity of the patient's immune response to the tumour, providing a more accurate guide to prognosis. From this point of view lymph-nodes are classified into three histologic patterns and designated as

stimulated, depleted and unstimulated (Herr et al, 1976). It has
been suggested that stimulated lymph-nodes may be the result of
immune response to the tumour with a favourable influence on the
survival.

REFERENCES

1.   Dergman, C. and Javadpour, N., The cell surface antigen A, B
     or O(H) as an indicator of malignant potential in stage A
     bladder carcinoma: preliminary report. J. Urol. 119, 49-51
     (1978).

2.   Falor, W. H. and Ward. R. M., Prognosis in early carcinoma of
     the bladder based on chromosomal analysis. J. Urol. 119, 44-48
     (1978).

3.   Herr, H. W., Bean, M. A. and Whitmore, W. F. Jr., Prognostic
     significance of regional lymph node histology in cancer of the
     bladder. J. Urol. 115, 264-267 (1976).

NEWER ASPECTS OF RESEARCH IN THE FIELD OF BLADDER TUMOURS

L ANDERSSON, T BERLIN, L COLLSTE, I GRANBERG-OHMAN
H GUSTAFSSON, B TRIBUKAIT and H WIJKSTROM

Departments of Urology and Medical Radiobiology
Karolinska sjukhuset and Departments of Morphology and
Urology, Huddinge Hospital, Stockholm, Sweden

This survey of recent research will deal with early events in urothelial cells when they undergo malignant transformation, and with new techniques for objective measurement of the cellular characteristics of malignancy.

It is generally accepted that carcinoma of the bladder is a field change in the urothelium, and that there are structural changes in the mucosa which are not visible on cystoscopy. Electron microscopy studies of urothelial cells have revealed a number of events occurring on transformation of benign cells to cancer, both in vivo and in vitro.

Hashimoto and Kitagawa (1974) introduced an in vitro technique to transform benign epithelium of rat bladder into carcinoma. Following incubation with butyl-nitrosamine and urea, the epithelial cells change their behaviour. They give rise to neoplastic outgrowth on implantation into syngeneic animals. Kahan et al (1977) performed scanning electron microscopy studies of rat bladder epithelial cells before and after nitrosamine incubation with Hashimoto-Kitagawa's technique. Following incubation the cells were covered by numerous pleomorphic microvillous structures and occasional coarse surface excrescences that were not observed in normal cells. In vitro studies of this kind have the special interest of showing changes which are closely associated in time with the malignant cell transformation.

There is also on record a number of similar in vivo studies, both in humans and experimental animals. Nelson et al (1978) and others have demonstrated a rough cell surface with pleomorphic microvilli and lack of cell-to-cell contact in transitional cell

carcinoma of the human bladder (Figure 1). These microvilli are
also seen on the surface of exfoliated tumour cells (Croft et al,
1978).

    In bladders containing a tumour it is sometimes possible to
identify by scanning electron microscopy (SEM) surface changes of a
similar nature to those in the tumour in areas where no tumour is
seen on cystoscopy or even on light microscopy examination of
biopsy specimens. This has importance for the future prognosis in
cases where conservative surgery is performed.

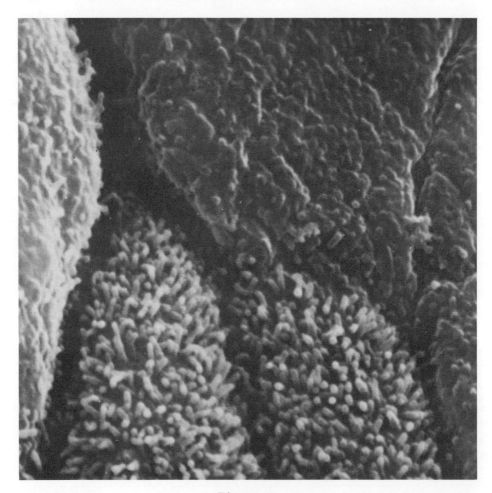

Figure 1

Scanning electron micrograph of bladder epithelium from the margin
of a transitional cell carcinoma of the bladder. To the left and
below are cancer cells with numerous pleomorphic microvilli
compared to adjacent non cancer cells (Courtesy of Dr C E Nelson).

The normal barrier function of the urinary tract walls may be altered in urothelial carcinoma. Merk et al (1977) investigated the transepithelial permeability in the normal and malignant urinary bladder, both in humans and in rats. In the normal epithelium distinct seam-like elevations between the cell boundaries are seen on SEM. The superficial cells are joined together by junctional complexes consisting of a network of strands encircling the cells and situated at that part of the intercellular cleft located near the bladder lumen.

In low grade and moderate bladder carcinoma there is an attenuation of the tight junctions between superficial cells and in high grade carcinoma there is often discontinuation of the tight junctions. This phenomenon is supposed to be the main cause of the increased mucosal permeability occurring in bladder carcinoma. It is probably also the explanation of the reduced cellular cohesion existing in carcinoma and giving rise to an accelerated exfoliation of cells.

Recently there has been increasing interest in topical chemo-therapy in carcinoma in situ of the bladder. It is possible that enhanced permeability of the malignant epithelium may permit better drug access even to the layer below the most superficial.

Attempts have also been made to identify surface alterations of malignant cells by chemical analysis of components dispersed by purified plasma membrane fractions or by extraction with KC1, a procedure known to release tumour-specific transplantation antigens. Carcino-embryonic antigen is one such substance. If even more specific antigens can be found we can hope to raise specific xeno-antisera that may afford useful immunodiagnostic reagents and may also enhance the immune response of the tumour host. Perlman, Troye and coworkers have recently isolated tumour antigens with the aid of immunoreactions (1978).

Even though much interest is being focused on identifying tumour markers to enable us to detect early tumour and tumour recurrence we must agree that as yet morphological techniques have been more reliable both to establish the diagnosis of urothelial carcinoma and to characterize its degree of malignancy. However, both histopathology of bladder specimens and, perhaps even more cytology of urine or bladder irrigation fluid are to some degree hampered by their inherent element of subjective evaluation.

In many centres today research is focused on the problem of finding methods for unbiased objective measurements of cell phenomena indicating malignant transformation. A number of flow cytometry techniques have made it possible to obtain information on the individual cells in large populations.

Cancer cells differ from normal cells in many respects such as nuclear size and shape, chromatin pattern, intensity of replication, etc. The cancer cell often displays a big, irregular nucleus with a dense chromatin pattern of irregular conformation. Bizarre mitoses are often seen with a higher than normal chromosome number differing from the diploid pattern.

DNA analysis of single cell nucleus gives an indirect measurement of the number of chromosomes in the cell. With the aid of rapid-flow cytofluorometry, Tribukait and co-workers (1978) have investigated bladder irrigation fluid and tumour biopsy suspensions from patients with urothelial carcinoma. A preparation containing

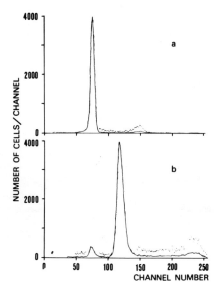

Figure 2

DNA-histograms from (a): well differentiated tumour, Grade I, and (b) poorly differentiated tumour, Grade III. Ordinate: Channel number corresponding to the amount of DNA. Abscissa: Number of cells per channel. The dotted lines represent a four-fold magnification.
The large peak to the left in (a) at channel number 75 represents diploid G_1-cells. The small peak at channel number 150 represents the tetraploid G_2-cells. Between these two peaks are the cells in S-phase. The small peak to the left in (b) represents normal G_1-cells. In the triploid region, at channel number 120, the G_1-cells of an aneuploid cell population can be observed. At channel number 240 the G_2-cells of this aneuploid cell population can be seen. Between these two peaks are the cells in S-phase, constituting 8.0% of the total aneuploid cell population.

an average of 20-40,000 cells, is analysed in a few minutes and the
result is presented as a DNA-histogram.

Figure 2 shows histograms from tumours of Grade I (a) and Grade
III (b) (WHO grading). The method allows quantitative determination
of the number of cells in different parts of the cell cycle. Thus,
measuring the proportion of cells in S-phase (DNA synthesis phase)
allows estimation of the proliferation rate in the tumour. It has
been shown that 80% of clinical category T1 tumours are diploid
with a low proliferation rate. In most cases tumours of category
T2, T3 and carcinomata in situ are aneuploid and show a high
proliferation rate. Grade I tumours are diploid, while Grade III
tumours practically always show aneuploidy, mainly in the triploid
region. In the clinically non-homogenous group Grade II tumours,
about 60% are diploid. The remainder show various degrees of
aneuploidy.

The implication of the degree of aneuploidy and proliferation
is about to be studied. Tumour cell populations having a DNA
content corresponding to the tetraploid region, in general seem to
have a lower proliferation rate compared to cell populations with
higher or lower degrees of aneuploidy. The latter tumours are more
likely to have an aggressive clinical course.

Melamed et al (1977) used the metachromatic fluorescent dye
acridin orange to distinguish cell and nuclear size, quantity of
DNA and RNA, and deviations in chromatin pattern. Acridin orange
is taken up by nucleic acids in different ways (Lerman, 1963). It
is bound to double-helical DNA by intercalation and to single
stranded RNA by stacking (Figure 3). The intercalated dye molecules
give green fluorescence in blue light while the molecules stacked
closely together give a red fluorescence.

In the device used by Melamed et al a suspension of cells to
be examined flows rapidly through a glass channel narrow enough for
the cells to flow in single file through a focused blue laser beam.
When the acridin orange stained cells flow through the laser beam
they emit a fluorescent pulse, that is separated into red and green
components. For each cell the two values are measured simultaneously
and recorded in a computer memory. Analysis of these computer-
plotted scattergrams enables estimation of RNA and DNA synthesis,
transition of cells from non-cycling to cycling phase, and under
certain conditions, of the structure of DNA. In the abnormal
chromatin of cancer cells the DNA resistance to heat is decreased.
A suspension of cells to be investigated is exposed to high
temperature and then stained with acridin orange. A higher than
normal denaturation of DNA gives a decreased proportion of green to
total fluorescence - indicating abnormal chromatin structure. Such
methods to detect early chromatin alterations are interesting
because chemical and functional changes of nuclear chromatin must
precede the visible changes.

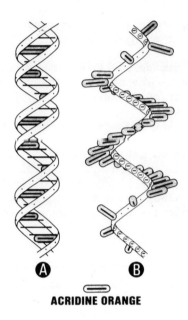

ACRIDINE ORANGE

Figure 3

Diagrammatic representation of binding by acridin orange to double-
helical DNA and to single stranded RNA. (Courtesy of Dr M R Melamed
et al and Cancer Research)

        In near diploid tumours where nuclear DNA quantity differs too
little from normal to be detected as abnormal on cytofluorometry,
chromosome analysis may give additional information as to the
biological properties of the tumour (Spooner et al, 1972; Sandberg,
1977; Falor et al, 1978). Granberg-Ohman et al (1978) compared
chromosome pattern and nuclear DNA content of tumour cells in 32
cases of transitional cell carcinoma of the bladder. Histological
grading was done according to WHO with the modification that grade
II was subdivided into "A" and "B" with increasing degree of dedifferentiation.

        In order to increase the number of metaphases the patients
were given 1.8 mg Vinblastine i.v. prior to operation. Fresh tumour
was minced and directly treated with hypotonic solution and routine
fixation. Analysable metaphases obtained by air-dry method were
counted and whenever possible karyotyped. The DNA content was
investigated by flow cytofluorometry. Eight GIIa tumours had cells
in the diploid region with occasional structurally abnormal "marker"
chromosomes. In the seven GIIb tumours the count was peridiploid,
ranging from 43-48. This could not be detected by cytofluorometry.
Some cases had "markers" in most cells analysed (Figure 4). All 17

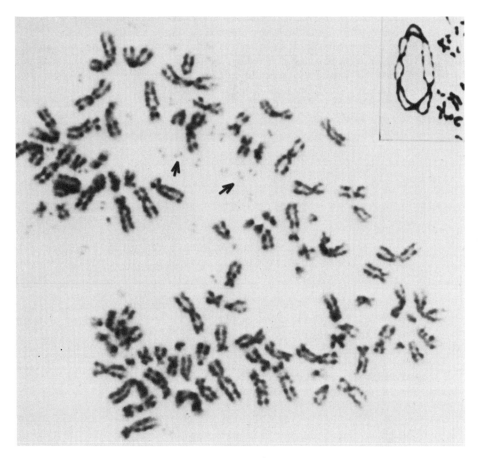

Figure 4

Male, 72 years, papillary bladder carcinoma grade III.

Modal metaphase containing 94 chromosomes and in addition plenty of
double-minutes (arrows). G-band. A few perimodal cells showed a
larger ring marker chromosome (detail of a metaphase in the upper
right corner).
Mode = Stemline = Predominating number of chromosomes.
Perimodal = Above or below the modal number. G-band = Giemsa-
Trypsin. Double-minutes = Small marker chromosomes, always
appearing by pairs.

GIII tumours were aneuploid. In polyploid tumours the chromosome
numbers varied widely within each tumour. By cytofluorometry,
however, more or less distinct modes could be detected. In all
cases "markers" were found and they most often seemed to be derived
from the groups A and B.

Even if the new research fields briefly reviewed have already given some promising preliminary results, they require continued follow-up by correlation with the clinical course of the tumour cases before we can evaluate their usefulness in solving the urgent problem of how to find the tumour early in its growth, when it is still potentially curable, and how to identify more accurately in this early phase, what degree of aggressiveness can be expected from this particular carcinoma.

REFERENCES

1. Croft, W. A., Nelson, C. E. and Nilsson, T., Scanning electron microscopy of exfoliated malignant and non malignant human urothelial cells. Scand. J. Urol. Nephrol. In Press (1978).

2. Falor, W. H. and Ward, R. M., Prognosis in early carcinoma of the bladder based on chromosomal analysis. J. Urol., 119, 44 (1978).

3. Granberg-Ohman, I., Tribukait, B., Wijkstrom, H., Berlin, T. and Collste, L., Chromosome and DNA Pattern in Bladder Cancer. To be published in Urol. Research.

4. Hashimoto, Y. and Kitagawa, H. S., In vitro neoplastic transformation of epithelial cells of rat urinary bladder by nitrosamines. Nature, 252, 497 (1974).

5. Kahan, B. D., Rutzby, L. P., Kahan, A. V., Oyasu. R., Wiseman, F. and LeGrue, S., Cell surface changes associated with malignant transformation of bladder epithelium in vitro. Cancer Res., 37, 2866 (1977).

6. Lerman, L. S., The structure of the DNA-acridine complex. Proc. Natl. Acad. Sci. US, 49, 94 (1963).

7. Melamed, M. R., Darzynkiewicz, Z., Traganos, F. and Sharpless, T., Cytology automation by flow cytometry. Cancer Res., 37, 2806 (1977).

8. Merk, F. B., Pauli, B. U., Jacobs, J. B., Alroy, J., Friedell, G. H.,and Wernstein, R. S., Malignant transformation of urinary bladder in humans and in N-(4-(5-nitro-2-furyl)-2-thiazotyl) formamide-esposed Fischer rats: Ultrastructure of the major components of the permeability barrier. Cancer Res. 37, 2843 (1977).

9. Nelson, C. E., Croft, W. A. and Nilsson, T., Surface characteristics of malignant human urinary bladder epithelium studied with scanning electron microscopy. Scand. J. Urol. Nephrol. In Press (1978).

10.   Perlman, P. and Troye, M., Unpublished data, 1978.

11.   Sandberg, A. A., Chromosome markers and progression in bladder
       cancer. Cancer Res. 37, 2950 (1977).

12.   Spooner, M. E. and Cooper, E. H., Chromosome constitution of
       transitional cell carcinoma of the urinary bladder. Cancer,
       29, 1401 (1972).

13.   Tribukait, B., Gustafson, H. and Esposti, P., Ploidy and
       proliferation in human bladder tumours as measured by flow
       cytofluorometric DNA analysis and its relations to histo-
       pathology and cytology. Cancer, In Press (1978).

CYTOLOGY OF BLADDER TUMOURS - ROUND TABLE

P L ESPOSTI, Radiumhemmet, Karolinska Sjukhuset,
Stockholm, Sweden
H J DE VOOGT, University Hospital, Leiden, The Netherlands
G GRECHI, Institute of Urology, University of Firenze,
Italy
J A MARTINEZ-PIÑEIRO, Autonomous University, Madrid, Spain
M VENTURA, Department of Urology, S. Andrea Hospital,
Vercelli, Italy

THE IMPORTANCE OF URINARY CYTOLOGY

Dr Esposti, opening the discussion, observed that the urinary
tract is lined with transitional cell epithelium or urothelium,
exhibiting several (up to seven or eight) layers of cells. The
exfoliated urothelial cells can easily be examined for cytological
diagnosis, using urinary sediment. However, experience at
Radiumhemmet (Esposti et al, 1970) showed that cellular preservation
was better and cytological details easier analysed in bladder
washings, using 0.9% NaCl solution. The centrifuged cell material,
fixed with methanol-acetic acid mixture, was stained according to
the Papanicolaou method. As the majority of the tumours of the
urinary tract are of urothelial origin and occur most often in the
bladder, cytological diagnosis has proved useful in the management
of tumours of the urinary bladder.

The accuracy of the cytological method must be evaluated by
clinical follow-up and by comparing cytological findings with the
histological reports from biopsy specimens. At Radiumhemmet the
histological classification of Bergkvist et al (1965) was adopted:
it consists of five grades (O-IV) according to the severity of
deviation of the cell pattern from normal urothelium. Such
histological grading provides a firm basis for judging the reliability of exfoliative cytology in the diagnosis of bladder
tumours. Following these principles and after more than ten years
of clinical experience one can conclude that a cytological report of
malignancy is highly reliable. In all cases without evident bladder

neoplasm and with repeated cytological reports of carcinoma, a
carcinoma in situ was eventually diagnosed histologically. As
regards "false negative" cytological reports, one must keep in mind
that urinary cytology does not permit recognition of the neoplastic
nature of papillary tumours grade O-I. The correlation between the
histological and cytological diagnosis is much closer in the frankly
invasive grade II, in grade III and in grade IV (anaplastic) tumours,
with a cytological accuracy of about 90%.

In cases of carcinoma of the bladder treated with super-
voltage irradiation, cytological follow-up is of diagnostic and
prognostic importance. A cytological diagnosis of persistent or
recurrent carcinoma after radiotherapy is feasible in most cases
with clinical signs of tumour growth. When cytological findings
become positive for carcinoma in cases free from tumours after
radiotherapy, a macroscopic recurrence of tumour must be expected to
occur in the majority of cases within one year.

The advantages offered by the cytological method are ease in
assessing intracellular details by high-power microscopy of the
smears and the possibility of repeating the cytological analysis
before, during and after therapy without discomfort for the patient.

Dr Grechi (Florence) speaking on behalf of Dr Mincione of
Florence and himself gave the urologist's point of view about the
importance of cytology in bladder tumours. Urinary cytology can be
routinely employed in patients with haematuria, in patients with
clinical and radiological suspicion of bladder tumour, in grading
the malignancy of a tumour and in follow-up studies of patients
treated for bladder neoplasms. In many cases cytology only ratifies
what is already evident from other diagnostic procedures. In a
limited number of cases where other diagnostic procedures have given
uncertain results, cytology may be of paramount importance. A
striking example is carcinoma in situ where carcinoma cells can be
found in the sediment isolated or in sheets against a clear background. The cytological method is helpful also in cases of severe
urothelial dysplasia, a lesion which, like carcinoma in situ, is
often associated with or precedes bladder tumours. The possibility
of recognising cytological bladder tumours depend on their
malignancy grade: while grade III and IV tumours according to the
classification of Bergkvist et al (1965) are easily recognised, the
borderline group of grade II tumours represents a diagnostic problem.
In grade O and I papillomas a report of suspected papillary tumour
can be given in 50% of cases, thanks to the presence of numerous
polymorphous and elongated epithelial cells, often arranged in
clusters. This cytological report of suspected papillary tumour,
however, can be given only when the occurrence of urinary calculi or
previous catheterisation, which induce similar cytologic alterations,
can be excluded. Finally, one should not forget the possibility of
using the cytological method as a screening method for high-risk

groups, such as chemical workers and heavy smokers. Since urothelial
lesions are often multicentric, urine cytology is a very suitable
test as it provides information about the whole urothelium.

REFERENCES

1. Bergkvist, A., Ljungqvist, A. and Moberger, G., Classification
    of bladder tumours based on the cellular pattern. Preliminary
    report of a clinical-pathological study of 300 cases with a
    minimum follow-up of eight years. Acta Chir. Scand. 130,
    371-378 (1965).

2. Esposti, P. L., Moberger, G. and Zajicek, J., The cytologic
    diagnosis of transitional cell tumours of the urinary bladder
    and its histologic basis. A study of 567 cases of urinary-
    tract disorder including 170 untreated and 182 irradiated
    bladder tumours. Acta Cytol. 14, 145-155 (1970).

PHASE CONTRAST MICROSCOPY OF THE URINARY SEDIMENT

Dr de Voogt (Leiden) emphasised the importance of Phase
Contrast Microscopy (PCM) for rapid screening of urinary sediment.
It takes no more time than a normal light microscope examination of
urinary sediment and enables the urologist to see whether atypical
or malignant cells are present. The principle of PCM is separation
of diffracted and non-diffracted light rays. Due to extinction by
interference, structural details of the object appear darker than
the surrounding medium. In this way epithelial cells in the urine
can be clearly seen. Five simple criteria can be used in order to
distinguish atypical and malignant cells from normal ones:
1) appearance of urothelial cells singly or in groups, 2) ir-
regularities in the arrangement of cell groups, 3) nuclear/
cytoplasmic ratio, 4) size and shape of nucleus, 5) presence of
nucleoli, their size and number.

The disadvantages of the method are those of less specificity
and sensitivity compared to the Papanicolaou and Giemsa stainings
and of difficulty in recognising epithelial cells when many erythro-
and leukocytes are present. Finally, the preparations cannot be
preserved for re-examination. By PCM a rapid screening can be done,
for instance during office hours, with a reliability that approx-
imates to the reliability of stained cytologic preparations.

Dr Ventura (Vercelli) proposed the use of different combined
cyto-histologic techniques: the classical cytological methods can
be completed with cariological studies, where the analysis is
focused on the nuclear morphology, after having destroyed the
cytoplasm, with phase contrast screening and finally with scanning

Electron Microscope. In the last case a small biopsy from the
bladder tumour is necessary. Like de Voogt, Ventura is impressed
with phase contract microscopy and feels that this method is
probably the most rapid and effective method of screening factory
workers when this is necessary.

     Professor Martinez-Piñeiro (Madrid) referred to the interest
which he and Dr Muntanola had shown in fluorescence cytology
starting in 1969 (1) with the use of ultraviolet light cystoscopy
(2,3) for the detection of neoplastic lesions not revealed by cold
light endoscopy. Shortly afterwards, in view of the shortcomings of
this procedure and supposing that the same acridine-orange dye used
for cystoscopy might equally well induce fluorescence in exfoliated
malignant cells in the urine they reviewed the literature and
discovered that fluorescence cytology had been previously applied
to a variety of tumours (4,5,6,7,8) with good results. The
preliminary experience in urology was not very favourable (9,10).
Gonzales Martin concluded, however, that fluorescence urinary
cytology yielded the same results as the Papanicolaou method, with
the additional advantage of its lower cost and technical simplicity
(11). Presently, after four years further large scale use, it is
felt that the main merit of acridine-orange fluorescence microscopy
lies in its capacity to establish the histochemical cell characteristics. In fact, acridine orange possesses a strong affinity for
nucleic acids, which when stained by this fluorochromatic dye, emit
a bright fluorescence under ultraviolet light (orange or reddish
for nucleolar and/or cytoplasmic RNA, and yellow for nuclear DNA).
Thus, the higher the nucleic acid content of a cell the higher its
affinity for amino-acridines (12) and the higher its fluorescence.
In this way the urothelial malignant cells possessing a high nucleic
acid synthesis and content will clearly stand out among the normal
cells in the dark ultraviolet microscopic field. The morphological
criteria of malignancy or atypia, consisting primarily of variations
in cell size, nuclear hyperchromatism, chromatin clumping, nuclear
size, number of nucleoli and nucleolar irregularity are thus
supplemented with histochemical criteria consisting of variations
in dye uptake and fluorescence, which are of great help in uncovering
dubious or masked cells. This accounts for the 90-95% accurate
cytological diagnosis in cases of proved bladder cancer in the
published series (11,13,14).

     These findings also support the value of fluorescence cytology
as a means of predicting the histological grade of malignancy of a
tumour. In an updated review of 794 patients 391 had persisting
tumour. Fluorescence cytology on voided specimens or on bladder
washings was positive in all patients. Table I shows the close
relationship between histological and cytological grade. Almost 85%
of patients with cytological grade IV had a high grade (G3) lesion
whilst 75% of patients with cytological grade IIIb (non conclusive
of malignity) has a low grade (G1) lesion. In the 403 patients with

TABLE I

CORRELATION OF HISTOLOGICAL AND CYTOLOGICAL GRADING IN 391 PATIENTS

WITH BLADDER TUMOUR INVESTIGATED BY FLUORESCENCE URINARY CYTOLOGY

Cytological Grade	Histological Grade					
	High (G3)		Medium (G2)		Low (G1)	
V 151 cases	128	84.8%	15	9.9%	8	5.3%
IV 174 cases	1	0.6%	119	68.4%	54	31%
IIIb 66 cases	1	1.5%	16	24.2%	49	74.2%

no evidence of tumour the cytology and its relationship to subsequent
recurrence is shown in Table II.

Although the potential of cytology to diagnose the presence, or
to herald the future appearance of bladder neoplasms has been
convincingly demonstrated in selected groups of patients, it is not
yet a widely accepted modality for the screening of unselected
populations, or for routine diagnostic purposes, due to the
relatively high cost, in terms of money and time, and to the
relatively high incidence of false negative results (around 20%) of
the most commonly used staining methods (16,17). This accounts also
for the reluctance of the urologists to replace cystoscopic
examination by urinary cytologic examination in the diagnosis and
follow-up of bladder cancer. The adoption of a more simple, cheaper
and less time-consuming technique, like fluorescence cytology, may
help to change their minds expecially as in this series the results
were accurate in 92.2%, with a false positive incidence of 7.8%.

TABLE II

CAPACITY OF FLUORESCENCE URINARY CYTOLOGY TO PREDICT RECURRENCE OF

BLADDER TUMOURS

	Subsequent Recurrence
I, II, IIIa - Benign - 213	0
IIIb - Suspicious - 102	59 (57.8%)
IV, V - Malignant - 88	69 (78.4%)

Professor Martinez-Piñeiro concluded that urinary cytology is of unsurpassed value for the:-

1. Screening of high risk populations such as industrial dye workers where large scale cystoscopy is impractical.

2. Detection of lesions where cystoscopy may not reveal an existing malignancy such as carcinoma in situ, carcinoma in bladders with chronic cystitis and cancers within a diverticulum.

3. Detection of lesions in patients presenting with haematuria, where the accuracy of a positive cytology is sufficient to indicate frequent re-evaluations and exhaustive investigation.

4. Follow-up of conservatively treated lesions, allowing the diagnosis of residual malignant urothelium or allowing one to predict the appearance of recurrences months before a cancer would ordinarily be found cystoscopically and thereby indicating the need for some chemoprophylactic treatment.

REFERENCES

1. Martinez-Piñeiro, J. A. and Arocena, F., El diagnostico de los tumores vesicales con luz ultravioleta. Actas Assoc. Esp. Urol. 3, 1, (1971).

2. Whitmore, W. F., Bush, I. M. and Esquivel, E., Tetracycline ultraviolet fluorescence in bladder carcinoma. Cancer, 17, 1528, (1964).

3. McDonald, D. F., Personal communication to Quint, T. H., Hett, J. A. and Wallace, F. Y. Fluorescence cystoscopy. J. Urol. 95, 208 (1966).

4. Schummelfeder, N., Histochemical significance of the polychromatic fluorescence induced in tissues stained with Acridine Orange. J. Histochem. Cytochem. 6, 392 (1950).

5. Friedman, H. P. The use of ultraviolet light and fluorescence dyes in the detection of uterine cancer by vaginal smear. J. Obstet. Gynaecol. 59, 852 (1950).

6. Bertalanffy, L. W., Masin, F., Masin, M., Use of acridine orange fluorescence technique in exfoliative cytology. Science, N.Y. 124, 1024 (1956).

8. Bertalanffy, L. W., Masin, M., Masin, F., A new and rapid method for diagnosis of vaginal and cervical cancer by fluorescence microscopy. Cancer, 2, 873 (1958).

9. Lin, W., Fluorescence microscopy in exfoliative cytology. Arch. Pathol. 71, 286 (1961).

10. Anderson, W. A. D. and Gunn, S. A., Cytology detection of cancer; considerations for its future: A comparative examination of the Papanicolau and Acridine Orange techniques. Acta. Cytol. 6, 468 (1962).

11. Gonzalez Martin, M., Citodiagnostico precoz del cancer vesico-uretral por micro fluorescencia. Doctoral thesis. Autonomous University. Madrid (1974).

12. Ackerman, N. B., Haldorsen, D. K., Wallace, D. L., Madsen, A. J. and McFee, F. S., Aminoacridine uptake by experimental tumours. J.A.M.A. 191, 115 (1965).

13. Martinez-Piñeiro, J. A., Gonzalez Martin, M., Arocena Lanz, F. and Escudero, A., Avances en el diagnostico del carcinoma vesical. Rev. Clin. Esp. 131, 273 (1973).

14. Martinez-Piñeiro, J. A., Muntanola, P., Gonzalez Martin, M. and Hidalgo, L., Fluorescence urinary cytology in bladder cancer. Eur. Urol. 3, 142 (1977).

15. MacFarlane, E. W., Some pathologic conditions affecting urine cytology. Acta Cytol. 7, 196 (1963).

16. MacFarlane, E. W., Ceelen, G. H. and Taylor, J. N., Urine cytology after treatment of bladder tumours. Acta Cytol. 8, 288 (1964).

17. Umiker, W., Accuracy of cytology diagnosis of cancer of the urinary tract. Acta Cytol. 8, 186 (1964).

SCANNING AND TRANSMISSION ELECTRON MICROSCOPY OF HYPERPLASTIC AND NEOPLASTIC HUMAN UROTHELIUM

S CASANOVA AND F CORRADO

Servizio di Anatomia Patologica e Divisione di Urologia I

Ospedale M. Malpighi, Bologna, Italy

INTRODUCTION

Recent experimental studies have shown that the occurrence of bladder cancer is preceded by preneoplastic urothelial lesions, whose development is related to a series of well defined cell-surface changes at scanning electrone microscopy (SEM). Some lesions, as demonstrated by Jacobs et al (3) can regress upon removal of carcinogenic stimulus, while others appear to be irreversible, even if the carcinogen is discontinued. The appearance of pleomorphic microvilli on surface cells seems to represent the hallmark of irreversible hyperplasia in rats.

Precancerous epithelial abnormalities may be observed in areas of bladder peripheral to visible tumour in man. At present few data are available regarding the surface morphology of these lesions.

By means of scanning and transmission electron microscopy we have examined cell surface changes of human urothelium in normal appearing areas peripheral to visible tumours, in order to detect the possible occurrence of ultrastructural features similar to those present in animal models.

MATERIAL AND METHODS

Samples were taken from tumours and from adjacent areas apparently free of tumours. Control specimens were obtained from bladders operated upon for non-malignant diseases.

The specimens were fixed as soon as possible in Karnovsky's

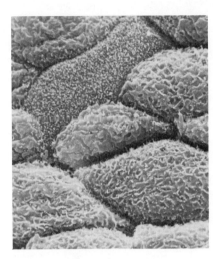 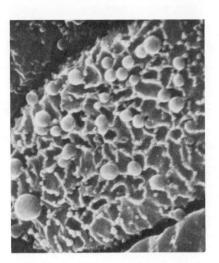

FIGURE 1 (left)   Scanning electron micrograph of the luminal surface
in a control human bladder. The luminal plasma membrane shows the
peculiar angular ridges. An intermediate cell is covered by regular
microvilli (SEM x 2,000). (Reduced 20% for purposes of reproduction)
FIGURE 2 (right)   Control human bladder. The superficial cells are
covered by a honeycomb network of rounded microridges and cytoplasmic
globules (SEM x 10,000). (Reduced 20% for purposes of reproduction)

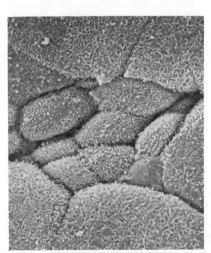 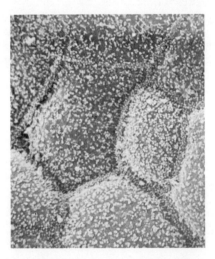

FIGURE 3 (left)   A normal differentiating area in a tumour-bearing
human bladder shows both angular microridges on mature superficial
cells and uniform microvilli on deeper intermediate cells (SEM x
2,000). (Reduced 20% for purposes of reproduction)
FIGURE 4 (right)   An area of urothelial hyperplasia adjacent to a
papillary carcinoma. Note the uniform microvilli and boundaries
between superficial cells (SEM x 3,000). (Reduced 20% for purposes
of reproduction)

fixative diluted I to I with phosphate buffer pH 7.4.

For electron microscopy, the specimens were postfixed in OsO_4 1% in veronal acetate buffer, dehydrated in alcohol and propilene oxide, and embedded in Epon-Araldite. Thin sections were obtained from selected areas and stained with uranyl acetate and lead citrate.

For scanning electron microscopy, the specimens were dehydrated in acetone and dried at the critical point using CO_2 as substitute; blocks coated with gold were examined in a JeoI U_3SEM at 25kV.

Parts from each specimen were processed for routine histological examination.

RESULTS

In all control bladders the urothelium showed three to six layers of epithelial cells, the superficial polyploid "umbrella" cells covering smaller intermediate and basal cells. The luminal plasma membrane of the umbrella cells displayed the peculiar angular appearance already described in rats and other mammals in four of our six controls. This aspect was particularly striking under the scanning microscope (Figure 1). At high magnification on thin sections, plaques of asymmetric unit membrane were present at the luminal surface.

In two controls the superficial cells exhibited rounded micro-ridges at the scanning microscope (Figure 2).

Specimens collected at the periphery of visible tumours showed different light microscopic changes.

Some areas exhibited maintainance of cell differentiation and the presence of microridges at the scanning (Figure 3), whereas others displayed pronounced hyperplastic changes with papillary or nodular hyperplasia. Scanning electron microscopy on the latter ones revealed regular microvilli on the luminal plasma membrane (Figure 4).

As the degree of dysplasia increased, the luminal surface of the urinary bladder assumed an irregular cobblestone appearance and displayed pleomorphic microvilli on the surface (Figure 5).

At the transmission electron microscope both regular and irregular microvilli were lined by an asymmetric unit membrane (AUM) and covered by a filamentous glycocalix.

The surface morphology of neoplastic areas showed papillary aggregates of cells protruding into the lumen; these cells were covered by microvilli (Figure 6).

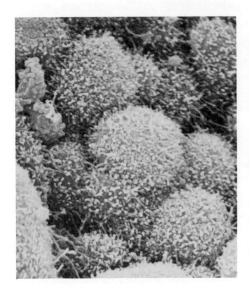 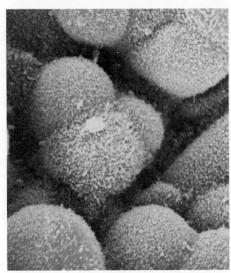

FIGURE 5 (left)   Superficial cells from an area of atypical hyperplasia show pleomorphic microvilli on the surface (SEM x 3,000).
FIGURE 6 (right)   Human bladder. Papillary carcinoma. Surface
cells protrude into the lumen showing both irregular arrangement and
pleomophic microvilli on the surface (SEM x 3,000).

DISCUSSION

The process of urothelial differentiation in rats seems to
involve the occurrence of luminal microvilli showing uniform size
and distribution; as differentiation proceeds the microvilli fuse
and form rounded microridges. Finally, the presence of AUM is
proved by the appearance of rigid angular folds (1).

Our data suggest that urothelial differentiation in man
parallels the features already described in rats. It further
demonstrates the presence of the SEM changes observed by Jacobs et
al (3) during experimental carcinogenesis, also in areas of hyperplasia peripheral to human bladder tumours.

In various experimental models pleomorphic microvilli and
surface glycocalix have been demonstrated to be correlated with
the transition from reversible to irreversible preneoplastic
lesions(2,3).

Pleomorphic microvilli have been described both by Newman and
Hicks (2) and by ourselves in tumour-bearing human bladder and by
Jacobs and coworkers (4) on cells exfoliated from human tumours.

On the contrary, we have observed glycocalix covering uniform micro-villi on surface cells in some cases of interstitial cystitis.

The occurrence of pleomorphic microvilli in man may reflect rapid epithelial growth rather than a specific feature of pre-neoplastic transformation, and further studies must be carried out in order to draw definite conclusions.

REFERENCES

1. Hodges, G. M., Hicks, R. M., Spacey, G. D., Scanning electron microscopy of cell-surface changes in methylnitrosurea (MNU) treated rat bladders in vivo and in vitro. Differentiation, 6, 143 (1976).

2. Newman, J., Hicks, R. M., Detection of neoplastic and pre-neoplastic urothelia by combined scanning and transmission electron microscopy of urinary surface of human and rat bladders. Histopathology, 1, 125 (1977).

3. Jacobs, J. B., Arai, M., Cohen, S., Friedell, G. H., A long term study of reversible and progressive urinary bladder cancer lesions in rats fed N-4-(5-nitro-2-furyl)-2-thiazolyl formamide. Cancer Res., 37, 2817 (1977).

4. Jacobs, J. B., Cohen, S. M., Arai, A., Friedell, G. H., SEM on bladder cancer cells. Acta Cytol., 21, 3 (1977).

IN SITU CARCINOMA OF THE BLADDER

G D CHISHOLM and D M WALLACE

Department of Urology, Western General Hospital and

Department of Surgery, University of Edinburgh, Edinburgh

In situ carcinoma has been defined by the UICC as pre-invasive carcinoma; it may occur in flat urothelium which appears "normal" or has formed a proliferative tumour which may be described as papillary or papilliferous. This may lead to confusion since, in pathological terms, tumours of either site can be reported as PIS (Wallace et al, 1975). However, these two forms appear to be significantly different and in this paper we examine these differences.

The incidence of a flat in situ tumour (TIS,PIS) compared with a papillary tumour (T1, PIS) is unknown due largely to the lack of biopsy information from apparently normal urothelium. It has generally been considered that T1 lesions are the commonest form of bladder tumour and that TIS (flat) in situ lesions occurring alone, are the least common. This view has been questioned from time to time. For example, in 1968, Schade and Swinney examined the apparently normal urothelium in patients with a proliferative carcinoma and found a high incidence of abnormality in biopsies taken from these bladders. This observation emphasised that without the appropriate information, the state of the bladder, apart from the obvious lesion, could not be known.

Thus, in practical terms, in situ carcinoma of the bladder may be considered under two headings: papillary carcinoma (T1, PIS) and in situ carcinoma (TIS, PIS).

SUPERFICIAL PAPILLARY CARCINOMA

The use of the term papilloma continues to cause confusion both in classification and in clinical description. Only a papillary lesion with no evidence of anaplasia (GO) can be called a papilloma and strictly speaking, this should not be included in a classification of malignant tumours. However, it is useful to retain this expression in a classification so that its place can be recognised and to prevent misuse of the word. All other papillary lesions are carcinomas varying only in their T category and their grade.

A question to be examined is whether or not a tumour can change its character. Melamed et al, (1964) have used the term "carcinoma in situ within a papilloma" for the papillary tumour with histological malignant change. He has suggested a course of events in the bladder: normal bladder mucosa $\longrightarrow$ papilloma $\longrightarrow$ papilloma with in situ change $\longrightarrow$ papillary carcinoma with either a) no invasion or b) invasion but not extending beyond the lamina propria. It is difficult to debate this suggestion without more knowledge of the natural history; this information can come only from more detailed studies of mucosal change in a wide variety of patients with bladder cancer.

FLAT IN SITU CARCINOMA

This tumour may be considered under three headings according to whether it is or is not associated with a bladder tumour and the separate problem of in situ carcinoma in the prostatic urethra.

1.   In Association with a Bladder Tumour

The incidence of in situ change in the bladder urothelium, separate from the primary tumour, may be as high as 40% with a similar proportion showing "atypia". In our studies of patients with all grades of bladder tumours who had biopsies of normal mucosa at the time of cystoscopy, the incidence of carcinoma in situ was 9% with 24% showing changes of hyperplasia or dysplasia only. Where the mucosa appeared abnormal but did not have a definite tumour, the incidence of carcinoma in situ rose to 38%.

In addition, these patients have a high incidence of both urethral and ureteric abnormalities, in the presence of a primary tumour, which supports the view that there is a generalised urothelial abnormality, or widespread premalignant change in these patients. Thus, a policy of regular follow-up, combined with 4-quadrant mucosal biopsies is recommended so that earlier radical treatment can be considered for those with widespread urothelial changes.

2.   Without Associated Bladder Tumours

This is a flat urothelial tumour occurring without either a
preceding or a concurrent papillary or invasive tumour. It is
undoubtedly one of the more perplexing of all forms of in situ
carcinoma because it may behave as a very aggressive tumours. It is
thought to be uncommon but this may be due to a lack of awareness
of the need to biopsy the bladder mucosa in a wide range of
circumstances. The UICC classification implies that the TIS lesion
is less aggressive than a T1 papillary lesion, but experience with
these tumours shows that this is not necessarily so.

In a study of 36 cases by Riddle et al, (1976) there were
several interesting clinical features. The age at presentation
ranged from 41 to 79. There was a male preponderance, 34 male :
2 female. Twenty three out of 36 patients had symptoms that were
mainly obstructive in character though this could be combined with
dysuria and haematuria. Many of these patients had had a
prostatectomy. The remainder in the series presented with a symptom
pattern in which pain (dysuria, penile pain or suprapubic pain) was
a central feature. Two patients had no symptoms and had positive
urinary cytology only.

The majority of patients had some colour change in the bladder
mucosa and this was described variously as "inflamed", "oedematous",
"mossy" or just "cystitis". An occasional patient had no specific
lesion.

There are insufficient patients, either in the series presented
by Riddle et al, (1976) or in other reports to draw firm conclusions
about management. A general conclusion from these studies is that
the patient with widespread mucosal change should be treated
aggressively (i.e. systourethrectomy) rather than a watching policy
until definite invasive tumour is identified. Some of the patients
have received radiotherapy as a primary treatment because, for various
reasons, surgery was contraindicated (Kulatilake et al, 1970).
Although these patients appeared to have a useful period of response,
most of these have died and it seems that the therapy did little to
alter the course of the disease.

In those patients where the in situ change is shown to be
localised, a choice of treatment exists. Cystodiathermy, intracavity chemotherapy, excision or no treatment may be sufficient.
However, these patients must be followed closely, with multiple
biopsies, and the surgeon should be prepared to consider radical
surgery at the first sign of progression.

3.   In Situ Carcinoma in the Prostatic Urethra

The report incidence of urethral involvement in association
with bladder carcinoma ranges from four to 18% while the finding of
in situ change in the ducts of the prostatic urethra may be even more
common when there is widespread in situ change within the bladder.
This must be regarded as a serious finding since it represents
malignancy involving an adjacent organ and early radical treatment
is recommended for these patients. It is important to recognise
the possibility of this locus for in situ change when in situ change
is being evaluated in the bladder (Seemayer et al, 1975).

SUMMARY

In situ carcinoma may be considered under the two headings
of superficial papillary carcinoma and flat in situ carcinoma. The
latter can be found in association with an obvious bladder cancer or
without it. It may also appear in the prostatic urethra. Flat
primary carcinoma in situ may present with a symptom pattern in which
pain is nearly always present. It may behave as a very aggressive
tumour, especially if it is widespread. In such a case total
cystectomy is the treatment of choice. In localised lesions TUR,
local chemotherapy or other conservative treatments may be
sufficient, provided the patient is followed closely.

REFERENCES

1.   Kulatilake, A. E., Chisholm, G. D. and Olsen, E. J. G.
      Proceedings of the Royal Society of Medicine, 63, 95-97 (1970).

2.   Melamed, H. R., Voutsa, N. G. and Grabstald, H. Cancer, 17,
      1535-1545 (1964).

3.   Riddle, P. R., Chisholm, G. D., Trott, P. A. and Pugh, R. C. G.
      Brit. J. Urol. 47, 829-833 (1976).

4.   Schade, R. O. K. and Swinney, J. Lancet, 2, 943-946 (1968).

5.   Seemayer, T. A., Knaack, J., Thelmo, W. L., Wang, N. S. and
      Ahmed, M. N. Cancer, 36, 514-520 (1975).

6.   Wallace, D. M., Chisholm, G. D., Hendry, W. F. Brit. J. Urol.
      47, 1-12 (1975).

PRIMARY AND SECONDARY CARCINOMA-IN-SITU

H J DE VOOGT

Reader in Urology, University Hospital Leiden

Rijnsburgerweg 10, Leiden, The Netherlands

During the period 1962-1976 in the Urology Department of the University Hospital Leiden a total of 394 patients were treated for carcinoma of the transitional epithelium. From these, 13 patients had what we called primary carcinoma-in-situ. They were mainly detected by urinary cytology and a specific symptomatology of pain on micturition, urgency and frequency. When we compared these with the findings of 23 randomly chosen patients with papillary carcinoma grade II and III (Bergkvist) we found that there was a distinct difference in signs and symptoms.

We also found seven patients who had presented first with papillary carcinoma and during follow-up biopsies also showed the histological picture of carcinoma-in-situ, though they usually did not have the above mentioned symptoms. Also the cytological pictures in these cases were different. We decided to call these secondary carcinoma-in-situ.

After discovering that conservative treatment in four cases of primary carcinoma-in-situ led in a very short time to progressive disease and the formation of solid infiltrating carcinoma from which the patients all died within a year, we decided to use much more aggresive treatment in these patients. This meant radical cysto-prostato-urethrectomy for the other nine patients.

During the period covered by this study 98 of the 394 patients were treated with radical cystectomy. Their clinical stages are shown in Table I.

TABLE I

CLINICAL STAGING IN 98 PATIENTS WHO UNDERWENT
RADICAL CYSTECTOMY

Tis	T1	T2	T3	T4
9	23	19	40	7

Histologically, primary and secondary carcinoma-in-situ are identical and apart from the changes in the epithelium itself, there are very distinct changes in the subepithelial stroma (oedema and dilated blood vessels).

Very often patients with papillary carcinoma have intermittent complaints in relation to micturition, and during follow-up cystoscopy areas of redness and velvety or cobble-stone appearance are seen. It was in this way that the seven patients with secondary carcinoma-in-situ were found. However, the question is whether more patients with papillary cancer have secondary carcinoma-in-situ as a precursor of their papillomas. Therefore, all tissue material from the 99 patients was examined again and we then detected areas of carcinoma-in-situ in 47 patients, 25 of which were not in conjunction with the papillary tumour, but at a distant site in the bladder. The localisation of the carcinoma-in-situ is shown in table II.

Finally in 81 preparations the stroma could adequately be evaluated and it turned out that 12 did not show any stromal changes, 25 had slight changes and in 44 the changes were severe.

TABLE II

LOCALISATION OF CARCINOMA-IN-SITU IN 47 BLADDERS
WITH PAPILLARY TUMOURS

Mucosa	Cell Nests of Brunn	The Prostate
12	-	-
19	19	-
13	13	13
3	-	3
47	32	16

CONCLUSION

Primary carcinoma-in-situ is a distinct disease entity with a characteristic clinical and cystoscopical picture and an aggressive biological behaviour with a tendency to develop into solid carcinoma.

Secondary carcinoma-in-situ is sometimes found during follow-up of a papillary carcinoma, but much more often in conjunction with recurrent and/or progressive papillomatous carcinoma. When, however, pain and complaints related to micturition due to stromal changes and denuding cystitis accompany this picture, this might be another indication to undertake radical cystectomy.

Editorial note (MP-M)   Carcinoma in situ is gaining interest among urologists, who are becoming increasingly aware of this condition. Many contributions were devoted to this topic in 1978 in meetings on bladder tumours organised by the WHO Collaborating Centre for urinary cancer in Stockholm and by the Italian Association for Treatment of Tumours in Bologna. The basis for a more frequent diagnosis lies in the expanding use of urinary cytology, but also on the practice of taking multiple biopsies of apparently healthy mucosa close to or far from the tumour.

The papers presented in Stockholm, in Bologna and in Erice clearly show that the small and localised lesions have a better prognosis than the diffuse ones and that primary carcinomas in situ responds better to conservative treatment than the secondary ones.

As shown elsewhere in this book, Edsmyr and other Scandinavian workers have observed that a high number of primary cases (100%) and secondary cases (84%) respond to monthly intravesical instillation of 80 mg Adriamycin. England et al in this course also showed that carcinoma in situ can be successfully treated with systemic cyclophosphamide. If these data are confirmed from a wider experience and a longer follow-up, chemotherapy will find a definite place in the treatment of carcinoma in situ. Constant surveillance and life-long follow-up remain essential, considering the high malignant potential of this disease.

COMPUTED TOMOGRAPHY OF BLADDER TUMOURS

C C SCHULMAN, X GIANNAKOPOULOS, J P BRION, N FREDERIC

Departments of Urology and Radiology, Brugmann Hospital
and Computed Tomography Unit, University of Brussels
Belgium

PRELIMINARY REPORT ON A NEW METHOD OF TUMOUR STAGING

The accurate clinical staging of bladder carcinoma is of the
foremost importance in determining the prognosis and modality of
treatment of the patient.

The prognosis is directly related to the extent of spread of
the disease and its clinical determination provides the best
information regarding the potential curability of the patient (1)
since the modality of the treatment is regarded as less important
than the stage of the tumour in determining the prognosis (2).

The clinical staging requires a physical examination, intravenous urogram, cystoscopy with transurethral biopsies and bimanual
examination under anesthesia. Complementary diagnostic regional
evaluation includes lymphangiography, liver scintigraphy, double
or triple contrast cystography, ultrasonography and selective pelvic
arteriography. Evaluation of distal metastases requires chest and
skeletal radiographies, isotope liver and bone scintigraphies.

Presently available clinical methods of staging bladder tumours
have limited value and their pitfalls have been frequently underlined (2). Clinicopathological correlation reveals that the staging
of bladder tumours is inaccurate despite the numerous diagnostic
procedures available. An overall inaccuracy of 56% is reported,
23% being clinically overstaged and 33% understaged (3).

A promising new method of the investigation of bladder tumours
with computed tomography (CT) is presented in this preliminary study.

PRINCIPLE AND METHOD

Computed tomography (CT) is the reconstruction of a tomographic section of the body using multiple x-ray absorption measurements. A CT unit transmits multiple x-ray beams from two scanning directions (rotation and translation) through the body. These are recorded by x-ray detectors. A computer is used to process the data and reconstructs the area scanned to generate a cross sectional image of the body. A special display is used to measure in numerical data relative densities or attenuation coefficients (Delta numbers) of any region of interest. The TV monitor is photographically equipped to provide a permanent record and all information is stored on magnetic tapes (4-5).

The diagnostic criteria employed in CT evaluation of the bladder are:-   a)   alteration of the normal shape,
        b)   visualisation of an intra- and/or extravesical masses,
        c)   disappearance of the outline of the perivesical fat space,
        d)   measurements of attenuation coefficients in a region of interest.

CLINICAL STUDY

Patients with bladder tumours were investigated by CT using the Ohio Nuclear Delta Scan which obtains two simultaneous 13 mm thickness slides in 2 minutes 30 seconds. Several techniques have been tried. Initially the examination was performed with the bladder full of urine. Later, contrast medium was used to opacify the bladder. These methods were not entirely satisfactory because of limited expansion of the bladder and obscuration of the intravesical projection of the tumour giving an insufficiently accurate image.

The most satisfactory results so far are obtained after complete distension of the bladder with gas (air - carbon dioxide) which allows the best demonstration of the normal bladder wall and of the intra- and extra-vesical extension of the tumoral process. This last information is regarded as the most useful in the evaluation of the spread of the disease.

CT allows one to visualise the intravesical protrusion of the tumour and its extravesical extension. The presence of fat and soft tissue around the bladder wall allows the distinction of structures of different densities and CT scanning is able to represent these images and to distinguish the density of the different structures since the attenuation coefficient of bladder tumour is greater than that of the normal and surrounding fatty tissues.

EXAMPLES

Example 1.   A 67 year old male was admitted for the evaluation of gross painless haematuria. The intravenous urogram was considered normal. Cystoscopy showed a polypoid tumour on the right wall of the bladder. The CT scan demonstrated a 3 cm diameter mass arising from the postero-lateral wall of the bladder, the mass did not penetrate through the thickness of the bladder wall (Figure 1). A trans-urethral resection of the tumour was performed and the pathological diagnosis was Grade I transitional cell carcinoma of the bladder.

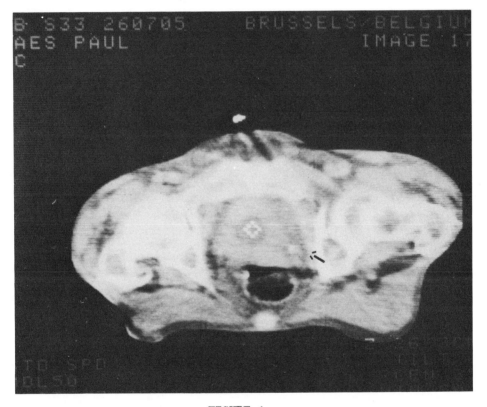

FIGURE 1

Polypoid bladder tumour on the right postero-lateral wall; the mass does not penetrate into the thickness of the wall (arrow).

Example 2.   A 61 year old male was found to have a filling
defect on the right side of the bladder on his intravenous urogram.
At cystoscopy, a tumour was observed on the left lateral wall of
the bladder. On bimanual examination under anaesthesia the bladder
was mobile with induration of the left side. Biopsies reported
Grade II transitional cell carcinoma.

A CT scan demonstrated a plaque-like tumour covering the entire
surface of the left lateral wall. The tumour did not seem to
extend outside the bladder and the perivesical fat was not invaded
by the tumour. (Figure 2A and B) Total cystectomy and ileal loop
diversion were performed. It was confirmed at surgery and
pathological examination of the specimen that the tumour did not
extend beyond the deep musculature. Lymph nodes were negative.

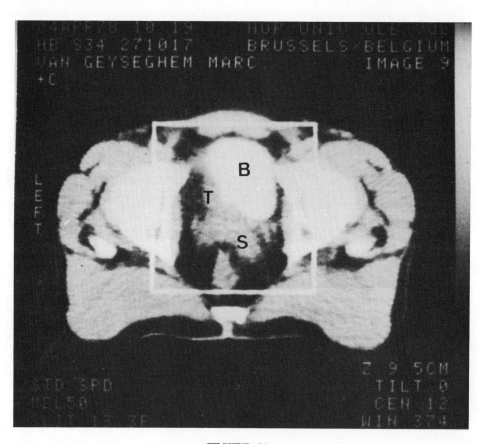

FIGURE 2A

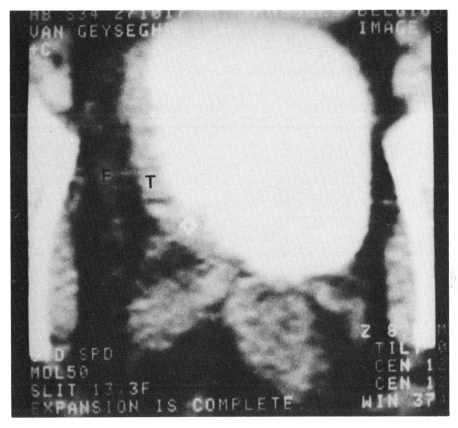

FIGURE 2B

Figure 2A and B. Plaque-like bladder tumour covering the entire left lateral wall, the process does not extend outside the bladder and the extravesical fat plane is free of invasion.
T : tumoral process, B : bladder, S : seminal vesicles

CONCLUSION

Although these are only preliminary results and the number of cases presently studied are not sufficient to give statistically significant data, it appears that this new non invasive technique will be most useful in differentiating invasive from non invasive tumours. The advantages of CT staging of bladder carcinoma are numerous. This non invasive method can be performed on an out-patient basis, repeated frequently to follow patients receiving chemotherapy and gives an accurate image of the intra- and more particularly extravesical spread of bladder tumours.

REFERENCES

1.   Jewett, J. H., Cancer of the bladder. Diagnosis and staging.
      Cancer, 32 1072 (1973).

2.   Schmidt, J. D. and Weinstein, S. H., Pitfalls in clinical
      staging of bladder tumours. Urol. Clin. North Am. 3, 107 (1976).

3.   Kenny, G. M., Hardner, G. J. and Murphy, G. P., Clinical
      staging of bladder tumours. J. Urol. 104, 720 (1970).

4.   Housfield, G. N., Computerised transverse axial scanning
      (tomography): Part I. Description of system. Brit. J. Radiol.
      46, 1016 (1973).

5.   Ledley, R. S., Di Chiro, G., Lussenhof, A. J. and Twigg, H. L.,
      Computerised transaxial x-ray tomography of the human body.
      Science, 186, 207 (1974).

TRANSRECTAL ULTRASONOGRAPHY: STAGING OF BLADDER TUMOURS

L DENIS

Department of Urology, A. Z. Middelheim

Antwerp, Belgium

INTRODUCTION

Transrectal ultrasonography is a reliable adjuvant technique to determine the mass, number and infiltration of bladder tumours.

Invasion is a critical turning point in the natural history of bladder tumours. Among the various techniques to evaluate this event a transurethral resection is widely accepted as the most reliable procedure. Transrectal ultrasonography can provide unique information prior to any surgery in selected instances of bladder tumours.

METHOD

The equipment consists of a transducer attached to a rotating probe and a regular video display unit (Aloka SSD 60C) (1). Radial B scan is the preferred mode at a frequency of 3.5 MHz with subsequent variations by gain adjustment and/or attenuation of sound.

The patient is placed in the left lateral decubitus with the legs flexed. The rectal probe is fitted in a condom which is filled with water. A full bladder facilitates the orientation. The bladder neck serves as an initial parameter after which step sections are taken every 0.5 cm. A total of 16 to 20 sections can be accurately examined by this technique. Polaroid black and white pictures are taken from every reconstructed section. Over 150 patients with a bladder tumour have been examined by this technique over a two year period.

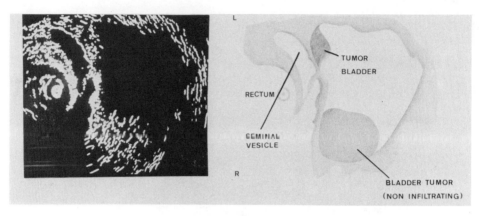

FIGURE 1

Sonogram (section - 1,5) of a bladder with two non invasive bladder tumours.

RESULTS

The normal bladder wall reflects as a uniform structure on sonographic display. Contour variations are due to differences in volume, patient position or extravesical pressure effect. The interface between the fluid medium and the bladder wall can be sharply outlined. Bladder tumours are identifiable as mass lesions located within the lumen adjacent to the bladder wall (Figure 1). The total tumour mass and/or the number of masses can be determined by the lay-out of all step sections. Invasion is characterised by disruption of the wall pattern, extension of the mass into the surrounding tissues or neighboring organs such as the prostate or the seminal vesicles. Unfortunately bladder tumour tissue has no distinctive sonic structure. We have been unable to correlate superficial or deep muscle invasion with our equipment.

DISCUSSION

Staging techniques in bladder tumours include cystoscopy, urography, bimanual examination under full anaesthesia and transurethral resection/biopsy. Transrectal ultrasonography is a painless, innocuous technique which brings important information in selected instances.

The exact localisation of multiple tumours or mass determination can be recorded in a preoperative investigation. Confirmation on a positive or negative pattern of invasion in a large tumour mass may direct the therapeutic approach. Ghost reflections by convoluted waves of the convex walls, extremely large tumours and air bubbles

in the dome cause problems for identification which are avoided
through experience.

REFERENCE

1.   Watanabe, H., Igari, D., Tanahasi, Y., Harada, K. and
     Saitho, M., Development and Application of New Equipment for
     Transrectal Ultrasonography. J. Clin. Ultras. 2, 91-98 (1974).

LYMPHANGIOGRAPHY IN ADVANCED BLADDER CANCER

R R HALL

Department of Urology, Newcastle General Hospital

Newcastle-upon-Tyne, England

INTRODUCTION

The importance of lymphangiography in the staging of advanced bladder cancer is accepted by many participants of this conference and is recommended by the U.I.C.C. for the complete classification of bladder tumours. A variety of authors have vouched for the accuracy of this radiological investigation. For example, the large series from the Royal Marsden Hospital (Turner et al, 1976) reported accurate correlation with histology in 90% of patients and concluded that the investigation was "essential in planning the treatment of infiltrating bladder tumours".

My own suspicions concerning the accuracy of lymphangiography were aroused by the illustration of a lymph node metastasis in an article by Professor Zingg in the British Journal of Urology in 1974. An almost identical lymph node from a similar position in one of my own patients was due to fat and not metastasis.

METHOD AND RESULTS

Over the past three years we have conducted our own study of the accuracy of lymphangiography in detecting nodal metastases in patients with stage T3 transitional cell carcinoma of the bladder. Twenty one lymphangiograms have been presented to four different radiologists for their interpretation and their observations compared with the histological examination of operative lymphadenectomy specimens. The results are shown in Table I.

TABLE I

ACCURACY OF LYMPHANGIOGRAPHY VERSUS LYMPHADENECTOMY

HISTOLOGY

8/21 cases : metastases >3mm diameter

1/21 cases : microscopic metastases

LYMPHANGIOGRAPHY

	Correct	False Negative	Identified wrong nodes
Radiologist A	3	3	2
Radiologist B	1	7	-
Radiologist C	2	6	-
Radiologist D	3	4	1

CONCLUSIONS

Until an alternative method is available for the diagnosis of lymph node metastases, it is reasonable to continue to use lymph-angiography looking for unexpected gross nodal involvement, indicating those patients where lymph node biopsy may save un-necessary radical surgery or suggest adjuvant therapy.

However, no system of tumour staging and certainly no cancer treatment should be based upon lymphangiography alone without histological confirmation.

CLINICAL SIGNIFICANCE OF URINARY CEA ESTIMATIONS IN THE FOLLOW-UP OF PATIENTS WITH BLADDER CARCINOMA

J RENAUD

National Cancer Institute, Antoni v. Leeuwenhok

Ziekenhuis, Plesmanlcan 121, Amsterdam, The Netherlands

INTRODUCTION

This paper deals with serial estimation of urinary CEA levels in relation to the clinical situation during follow-up in 97 patients (78 males and 19 females) who suffered or had previously suffered from bladder carcinoma.

METHODS AND RESULTS

The tumours were classified and staged according to the UICC criteria. The urine was collected during cystoscopy and divided in two parts, one for culture and one for CEA estimation. The upper limit of normal for CEA, measured by radio immune assay, is 30 ng/ml. 70 patients, after treatment of their bladder carcinoma, had a normal CEA level on several occasions and were tumour free at the time CEA was measured.

False negative results (CEA values lower than 30 ng/ml) can be found in the presence of a bladder tumour and a single negative result of a CEA assay in urine does not add essential information on the patient's clinical condition. From the results of this study it appears, however, that negative results do have a value if they follow previously elevated values.

Cystoscopy is regularly carried out during follow up of bladder carcinoma. If urinary CEA is estimated between two cystoscopies this may lead to earlier discovery of recurrence of the bladder tumour.

Raised levels of CEA were nearly always related to tumour growth in the bladder, once urinary infection was excluded. False positive results were however seen in several patients with doubtful abnormalities in the bladder or in whom no lesion could be found.

An important complication in the interpretation of urinary CEA levels is the appearance of urinary infection. CEA levels rise in association with infection but return to normal levels very soon after it is treated. The data obtained shortly after cure of an infection can therefore be considered reliable.

In patients whose urinary CEA returns to normal after successful therapy, recurrence of the tumour is often reflected by a rise of urinary CEA. In our group of 97 patients 10 showed a rise of urinary CEA level during follow up after an initial normal value. These increased values corresponded with re-growth of tumour, as confirmed by cystoscopy in seven patients. In three patients no lesion could be found.

CONCLUSIONS

CEA levels which decrease from elevated to normal or vice versa reflect progression or regression of malignant processes in the bladder until proved otherwise. The urinary CEA assay can therefore be helpful in assessing the adequacy of treatment in patients with bladder carcinoma. As such it will be an indispensable adjunct to cystoscopy and other clinical means to judge the patient's condition. Regular measurement of urinary CEA may prevent a delay in further treatment.

GLYCOSAMINOGLYCANS (GAG) IN THE NORMAL AND NEOPLASTIC URINARY

BLADDER - PRELIMINARY RESULTS

H RÜBBEN, H G STUHLSATZ, W LUTZEYER

Abteilung Urologie der Klinischen Anstalten der RWTH

Aachen, Goethestr. 27/29, 5100 Aachen, West Germany

ABSTRACT

Glycosaminoglycans (GAG) were isolated biochemically in normal and neoplastic urinary bladder epithelium and the results compared to those of histochemical investigation. The results showed that histochemical stains are not specific for GAG, that normal urothelial epithelium contains only traces of GAG and that transitional cell carcinomas contain GAG, whose composition differs from connective tissue GAG.

PROBLEM

GAG are shown by histochemical stains within epithelial layers (3); they should be involved in the local defence mechanism against bacterial infections (4) as well as in the process of developing neoplastic disease (1). Our investigation was undertaken to show biochemically the presence of GAG within the transitional-cell epithelium of the normal and the neoplastic bladder.

METHOD

The epithelial, submucosal and muscular layers of normal urinary bladders and urothelial carcinomas were isolated.

Formalin fixed preparations served as controls for histochemical stains (PAS, colloidal iron, alcian blue 8 GS). Biochemical analyses was done by proteolysis with papain, chromatography on Dowes 1X2 microcolumns, elution with 0,15; 0.50; 1.50 and 3,00 molar NaCl solutions and dialysis and hydrolysis of the four fractions. Glucosamines and galactosamines were isolated by means of an amino acid analyser (TSM Technicon) (2).

RESULTS

Biochemical analysis of normal urinary bladder showed only traces of GAG in the epithelium. In the submucosa relatively high concentrations were detected in all cell fractions and in the muscle layer the concentrations were intermediate. Well and moderately well differentiated tumours showed relatively high concentrations of GAG in the 3,00 molar NaCL fraction and low concentration of GAG in the 1,5 fraction. Poorly differentiated tumours showed relatively high concentration of GAG in all fractions with an increase of glucosamine-containing GAG and a decrease of galactosamine-containing GAG in 1,5 fraction in comparison to connective tissue GAG.

Results of histochemical stains could not be correlated with biochemical analyses. Positive staining could be observed in areas shown to be free of GAG biochemically such as normal epithelium.

CONCLUSION

Histochemical stains are not specific for GAG. The surface coat involved in the bacterial defence mechanism does not consist primarily of GAG. Urothelial cancer contains GAG, whose composition differs from connective tissue GAG.

REFERENCES

1. Bhavanadam, V. P., Davidson, E. H., Characterisation of the chondroitin sulfate produced by B16 mouse melanoma cells. Carbohydrate Res. 57, 173 (1977).

2. Greiling, H., Stuhlsatz, H. W., Cantz, M., Gehler, J., Increased urinary excretion of keratansulfate in fucosidosis. J. Clin. Chem. Clin. Biochem. (1978) In Press.

3. Hulkill, P. B., Vidone, R. A., Histochemistry of mucus and other polysaccharides on tumours. 1. Tumours of the bladder. Lab. Invest. 14, 1624 (1965).

4. Parsons, C. L., Greenspan, C., Moore, St. W., Mulholland, S. G., Role of surface mucin in primary antibacterial defense of bladder. Urology, 9, 48-52 (1977).

COLLAGENASE ACTIVITY IN HUMAN BLADDER CANCERS

G KUNIT, G WIRL and J FRICK

Institute of Molecular Biology of the Austrian Academy of
Sciences and the Department of Urology, General Hospital
A 5020 Salzburg, Austria

INTRODUCTION

Although it has been known for about 10 years that explants of
malignant tissues show the ability to liquify collagen gels (1,2,3),
and are capable of releasing collagenase into the culture medium
(4,5), there are relatively few published studies that have dealt
directly with the activity of collagenase in vivo. Yamanishi and
his associates have shown variable amounts of extractable collagenase
in human skin cancers (6,7) and other workers have reported increased
levels of collagenase in several highly invasive animal tumours (8,
9,10).

In a number of these experimental situations the high yield of
this enzyme in invasive tumours is subject to modulation in a manner
that is entirely consistent with the notion that collagenases are
secreted by tumour cells and serve an important physiological
function in the breakdown of the collagenous matrix of host tissue
surrounding tumour growth. Collagenases may not only help to
traverse the endothelial basement membrane in vascular invasion but
also can destroy the collagen component of massive layers of
connective tissues like that of the dermis.

In view of the extensive but localised degradation of collagen
structures that accompanies invasion by several tumours (11,12,13),
we have examined the highly invasive human bladder tumour for the
possible involvement of collagenase. Our report briefly summarises
our findings.

METHODS

Tumour fragments were obtained from 28 patients who underwent partial or total cystectomy. The diagnosis in each case was clearly established on the basis of generally accepted histological criteria. The staging of the carcinomas followed the method of Jewett and Strong (14).

In all cases tissue specimen were carefully washed, minced, weighed and homogenised in 10 volumes of buffered sucrose as described previously in detail (15). Centrifugation of the tumour homogenates resulted in the supernatant and the residue that was reextracted with 5 M urea. After ammonium sulphate fractionation the activity of collagenase in both fractions was quantitated by measuring the release of soluble, radioactive collagen peptides from C^{14}- labelled collagen in solution. Some tumours were found to contain both active and latent collagenase. In these cases inactive enzyme was activated by 10 min. treatment of the supernatant at $25^{0}C$ with 50 μg trypsin/ml.

RESULTS

The results of assays for collagenase in the urea extract are presented in Figure 1. They failed to show detectable amounts of this enzyme in control tissues and stage A tumours. In contrast all the C- and D-tumours contained high amounts of collagenase. In the group including both B1 and B2 tumours only two of eight cases showed collagenase activity. In the group B-C including four patients, intermediate levels of collagenase were found.

Soluble collagenase, as represented in Figure 2, was detected in the majority of tumours only in groups C and D but was generally lower than the collagenase in the residue after centrifugation. Following activation with trypsin collagenolytic activity was demonstrated in the sucrose extract of the borderline group B-C and markedly enhanced activity was found in C- and D-staged tumours. Assay of this fraction from stage A and B tumours and in the control group failed to elicit collagenolytic activity.

DISCUSSION

In interpreting our results we conclude that highly invasive bladder cancers, in contrast to stage A tumours and most of the stage B tumours, possess high levels of enzymes which are capable of degrading collagen. These findings support the concept that collagenases may play an important role in the invasive properties of tumours. However we can give no answer to the important question of whether collagenase activity is an inherent property of the tumour

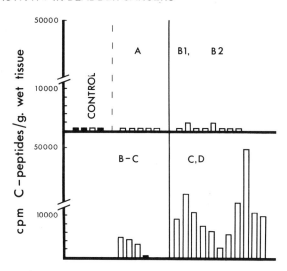

Figure 1.   Levels of sediment-bound collagenase in normal and neoplastic bladder tissues. The sediment obtained after homogenisation
and centrifugation was extracted with 5 M urea for two hours. After
dialysis and (NH$_4$)$_2$SO$_4$ precipitation the enzyme activity was
determined, incubating with substrate at 25°C for eight hours. Each
value represents one case.

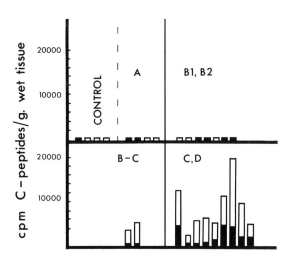

Figure 2. Levels of soluble collagenase in normal and neoplastic
bladder tissues. Collagenase activity was determined before (▆)
and after treatment of fraction I with trypsin (▭). Each column
represents a different case.

cells themselves or is contributed by the cells of the host, such as fibroblasts (16) of inflammatory cells (17) participating in the stromal reaction against the tumour.

If the results of these studies are verified by other investigators it may be possible to use collagenase as a biological marker in differentiating between superficial lesions of a given grade and those that have gone on to invade the bladder wall deeply, that is between B and C- staged tumours.

REFERENCES

1.   Riley, W. B. and Peacock, E. E.   Proc. Soc. Exp. Biol. Med. 124, 207 (1967).

2.   Taylor, A. C., Levy, B. M. and Simpson, J. W.   Nature, 221, 336 (1970).

3.   Dresden, M. H., Heilman, S. A. and Schmidt, J. D.   Cancer Res. 32, 993 (1972).

4.   Strauch, L.   In Tissue Interactions in Carcinogenesis.   Ed. Tarin, D.   Academic Press, New York, p 339-433 (1972).

5.   Abramson, M., Schilling, R. W., Huang, C. and Salome, R. G. Ann. Otol. Rhinol. Laryngol. 84, 1 (1975).

6.   Yamanishi, Y., Dabbous, K. M. and Hashimoto, K.   Cancer Res. 32, 2551 (1972).

7.   Ohyama, H. and Hashimoto, K.   J. Biochem. 82, 175 (1977).

8.   Wirl, G.   Connect. Tissue Res. 5, 171 (1977).

9.   Steven, F. S., and Itzhaki, S.   Biochim. Biophys. Acta. 496, 241 (1977).

10. Biswas, C., Moran, W. P., Bloch, K. J. and Gross, J.   Biochem. and Biophys. Res. Commun. 80, 33 (1978).

11. Tarin, D.   Int. J. Cancer, 2, 195 (1967).

12. Woods, D. A. and Smith, C. J. J. Invest. Dermatol. 62, 259 (1969).

13. Chowaniec, J. and Hicks, R. M.   Brit. J. Cancer, 35, 254 (1977).

14. Jewett, H. J. and Strong, G. H.   J. Urol. 55, 366 (1946).

15.   Wirl, G. Hoppe-Seyler's Z. Physiol. Chem. 356, 1289 (1975).

16.   Bauer, E. A., Gordon, J. M., Reddick, M. E., Eisen, A. Z.
      J. Invest. Dermatol. 69, 363 (1977).

17.   Abramson, M. and Huang, C. The Laryngoscope, 87, 771 (1977).

THE COPENHAGEN BLADDER CANCER PROJECT 1968-1974

P A GAMMELGAARD and B L SØRENSEN

Herlev Hospital
University of Copenhagen
Denmark

INTRODUCTION

In the period 1968-1974 all patients admitted to three
urological departments in Copenhagen were examined and treated
according to identical principles.

In all there were 746 patients. The aim of the trial was to
examine the incidence of the disease in different stages related to
survival. Details were obtained of numerous clinical parameters
including T and G category, number, type and size of tumours and of
survival.

Since the three urological departments treat almost all cases
of bladder cancer in their respective areas the results must be
considered representative of the area as a whole.

In accordance with the Swedish pattern, patients with the less
differentiated tumours and tumours with deep infiltration were
treated with high voltage irradiation (6000 rads) except where the
extreme age of some patients did not permit such a dose.

RESULTS

The distribution of T category and of histological grade
(Bergkvist) in relation to survival is shown in Tables I and II.

113

TABLE I

T CATEGORY AND 5 YEAR SURVIVAL

	T1	T2	T3	T4	Not Known
Patients	460 (62%)	169 (23%)	76 (10%)	35 (5%)	6
% 5 yr Survival	60	39	20	0	

There is a significant difference in survival in the various groups in table I and table II. The figures show the crude survival.

The presence of solitary or multiple papillary tumours did not influence survival but the solid tumours carry a much worse prognosis as do adenocarcinomata and squamous cell lesions.

The size of the tumour is also important, the prognosis being better if the diameter of the tumour is less than three centimeters.

Of the patients 219 were treated with high voltage irradiation. All had deeply invading tumours or very poorly differentiated tumours. Tables III and IV show the distribution of patients who received radiotherapy and their survival.

TABLE II

HISTOLOGICAL CLASSIFICATION AND 5 YEAR SURVIVAL

TCC, Papillary Grade:		Patients	% Survival
	0-I	92 (12%)	78
	II	348 (47%)	58.5
	III	219 (30%)	28.2
	IV	26 (3%)	23.1
Other Types:	Solid	14 (1.5%)	
	Adeno	6 (1%)	0
	Squamous	24 (3%)	
	Not Known	17 (1.5%)	

TABLE III

T CATEGORY AND 5 YEAR SURVIVAL IN PATIENTS

TREATED WITH RADIATION

Category	T1	T2	T3	T4	Not Known	Total
Patients	52	77	61	22	2	219
% 5 yr Survival	24	24	23.2	21.3	0	22.1

TABLE IV

HISTOLOGICAL GRADING AND 5 YEAR SURVIVAL IN

PATIENTS TREATED WITH RADIOTHERAPY

Grade	0-I	II	III	IV	Other	Total
Patients	1	25	144	21	28	219
% 5 yr Survival		21	18.5	28.6	0	22.1

After radiotherapy there is a much less clear distinction between T-category, histological Grade and Survival.

In the continuous endeavour to improve the survival of these patients, especially of those 40% who have tumours with deep infiltration, i.e. T2, T3 and T4 tumours, it is desirable to organize clinical trials comparing two or more different regimes, comprising surgery, radiotherapy and chemotherapy. This is possible in Denmark with about 1000 new cases of bladder cancer each year and a committee has been appointed to co-ordinate this on a National basis.

SUMMARY

An analysis of 764 patients with bladder cancer treated in Copenhagen from 1968-1974 has shown that important prognostic factors at the time of diagnosis indicate T-category, histological grade and type and size of tumour.

In 219 patients referred for Radiotherapy there was much less difference in survival in the criteria assessed and a plea is made for clinical trials of combined therapy in the hope that the prognosis for these patients, most of whom have infiltrating tumours, can be improved.

FACTORS INFLUENCING PROGNOSIS IN PATIENTS WITH BLADDER TUMOURS

M HORŇAK

Department of Urology
University Medical School
Bratislava, Czechoslovakia

INTRODUCTION

In 1969 Whitmore (1) enumerated the features that may bear upon the tumour behaviour, without attempting to assess their relative importance. The value of the histological features of grade, stage and multicentricity is generally known.

In this report the influence of some clinical and gross criteria of the tumours on five year survival is demonstrated. The clinical material involves 120 patients treated for bladder tumours. In all cases the patients were previously untreated. All have been followed up for at least five years.

TABLE I

FIVE YEAR SURVIVAL INDEPENDENT OF THE METHOD OF TREATMENT

RELATED TO DELAY IN DIAGNOSIS OF 1,120 PATIENTS

Delay in Diagnosis Duration of Symptoms before Diagnosis	Survival	
	No.	%
$<$ 1 month	20/37	54.1
2 - 6 months	12/37	32.4
7 - 12 months	8/16	50.0
1 - 3 years	8/24	33.4
$>$ 3 years	1/6	16.7
TOTAL	49/120	40.8

117

CLINICAL RESULTS

Table I shows the five year survival, independent of the method of treatment, according to the delay in diagnosis. Only a delay of greater than one year in seeking treatment is associated with a decreased chance of survival. Similar findings were reported by Wallace and Harris in 1965 (2) who believed that the biological potential of the tumour, and its relationship to the host, was probably more important than delay in establishing the correct diagnosis. Naturally, these findings must not reduce the endeavours of physicians to make the diagnosis and to treat the patient as soon as possible.

Further, the five year survival irrespective of the mode of treatment has been compared with the localization of the tumour. Table II shows that tumours of the base of the bladder and of the bladder neck exhibited the worst survival.

The correlation between five year survival and the macroscopic appearance is shown in Table III. The survival of patients with papillary tumours is much more favourable than it is for patients whose tumours are solid.

SUMMARY

One hundred and twenty patients with bladder cancer were evaluated. It was discovered that delay in treatment greater than one year after the onset of symptoms, the presence of tumour on the bladder neck or base and the presence of a solid or ulcerated tumour were adverse prognostic factors.

TABLE II

FIVE YEAR SURVIVAL INDEPENDENT OF THE METHOD OF TREATMENT

ACCORDING TO LOCALIZATION OF TUMOUR IN 118 PATIENTS

Localization of tumour	Survival	
	No.	%
Bladder neck	2/17	11.7
Base	7/26	27.0
Posterior wall	4/6	66.6
Lateral walls	33/64	51.5
Dome	3/5	60.0
TOTAL	49/118	41.5

TABLE III

FIVE YEAR SURVIVAL INDEPENDENT OF THE METHOD OF TREATMENT

ACCORDING TO MACROSCOPIC APPEARANCE OF TUMOUR IN 118 PATIENTS

Appearance of tumour	Survival	
	No.	%
Papillary	33/51	64.7
Nodular	12/43	27.9
Ulcerated	3/19	15.7
Other	1/5	20.0
TOTAL	49/118	41.5

REFERENCES

1. Whitmore, W.F. Jr., The treatment of bladder tumours. Surg. Clin. N. Amer., 49, 349-370 (1969).

2. Wallace, D.M. and Harris, D.L., Delay in treating bladder tumours. Lancet., 2, 332-334 (1965).

URINARY TRACT INFECTION IN PATIENTS WITH BLADDER TUMOR

L WAHLQVIST

Department of Urology

University of Umeå, Umeå, Sweden

Urinary tract infection in patients with bladder carcinoma may be the indirect cause of death through induction and/or promotion of the tumour, or may be the direct cause of death. Patients in whom urinary tract infection was the direct cause of death were studied retrospectively. The autopsy records from cases operated upon for bladder carcinoma with or without a conduit urinary diversion were analysed.

In the last urinary culture before death a significant bacteriuria was found in 51% of the 157 non diverted and in 85% of the 55 diverted cases. Macroscopical signs of infection in the kidneys were found in 35% of the cases without and in 67% of those with diversion.

The most serious sign of renal infection was renal abscess. In cases without any cancer found at autopsy abscesses were found in 11% of 96 renal units without and in 44% of 41 units with diversion. The difference is statistically significant. In non-diverted cases without cancer at autopsy abscesses were found in 19% of dilated renal units and in 7% of "normal" units; 24% of the cases without any cancer at autopsy had died of pyelonephritis.

A high incidence of significant bacteriuria was found in patients with bladder carcinoma before they died. At autopsy there was a high frequency of severe renal infection, especially in cases with cutaneous ureteroileal diversion.

The findings indicate that urinary tract infection is more frequent than we suspected. Bergman (1978) has shown that the radiological signs of pyelonephritis appear late and increase in frequency with the time after diversion. He found that signs and symptoms as well as C-reactive protein and erythrocyte sedimentation rate are unreliable as indicators of pyelonephritis. E.coli and Proteus mirabilis were the dominating causes of bacteriuria in diverted patients. Bergman also showed that antibody titres against E.coli and Proteus mirabilis respectively were raised when the patient had pyelonephritis.

CONCLUSION

Patients with pyelonephritis often have symptoms in the lower urinary tract. Diverted patients have no such symptoms. There is a high frequency of renal infection at autopsy of cases operated upon for bladder carcinoma with or without conduit diversion. One fourth of the cases without any cancer at autopsy had died of pyelonephritis.

REFERENCE

1.   Bergman, B., Studies on patients with ileal conduit diversion with special regard to renal infection. Scand. J. Urol. Nephrol. supplement 47 (1978).

ADENOCARCINOMA OF THE BLADDER

G JAKSE

Department of Urology
University of Innsbruck
Innsbruck, Austria

HISTOGENESIS

Formiggini, Patch and Rhea clearly showed that mucous epithelium and mucinous glands are not normally present in the mucosa of the urinary bladder and a number of theories have been developed to explain the origin of vesical adenocarcinoma (3,12).

Primitive cells harboured in cloacal rests may persist after the development of the septum between the primitive bladder and rectum and may be the source of glandular epithelium. But the most favoured theory is that by chronic irritation the urothelium undergoes metaplastic changes. The metaplasia starts with epithelial downgrowths and goes ahead with formation of cysts in which mucus production may occur. This theory has been reinforced by clinical and experimental observations. For example in more than 90% of bladder extrophies the tumour which develops is an adenocarcinoma, also in biharziasis an adenocarcinoma is more frequent than in other populations (8). Experimentally Giani and Hills were able to produce adenoid metaplasia by chronic urinary tract infection and by an irritating foreign body respectively (4,6). However, until now there have been only three reports in the literature, where it could be proven histologically that glandular metaplasia of the urinary bladder preceded by five to 15 years the occurrence of an adenocarcinoma (2,13,14). Because of these observations some authors believe that glandular metaplasia should be considered as a premalignant lesion.

CLINICAL FEATURES

Adenocarcinoma of the urinary bladder has to be differentiated very clearly from adenoid carcinomas of other origin, because of the different histogenesis and different therapeutic approach required. This differentiation has to be made on clinical as well as pathological grounds as Thomas and coworkers showed in their very careful review of 174 collected cases of adenocarcinoma of the bladder in which only 52 fulfilled the histological and clinical criteria (15). A clinical analysis according to age and sex and symptoms reveals no difference from transitional cell tumours; also mucus is rarely found in the urine. Histopathologically adeno-carcinoma is a pure glandular tumour with all grades of differen-tiation and mucin production. Metaplasia of the adjacent urothelium is noted frequently. A transitional cell carcinoma with adenoid metaplasia must be carefully excluded. In about 60% of patients the tumour is solitary. Infiltration is found in about 90% but metastasis occurs according to Mostofi in only 20% (9).

The diagnosis of primary adenocarcinoma of the bladder should only be made when the above mentioned criteria are present and an adenocarcinoma at another site has been excluded.

TABLE I

ORIGIN OF ADENOCARCINOMA OF THE BLADDER

SECONDARY ADENOCARCINOMA

prostatic carcinoma - acid phos., rarely mucinous, rectal palpation
ovarian cystadenocarcinoma - suprapubic mass, "Psammom" bodies
colorectal carcinoma - stool anomalous, CEA
carcinoma of the uterus - vaginal bleeding, metrorrhagia
carcinoma of the seminal vesical - rectal palpation, oliguria

URACHAL CARCINOMA

intramural tumour, intact urothelium, no metaplasia
bladder vault, suprapubic mass

TRANSITIONAL CELL CARCINOMA

adenomatous metaplasia

BENIGN GLANDULAR LESIONS

hyperplastic paraurethral glands, severe cystitis glandularis
adenofibroma, endometriosis, nephrogenic adenoma

The importance of clinical evaluation in diagnosis is stressed by Mostofi, who was able to demonstrate that stool symptoms were always present prior to the urinary tract symptoms in all cases of colorectal tumour which invaded the bladder (9). The role of CEA in differentiating between these tumours has to be evaluated. According to Tiltman and Maytom, colorectal tumours can be distinguished from primary adenocarcinoma by the presence of sulphated acid mucopoly-saccharide in the pathological specimens (16).

As Begg stated the urachal carcinoma is strictly speaking not a primary bladder tumour because it originates from the distal part of the urachal remnant (1). A suprapubic mass may be noted as the first symptom. It can also be differentiated from a primary adenocarcinoma by its site on the bladder dome or anterior wall and by the fact that the urothelium over or adjacent to the tumour is intact and that metaplastic changes are absent in most cases.

CLINICAL MATERIAL

Of 715 bladder tumours, treated at the Department of Urology, Mainz/Germany, where I had the chance to review their histories, there were 18 adenocarcinomas, of which five were of urachal origin. The average age was 60 and the sex distribution was 5:1 for men. In one patient a bladder exstrophy was present. In five patients the tumour was localised on the posterior wall, in six it was on the lateral wall, in one on the trigone; one patient showed multiple tumours. In none of the patients could metastasis be found at diagnosis. The histology showed a superficial tumour (Category T1) in one patient only.

THERAPY AND PROGNOSIS

Various therapies were applied as demonstrated on Table II. In five patients a cystectomy was done, which gave a favourable outcome if we include the patients who died without evidence of recurrent tumour.

According to Mostofi the prognosis of the primary adenocarcinoma is poor and resembles that of infiltrating transitional cell carcinoma of grade II-III, with a five year survival of about 25% (9). Mostofi does not consider cystectomy the treatment of choice, because he could follow some patients who did well without radical treatment.

However, in the series of Thomas and coworkers including the patients above mentioned it can be clearly demonstrated that the prognosis is closely correlated to the treatment given, cystectomy being superior to any other therapy (Figure 1). This is in agreement with the

TABLE II

ADENOCARCINOMA OF THE BLADDER - TREATMENT

		TUR +/- Radiotherapy			Cystectomy	
Stage	n	Alive	Died	n	Alive	Died
T1	1	6 mo.	-	-	-	-
T2	3	27 mo.	22 mo., 8 mo.	1	-	16y*
T3	2	-	22 mo., 6 mo.	3	15 mo., 20 mo	23 mo.*
T4	1	-	6 mo.	1	-	14 mo.

* died without tumour

report from the Mayo clinic, where a five year survival rate of about 80% could be obtained by cystectomy (11,15).

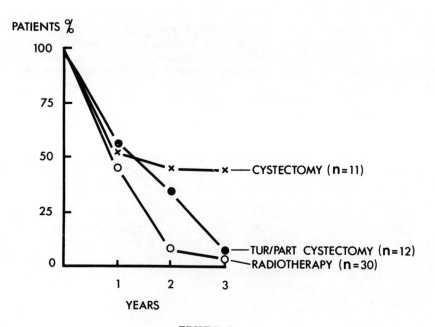

FIGURE 1

ADENOCARCINOMA OF THE URINARY BLADDER*
*Thomas et al. (1971), Dept. of Urology, Mainz (1978)

In contrast to the recommended cystectomy for primary adenocarcinoma, the patient with secondary adenocarcinoma such as
colorectal carcinoma is usually treated by a simple resection of the
invaded bladder wall.

The therapy of choice for urachal carcinoma is partial cystectomy
with removal of an appropriate peritoneal flap and the umbilicus.

A transurethral resection might be feasible in superficial
adenocarcinoma; however in more than 90% the tumour is already at an
advanced stage when the patients are first seen.

Radiotherapy - high voltage or radon seeds - with TUR or alone
has proved to be without any effect concerning long time survival, as
Hendricks et al and Jacobo et al demonstrated (5,7).

Chemotherapy has rarely been used, and Nevin and Hoffman report
that intrarterial therapy with 5-Fluorouracil following radiotherapy
was successful in three patients with stage C and D tumour resulting
in complete remission for more than 36 months (10). Cisplatinum has
been used by Yagoda in adenocarcinoma with metastasis to the regional
lymph nodes, but no benefit was seen (1).

REFERENCES

1. Begg, C., The colloid adenocarcinoma of the bladder vault
    arising from the epithelium of the urachal canal: with a
    critical survey of the tumours of the urachus. Brit. J. Surg.
    18, 422-466 (1931)

2. Edwards, Ph. D., Raymond, A. H., Jaeschke, W. H., Conversion
    of cystitis glandularis to adenocarcinoma. J. Urol. 108,
    568-570 (1972)

3. Formiggini, B., Contibuto allo studio istologico della mucosa
    vesicle estrofica. Riforma med. 36, 252 (1920)

4. Giani, R., Neuer Experimenteller Beitrag zur Entstehung der
    Cystitis Cystica. Zentr. Allgem. Pathol. Anat. 17, 900 (1907)

5. Hendricks, E. D., Massey, B. D., Nation, E. F., Gallup, Ch. A.,
    Massey, B. D. Jr., Edwards, J.W., Radon in treatment of
    infiltrating carcinoma of the urinary bladder. Urology, 5,
    465 (1975)

6. Hills, G. S., Experimental production of pyeloureteritis cystica
    and glandularis. Invest. Urol., 9, 1 (1971)

7. Jacobo, E., Loening, S., Schmidt, J.D., Culp, D.A. Primary

adenocarcinoma of the bladder: a retrospective study of 20
patients. J. Urol., 117, 54 (1977)

8.   McIntosh, J. F., Worley, G., Adenocarcinoma arising in exstrophy
     of the bladder: report of two cases and review of the literature.
     J. Urol., 73, 820 (1955)

9.   Mostofi, F. K., Thomas, R. V., Dean, A. L., Mucous adeno-
     oaroinoma of the urinary bladder. Cancer, 8, 741 (1955).

10. Nevin, J. W., Hoffman, A. A., Use of arterial infusion of
     5-Fluorouracil either alone or in combination with supervoltage
     radiation as a treatment for carcinoma of the prostate and
     bladder. Amer. J. Surg. 130, 544 (1975).

11. O'Dea, M. J., Malek, R. S., Utz, D. C., Adenocarcinoma of the
     bladder : experience with twenty five cases. AUA, 72 Meeting.
     Chicago, (1972)

12. Patch, F. S., Rhea, L., The genesis and development of Brunn's
     next and their relation to cystitis cystica, cystitis
     glandularis and primary adenocarcinoma of the bladder.
     Canad. Med. Ass. J. 33, 597 (1958).

13. Shaw, J. L., Gislason, G. J., Imbriglia, J. E., Transition of
     cystitis glandularis to primary adenocarcinoma of the bladder.
     J. Urol., 79, 815 (1958)

14. Susmano, D., Rubenstein, A. B., Dakin, A. R., Lloyd, F. A.,
     Cystitis glandularis and adenocarcinoma of the bladder. J.
     Urol., 105, 671 (1971)

15. Thomas, D. G., Ward, A. M., Williams, J. L., A study of 52
     cases of adenocarcinoma of the bladder. Brit. J. Urol. 43, 4
     (1971).

16. Tiltman, A. J., Maytom, P. A. N., Adenocarcinoma of the
     urinary bladder. S. Afr. Med. J., 51, 74 (1977)

17. Yagoda, A., Watson, R. C., Gonzalez-Vitale, J. C., Grabstald, H.,
     Whitmore, W. F., Cis-dichlordiammineplatinum in advanced bladder
     cancer. Cancer Treat. Rep., 60, 917 (1976)

Editorial Note (PHS)

In an active discussion Anderson (Leeds) observed that in a
series of 1800 patients reported from Sheffield only 25 had squamous
carcinoma, whilst Koch (Copenhagen) noted that the incidence of
squamous and adenocarcinoma combined in the Danish series was 7%.
Rocca-Rossetti(Trieste) had been surprised to find that whereas in
Sardinia 20% of carcinoma was of the squamous type, the incidence
of such tumour in Trieste was only 1.6%. Amaku (Lagos) observed
that squamous carcinoma was common in Nigeria usually occurring in
young men soon after the age of 30 years and usually in an advanced
stage. He felt that most were secondary to schistosomiasis and
observed that it was commonly impossible to treat such patients as
they were not prepared to accept total cystectomy. Although
chemotherapy had not been used in such patients, two had been
treated with radiotherapy with early death. Hall (Newcastle) had
seen nine cases of squamous carcinoma in four years and had used
Bleomycin in four patients.

Whilst participants accepted that cystectomy was the best
treatment for adenocarcinoma, mention was made of the potential
benefit of intra-arterial infusion of 5-FU in this condition. There
was less agreement on the value of cystectomy in those with squamous
carcinoma.

Riddle (London) observed that 18% of his patients after
cystectomy were shown to have cancer of the prostate.

England (London) noted that bacteriological examination of
tumours show that 30% were infected in those with sterile urine.
De Voogt (Leiden) asked whether proplylactic antibiotic therapy was
of help after diversion. Wahlqvist (Umea) replied that the patients
reported had not been treated actively but were now treated
aggressively as soon as infection was suspected. He felt the
situation had improved with this change of policy. Zingg (Bern)
asked where the urine was collected from, as 7% bacteriuria was
found on catheterisation of conduits. Wahlqvist replied that the
urine was collected at the stoma since searching for "significant"
bacteriuria was irrelevant in patients with no bladder. He felt
that any bacteriuria in a conduit was of significance. Oliver
(London) observed that this matter was of great potential importance
if the use of cytotoxic chemotherapy became more common as urinary
infection was seen within three to four days of treating patients
with CISCA (Cis-platinum, Cyclophosphamide and Adriamycin).

Amaku observed that primary carcinoma of the urethra was rare -
representing only 0.003% of 12,455 malignancies at Ibadan. Surgical
excision involving amputation of the penis offered the best hope of
cure but this was not accepted by the patients. Barnard (Manchester)

commented on the incidence of secondary urethral carcinoma after
cystectomy and observed that even though he undertook primary
urethrectomy for all patients whose tumours were multiple or
involved the bladder neck or prostate, 14% of the remainder
subsequently developed urethral lesions. <u>Hall</u> mentioned that even
with urethrectomy one sometimes subsequently saw invasion of the
corpora cavernosa. One participant questioned whether the high
incidence of urethral tumour was due to the operation since only
three such lesions had been seen in 95 patients treated by
radiotherapy.

INTRODUCTION TO IMMUNOLOGY AND IMMUNOTHERAPY OF BLADDER TUMOURS

J A MARTINEZ-PIÑEIRO

CS La Paz, Servicio De Urologia, Av. Generalissimo

Madrid, Spain

A specific antitumour immune response has been repeatedly
demonstrated in man and in experimental animals, which is mediated
by T and B lymphocytes and by monocytes. Firstly these cells
recognise tumour associated antigens and secondly they launch a
complex immune response against them, whose aim is the elimination
of the foreign antigen, i.e. the neoplastic cells; unfortunately
such an immune response often fails to destroy the tumour.

There is also evidence suggesting that a tumour is immunosuppressive in itself, affecting both the specific anti-tumour
immunity and the general host immunity, through the interaction of
soluble blocking factors and/or the activation of clones of suppressor cells, which are distinct subpopulations of either T- cells
or monocytes. This tumour escape mechanism accounts for both the
failure to reject an incipient tumour and the decline in immune
response with progressive disease.

Presently it is admitted that a deficient immunity is a bad
prognostic sign and that immunologic testing should be considered as
one of the routine assessments in oncologic patients. In a series
of 191 bladder tumours studied in my Service by means of the DNCB
test, we found a normal cell-mediated immune response only in 16.7%
of the patients; the degree of immunologic impairment did not
correlate however with the stage of the disease as can be seen in
Table I, contrary to what had been reported previously by ourselves
and by others in smaller series.

The three year follow up of 106 of these patients has demonstrated a significant correlation between immunological depression and
death due to progression of the tumour. Of 11 deaths, 10 occurred

TABLE I

CELL-MEDIATED IMMUNE RESPONSE (DNCB TEST)

		Normal	%	Abnormal	%	Anergy	%
Tis	34	8	23.5	7	20.6	19	55.9
T1	62	13	21	13	21	36	58
T2	31	2	6.4	8	25.8	21	67.7
T3	44	7	15.9	12	27.3	25	56.8
T4	20	2	10	7	35	11	55
				47	24.6	112	58.6
Total	191	32					
				159	83.24		

in patients with an abnormal DNCB test and only one in a patient with a normal response (Table II). Similar findings have been reported by several groups, providing the rationale for the current trend towards immunotherapy for cancer, which aims to restore the deficient immune response to normal.

TABLE II

CORRELATION BETWEEN DEATH DUE TO PROGRESSION AND IMMUNOLOGIC

COMPETENCE (3 YEAR FOLLOW-UP)[*]

Stage	No. of Patients at risk	Deaths due to prog- ression	Immune Response			
			Normal	%	Abnormal	%
Tis T1 T2	80	0	0/33	0	0/47	0
T3	16	5	1/6	16.7	4/10	40
T4	10	6	0/1	0	6/9	66.7
Total	106	11	1/11	9.1	10/11	90.9

[*] Corrected figs. by subtraction of postop. and intercurrent illness deaths.

TABLE III

CELL MEDIATED IMMUNE RESPONSE IN IRRADIATED PATIENTS

DNCB test	Receiving BCG - 25 Patients		Not receiving BCG - 17 Pts.	
		%		%
Remained normal before and following HER	3	12	3	17.6
Remained abnormal or deteriorated following HER	12	48	12	70.6
Improved following HER	10	40	2	11.8

The need for some means of immunotherapy is further emphasized by the fact that most anti-cancer treatments are immunosuppressive in themselves; it is well known that cytostatics, hormones, irradiation and even surgery and anaesthesia are immunosuppressive agents and it has been argued that if they fail to eradicate the tumour they may actually enhance its growth. The correction of therapy-induced immunosuppression may be considered therefore an additional reason for immunotherapy.

In this sense, BCG vaccine has been employed by us to counteract the effect of high energy irradiation (H.E.R.) in bladder cancer patients, with encouraging results. Table III shows that the percentage of patients whose cell-mediated immune response improved

TABLE IV

CELL MEDIATED IMMUNE RESPONSE IN PATIENTS BEFORE AND AFTER

IMMUNOSTIMULATION WITH LEVAMISOLE OR BCG

DNCB Test

		Normal	%	Abnormal	%	Anergy	%
Levamisole Group 44 patients	Before	0	0	14	31.8	30	62.2
	After	10	22.7	21	47.7	13	29.5
BCG Group 91 patients	Before	12	13.2	23	25.3	56	61.5
	After	59	64.8	16	17.6	16	17.6

following HER was significantly higher in the group receiving immunotherapy and that the percentage of patients with abnormal response was also much lower in the group treated by BCG.

Apart from BCG, Levamisole has been widely used in different cancers as a non-specific stimulating agent with variable results. A retrospective study by our group, comparing the effects of Levamisole and BCG in bladder cancer patients, has shown a clear advantage for the latter (Tables IV and V); therefore we have abandoned Levamisole.

TABLE V

Tis - T1 BLADDER TUMOURS

Recurrences by treatment

| Levamisole | - | 8/17 | - | 47% |
| BCG | - | 6/29 | - | 20.6% |

Generally speaking, the strategy of immunotherapy is to back the host defense mechanisms, either by means of a specific stimulation of the immune response, or by non-specific means, trying to make existing immune responses more effective. However, to be really effective, immunologic stimulation has to take place after the tumour bulk has been reduced to a mass which can be controlled by the immune system. This means that immunotherapy should be added to integrated therapeutic programmes immediately after tumour ablation and before the residual cancer might have again grown to a volume which can no longer be kept under control.

IMMUNE RESPONSE IN BLADDER CANCER

S BROSMAN

Department of Urology
Harbor General Hospital
University of California, Los Angeles, USA

The interaction between the host and cancer can be evaluated in terms of peripheral or local cellular response and the presence of delayed cutaneous hypersensitivity. Most investigations in immuno-biology have focused on peripheral cells because of the ease with which they can be obtained.

MATERIALS AND METHODS

Patients with histologically proven bladder cancer were divided according to the stage of their disease. The pathologic stage was used wherever possible. Patients were divided into those with super-ficial tumours (Stage O, A; TO, T1), invasive disease (Stage B, C; D1; T2, T3, T4) and those with metastases (Stage D2; M1).

Immune function testing was performed prior to and following completion of standard therapy. Whenever possible, sequential testing was performed at three month intervals. Tumour recurrence and survival was evaluated in all patients (Figure 1).

The battery of studies available for assessing the immune response is listed in Table I. In this particular study, the immune response was studied with skin testing, quantitation of T-cells and Fc receptor bearing cells, phytohaemagglutinin stimulated T-cell cytotoxicity (PDCC), and antibody dependent cytotoxicity (ADCC). The latter is a measure of non-T-cell cytotoxicity.

Three types of skin testing were used: 1) response to primary contact sensitisation with 2,4 - dinitrochlorobenzene (DNCB), 2) recall response to prior sensitisation using a battery of four

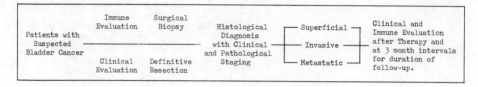

FIGURE 1

Protocol for bladder cancer patient showing the timing of immune
cell studies.

antigens (candida, mumps, PPD, streptokinase-streptodornase) and
3) inflammatory response to the primary irritant Croton Oil. The
Croton Oil test was included as a measure of the inflammatory
response and does not involve any known immunologic reaction in
contrast to the primary DNCB sensitisation and secondary recall
antigen immune responses.

The techniques of DNCB skin test application have been published
elsewhere (1). A negative score implied that no discernible reaction
occurred at any of the application sites. Only those patients who
responded to the initial sensitisation or a challenge dose of 25 mcg
were considered to be positive responders.

TABLE I

IMMUNE EVALUATION IN BLADDER CANCER PATIENTS

Skin Testing

    DNCB (Dinitrochlorobenzene)
    Recall antigens (Mumps, monilia, purified
        protein derivative (PPD), Streptokinase-
        Streptodornase)
    Croton Oil

Lymphocyte Function

    Quantitation

        T-cells
        Fc receptor bearing cells (B-cells)
    Cytotoxicity
        PDCC (PHA dependent cytotoxicity, T-cells)
        ADCC (Antibody dependent cytotoxicity, B
                or K cells).

Recall antigens were applied as intradermal injections on the inner aspect of the right forearm. Each skin test was considered positive if there was an area of 5 mm or more with erytherma and/or induration 48 hours following the injection. The Croton Oil reaction was read at 48 hours and considered positive if there was erythema with or without vesiculation.

Lymphocyte quantitation was performed by rosette formation assays and immunofluorescent detection of cell surface immunoglobulin (2).

The techniques for the cytotoxicity assays have been previously described (2). The normal range was determined by studying individual cell samples from healthy age-matched controls (50-80 years of age) and younger controls (19-49 years of age). No differences were detected between the two groups of controls and a mean score and standard deviation was established.

The data was categorised into those scores more than one standard deviation above the mean of a healthy control population scores within one standard deviation of the control mean. Statistical analysis was performed using chi square tests.

RESULTS

Skin Testing Response and Tumour Stage (Figure 2)

One hundred and seventy-three bladder cancer patients were skin tested one or more times and followed closely to establish clinical and laboratory correlations of immunologic tests. The data presented refers to the patients' initial skin test response. The results were judged to be significant if the P value was less than 0.05.

As a group, bladder cancer patients showed a trend towards a greater percentage of negative skin tests (of each type) with increasing quantities of tumour. All skin test groups were depressed compared to the non-cancer controls. Only DNCB and streptokinase-streptodornase response correlated closely with stage of disease. The difference in responses between groups of patients with super-ficial and those with invasive or metastatic bladder cancer was highly significant using the chi square test for trend (DNCB, $p < 0.025$; streptokinase-streptodornase, $p < 0.001$). Croton Oil response was markedly depressed for all stages of disease when compared to a control population ($p < 0.001$) but did not vary significantly between stages of disease.

There was agreement between DNCB inflammatory and Croton Oil response in 56% of patients. DNCB inflammatory responses were

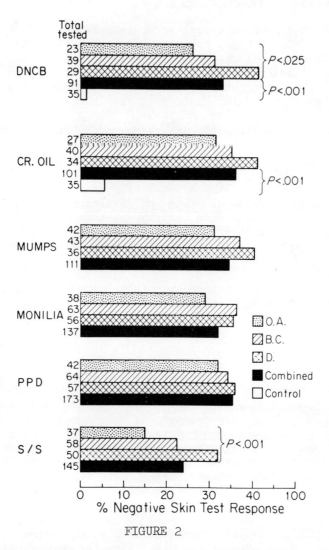

FIGURE 2

The percentage of negative skin test responses in bladder cancer patients as tested with DNCB, Croton Oil, Streptokinase-Streptodornase, monilia, mumps and PPD. Each stage of disease is represented.

positive and Croton Oil was negative in 22% of the patients and the reverse was true in 22%.

These findings could be explained by changes affecting the inflammatory response and affecting delayed hypersensitivity induction and response to DNCB.

Effects of Tumour Reduction on Skin Test Response and

Immune Cell Function

The effect on host immunity of tumour reduction by surgery (or surgery plus radiotherapy) was determined by comparing the first skin test results in tumour-bearing patients versus results in patients whose neoplasm had been removed within the previous six months (Figure 3). In the combined group of patients, there was a significant decrease in DNCB negative responses after tumour removal ($p < 0.01$), but this improvement was primarily reflected in patients with invasive or metastatic disease who had a tumour reductive procedure.

In general, the DNCB response tends to remain stable. Patients who were initially positive to DNCB remained positive and vice versa. Very few patients demonstrated a cross-over in response.

Following tumour removal, the combined group of cancer patients had fewer negative responses to Croton Oil ($p < 0.05$). This was particularly true in patients with large tumour volumes who were rendered tumour free.

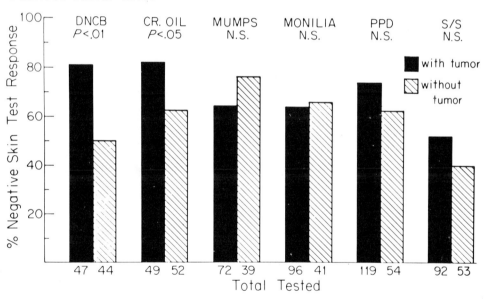

FIGURE 3

The percentage of negative skin test responses in bladder cancer patients as tested with DNCB, Croton Oil, Streptokinase-Strepto-dornase, monilia, mumps and PPD. All stages of bladder cancer are combined, but divided into two groups - those with tumour and those without tumour at the time of skin testing.

There was no statistical difference in any of the recall antigen
responses after surgery.

Immune Cell Function and Tumour Stage (Figure 4)

The first test result for T-cell, Fc receptor-bearing (Fc)
cells, ADCC and PDCC was used to make comparisons on the percentage
of tests that were more or less than one standard deviation from the
mean of a group of age-matched normal subjects.

The data indicates that the cancer population differs from the
controls. Rather than finding a large proportion of patients with
either depressed or elevated results, we found that the cancer
patients have a wide variability of response. There may be as many
patients who have elevated responses as there are with depressed
responses. What distinguishes the cancer patients from the controls
is the greater extent of the variability in their responses rather
than the numbers of elevated or depressed responses.

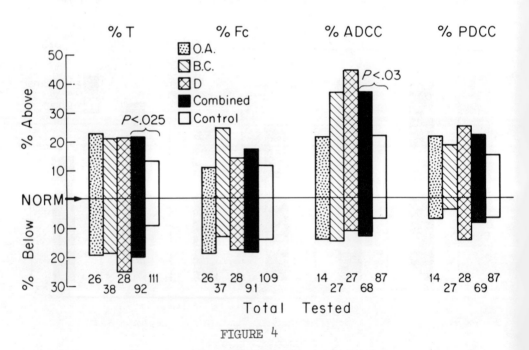

FIGURE 4

The percent of bladder cancer patients as tested with immune cell
studies (T-cells, Fc receptors, ADCC and PDCC cytotoxicity) whose
test results vary more than one standard deviation above or below
the norm. Each stage of disease and a group of healthy age-matched
controls by a single bar, is represented.

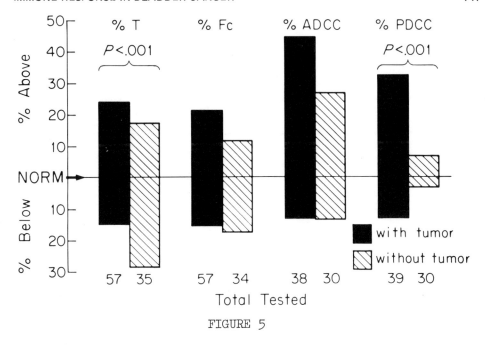

FIGURE 5

The percentage of bladder cancer patients as tested with immune cell studies (T-cells, Fc receptors, ADCC and PDCC cytotoxicity) whose test results vary more than one standard deviation above or below the norm. All stages of bladder cancer are combined, but divided into two groups - those with tumour and those without tumour at the time of blood evaluations.

Bladder cancer patients with all stages of disease combined had greater variability above and below the norm in T-cell percentages than non-cancer controls (p < 0.025). Stage D patients showed more variability compared to the controls (p < 0.03) than did patients with lesser stages of disease. Compared to each other, the different stages of disease showed no statistically significant differences in their variability.

Fc receptor cell percentages were not significantly elevated or depressed in the combined group of cancer patients. Neither was there any correlation between stage of disease and Fc receptor cell percentages.

As a combined group, the cancer patients demonstrated significant variations in ADCC from the controls (p < 0.03). Differences between each stage and the controls were most variable in Stage D patients (p < 0.05). There was no significant difference between each of the stages themselves.

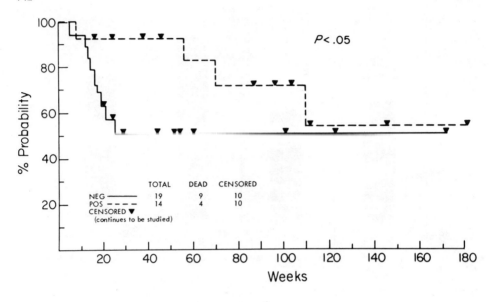

FIGURE 6

The probability (as expressed in %) of stage O,A bladder cancer patients to remain tumour free over a period of weeks. The patients have been divided into two groups - those who have a positive (----) response to DNCB and those who have a negative (——) response to DNCB at the time of their initial skin test. Patients who continue to be studied are represented as a censored observation = ▼ at the approximate date of last known status.

PDCC scores showed no significant differences between the cancer patients as a group and the controls, between individual stages and controls, or between the individual stages themselves.

In vitro immune function tests compared before and after tumour removal demonstrated significant decreases in the variability of T-cell quantitation ($p < 0.001$) and cytotoxicity ($p < 0.001$) (Figure 5).

Correlation of Immune Competence with Tumour Recurrence
and Prognosis

Thirty-three patients with low grade, stage O,A bladder cancer were studied to determine if DNCB response could predict the probability of tumour recurrence (Figure 6). The data was analysed according to the Kaplan-Meier Product Moment Statistical Technique. At one year, 92% of the 14 responders were tumour free and 51% of

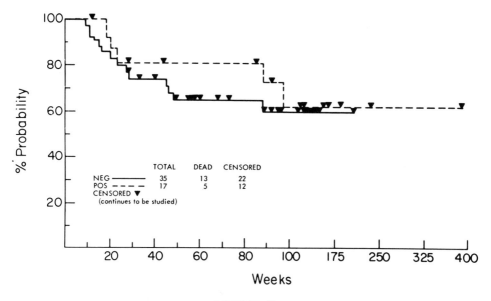

FIGURE 7

The probability (as expressed in %) of stage B, C bladder cancer
patients to survive over a period of weeks. The patients have been
divided into two groups; those who have a positive (----) response to
DNCB and those who have a negative (———) response to DNCB at the
time of their initial skin test. Patients who continue to be studied
are represented as a censored observation ▼ at the approximate date
of last known status.

the 19 non-responders were tumour free. The number of responders
who developed recurrences increased during the second year. After
110 weeks of follow-up, there was no difference in DNCB response
between the numbers of patients with recurrences.

Neither Croton Oil or recall antigen response correlated with
the tumour free period. Immune blood studies did not prove to be
significant prognosticators in this superficial disease group.

The disease free interval was measured in 52 patients with
invasive cancer who were treated with a short course of radiation
(1600 rad) followed by radical cystectomy (Figure 7). At one year,
81% of the positive DNCB responders were tumour free compared to
65% who were non-responders and tumour free. After two years, there
was no difference in tumour recurrence between the two groups. There
was no prognostic correlation found with Croton Oil, recall antigens
or immune blood studies.

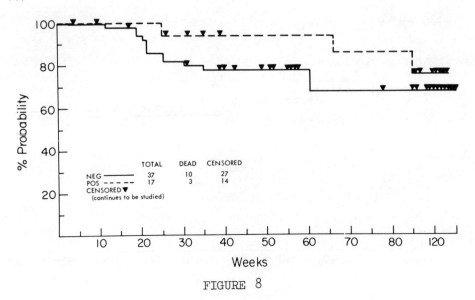

FIGURE 8

The probability (as expressed in %) of stage B, C bladder cancer
patients to survive over a period of weeks. The patients have been
divided into two groups; those who have a positive (----) response
to DNCB and those who have a negative (———) response to DNCB at the
time of their initial skin test. Patients who continue to be
studied are represented as a censored observation ▼ at the approximate date of last known status.

        The probability of survival was studied in 54 patients with
invasive disease (Figure 8). There were 37 DNCB non-responders who
had a 78% chance of survival for one year. Of the 10 deaths in this
group, eight died within the first year. In the 17 DNCB responsive
patients, there was a 94% chance of survival for one year with one
death occurring in that first year. There was no prognostic
significance to DNCB response during the 140 week follow-up period.

        Neither Croton Oil, recall antigens or immune blood studies
correlated with survival in this disease group.

        Similar analyses were performed in patients with metastatic
disease to determine if host immunocompetence would relate to
survival. There was no significant difference in survival between
DNCB responders and non-responders, recall antigen response and
immune cell function.

DISCUSSION

The data in this study demonstrate that delayed hyper-sensitivity is altered in bladder cancer patients and this is related to the stage of their disease. No correlation could be found between delayed hypersensitivity and prognosis. The tumour-free interval is longer in patients with superficial or invasive disease if they are DNCB responsive but tumour recurrence and survival is the same in DNCB responders and non-responders.

Assessment of DNCB skin test results, together with tumour staging by conventional means indicates two major conclusions: 1) poor response to DNCB in patients with invasive or metastatic disease correlates with the extent of disease but not prognosis, and 2) among the patients with apparently equal extent of disease poor DNCB response indicates a shorter tumour-free period because of some other factor or system that is not assessed in conventional staging procedures. When the observations made by Croton Oil testing are also taken into account, a third conclusion is evident; ie. bladder cancer alters the non-immune host inflammatory system in addition to the delayed hypersensitivity immune system.

Croton oil induces a non-immune inflammatory response and this response has been noted to be impaired in patients with neoplastic disease (3,4). There is a disagreement about whether this does (3) or does not (4) parallel the reduction in DNCB response. Our data show that there is a depressed Croton Oil response in patients with bladder cancer and indicates that this inflammatory response parallels the DNCB immune response according to stage of disease.

There was a concordance between Croton Oil response and DNCB inflammatory response in 56% of patients. The other 44% discordancy (positive DNCB, negative Croton Oil and vice versa) suggests that two important host defense systems are altered in bladder cancer patients, those involving T lymphoid cell function as well as the non-immune inflammatory system.

Delayed hypersensitivity testing by intradermal injection or application of appropriate recall antigens is imprecise because of the variability of intensity and range of prior exposure that will occur in a population. Our data indicated that streptokinase-streptodornase was the only recall antigen which correlated with stage of disease.

In vitro lymphoid tests permit enumeration of T and B cells in the peripheral blood and evaluation of the blastogenic response of (primarily) T cells to antigens such as phytohaemagglutinin (PHA) and Concanavalin A (ConA) and measurement of cytotoxicity. Cancer patients, especially those with metastases, have been reported to have fewer T and B cells in the peripheral blood than normal subjects

(5,6). Lymphocytes from many patients have also been found to have decreased reactivity to the T cell mitogens PHA or ConA and to be poor killers in an antibody dependent and direct cytotoxicity cellular assay (7). Although the reasons are not clear for the decrease in the number of circulating T and B cells in bladder cancer as well as in other cancers, there is speculation that this may be the result of recruitment or sequestration by activated lymphoid organs (8). Similarly, the inability of cancer patients to respond in mitogen and cytotoxic assays could be due to the selective depletion of lymphocyte subpopulations, T or B suppressor cell activity, or antigen-antibody complex binding of functional receptors (8).

In bladder cancer patients as a group, the battery of in vitro tests used to quantitate T and B cells and measure lymphoid cell cytotoxicity have shown no correlation with stage of disease, tumour-free period or survival. There are significant differences when cancer patients are compared to healthy age-matched controls. There is greater variability above and below the norm in T cell percentages and ADCC in the cancer patients. This is most evident in patients with metastatic disease. Although the variability in immune function tests tended to decrease following tumour removal, only PDCC showed a statistically significant change toward normal within six months after surgery.

The blood tests of patients skin tested with DNCB were analysed to determine if any correlation existed between these two types of immune function testing. There was none. Non-responders to DNCB were just as likely to vary above and below the norm as DNCB responders.

The initial hope that the specific and non-specific immune system changes in neoplasia could be easily assessed by one-step laboratory testing of the complex system that includes many different peripheral blood cells has not been substantiated. Testing of more precisely defined lymphoid and monocyte subpopulations for baseline activity and response to minimal and maximum (load) stimuli should lead to better insight into the depressive (or exhaustion) effects of neoplasia on certain immune functions. In vitro assays allow careful control of test conditions and should permit assessment of inhibitory or stimulatory factors from sera, blood cells, or tumours. Testing systems are likely to pass through several generations of development and refinement. The process is well underway but far from completion.

SUMMARY

1.   The skin test response, particularly the delayed hypersensitivity of DNCB, correlates with the stage of bladder cancer.

2.   Skin test responses do not tend to change with the course of disease. Patients with low grade superficial tumours are an exception. When their tumour is removed, skin test response revert to normal.

3.   Skin testing is not prognostic for tumour recurrence or survival.

4.   Immune function tests and skin tests are affected by radiation therapy, chemotherapy and surgery which produce a depression of host response.

5.   Immune function tests do not correlate with stage of disease or skin testing and are not prognostic for tumour recurrence or survival.

6.   Immune function tests are not elevated or depressed more than controls but are more variable both above and below the norm than non-cancer patients.

REFERENCES

1. Catalona, W. J., Taylor, P. T., Rabson, A. G. and
    Chretian, P. B., A method for dinitrochlorobenzene contact
    sensitisation. N. Eng. J. Med. 286, 399 (1972).

2. Elhilali, M. M., Britton, S., Brosman, S. and Fahey, J. F.,
    Critical evaluation of lymphocyte functions in urological
    cancer patients. Cancer Res. 36, 132 (1976).

3. Johnson, M. W., Maibach, H. I. and Salmon, S. E., Skin re-
    activity in patients with cancer: impaired delayed hyper-
    sensitivity or faulty inflammatory response. N. Eng. J. Med.
    284, 1255 (1971).

4. Roth, J. A., Eilber, F. R., Nizze, J. A. and Morton, D. L.,
    Lack of correlation between skin reactivity to dinitrochloro-
    benzene and Croton Oil in patients with cancer. N. Eng. J. Med.
    293, 388 (1975).

5. Wybran, J. and Fundenberg, J. H., Thymus-derived rosette-
    forming cells in various human disease states: cancer, lymphoma,
    bacterial and viral infection and other disease. J. Clin.
    Invest. 52, 1026 (1971).

6. Hersh, E. M., Immunology of cancer. Cancer Bul. 31, 67 (1975).

7. Rocklin, R. W., Clinical application of in vitro lymphocyte
    tests. Prog. Clin. Immunol. 2, 21 (1974).

8. Greaves, M. F., Owen, J. J. T. and Raff, M. C., T and B
    lymphocytes: origins, properties and roles in immune responses.
    Excerpta Medica Amsterdam. New York: American Elsevier
    Publishing Co., Inc., pp. 315 (1973).

MONOCYTE FUNCTION IN BLADDER CANCER

M C BISHOP and J RHODES

Department of Urology

Addenbrooke's Hospital, Cambridge, England

ABSTRACT

A rosette assay was used to test Fc receptor expression of
normal human monocytes cultured in a variety of media. Monocyte
activity was suppressed by a heat stable ultrafiltrate of normal
serum and of supernatants from cultured explants of malignant
tumours, mainly superficial transitional cell carcinoma of the
bladder removed by transurethral resection. The data supports an
hypothesis that tumours develop by suppressing host macrophages
at a particular site. This is achieved by subverting the normal
physiological humoral control of monocyte activity in peripheral
blood.

INTRODUCTION

There is now a considerable amount of evidence for the
defensive role of peripheral blood monocytes and tissue macrophages
in host surveillance against tumours (1,2). Their significance in
human cancer has been considered in terms of a number of in vitro
measurements of varying complexity. These include estimation of
the peripheral blood monocyte count; a series of tests based on
non-specific lysis of sensitised cells; measurement of serum
lysozyme, a product of active macrophages; and the determination of
the fraction of host monocytes in the tumour cell mass (3).
Furthermore, measurements of the chemotactic response of blood
monocytes has been measured and found to be depressed. This mirrors
the results of in vivo experiments on tumour bearing animals in
which the capacity to mobilise macrophages into inflammatory sites
may be defective (4).

149

Monocyte function in bladder cancer has only been studied through the chemotactic response (5). This paper describes the results of another in vitro test from which an hypothesis has been derived to explain how tumours in general, and transitional cell carcinomas in particular, maintain their growth.

METHODS

Monocytes and macrophages possess membrane receptors for the Fc portion of the IgG molecule. Such receptor expression varies with the degree of monocyte activation by a variety of stimuli and is conveniently measured by a rosette assay in which sensitised bovine erythrocytes become attached to monocytes in proportion to the number of Fc receptors (6).

Normal mononuclear cells were isolated from defibrinated blood centrifuged over a Ficoll-Triosil gradient and incubated in a defined medium on tissue culture slides. The adherent monocytes were then separated from non-adherent lymphocytes. Samples of solid tumours were obtained. These consisted mainly of the exophytic parts of non-invasive transitional cell tumours of the bladder removed by transurethral resection. The group also included a small number of tumours from patients with carcinoma of the bronchus and breast. Biopsies of macroscopically normal bladder mucosa were also obtained from patients with obvious tumour in another part of the bladder. The tissue fragments were minced and incubated for 24 hours at 37°C. Cell-free supernatants were then obtained by centrifugation. Normal monocytes were then cultured in an artifical defined medium (RPMI 1640) supplemented with serum, tumour supernatants, or their heat-stable ultrafiltrates (molecular weight of fractions less than 25,000 heated to 56°C for 35 minutes). After culture for 24 hours the cells were washed and the assay for Fc receptor expression performed using a panel of ox erythrocytes bearing increasing amounts of a specific antibody. The presence of foetal calf serum in the final culture medium provided maximum stimulation of receptor activity and allowed the effect of various inhibitors to become more obvious. Two groups of experiments with and without addition of foetal calf serum, are described.

RESULTS

Group 1 (Figure 1) Fc receptor expression increased in proportion to the rise in concentration of sensitising antiserum when monocytes were cultured in cell-free conditions. This rise was inhibited when monocytes were cultured in normal serum or its ultrafiltrate. However, it was considerably enhanced by an ultrafiltrate of serum from individuals with cancer.

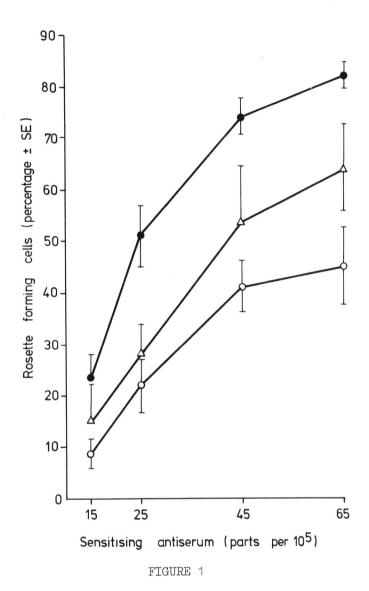

FIGURE 1

The percentage of rosette-forming monocytes as a function of
erythrocyte sensitisation after 24 hours culture in artificial
medium with addition of:-
    Normal human serum (o)
    An ultrafiltrate of serum from cancer patients (•)
    Serum free conditions (Δ).
    (14 patients and 14 controls, mean ± S.E.M.)

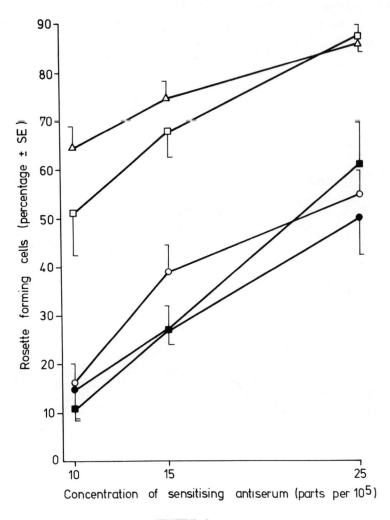

FIGURE 2

The percentage of rosette-forming monocytes as a function of
erythrocyte sensitisation after 24 hours culture in artifical
medium containing 10% foetal calf serum with addition of:-
    Tumour supernatant (●)
    Heat inactivated ultrafiltrate of tumour supernatant (■).
       (m. wt. less than 25,000)
    Heat inactivated ultrafiltrate of normal serum (o)
       (m. wt. less than 25,000)
    Normal bladder mucosa supernatant (□).
    No addition (△).

Group 2 (Figure 2) Maximal stimulation of monocytes with foetal calf serum in the culture media was inhibited by supernatants and their heat-stable ultrafiltered fractions from tumour and normal serum. Supernatants from normal bladder nucosa showed some inhibitory activity.

DISCUSSION

Rhodes (1977) previously showed that the activity of monocytes as judged by Fc receptor expression was enhanced in patients with malignant disease. In the present work normal monocytes have been studied. Since their activity is also increased by serum from cancer patients the effect is clearly of a humoral substance on un-modified cells. Such activation is inhibited by a heat stable low molecular weight fraction from normal serum and from supernatant of tumour explants - mainly from transitional cell carcinoma of the bladder. It is of interest that supernatant from apparently normal bladder mucosa had some inhibitory activity. This would be consistent with the known malignant tendency of the whole urothelium in patients who apparently have one focus of tumour.

Monocyte activation by serum from cancer patients cannot be entirely accounted for by a decreased level of inhibitor, since the degree of activation is greater than that occurring in serum-free conditions. There must therefore be a positive stimulus for activation. This could be manifest through lymphokines or "macrophage activating factor".

These results showing enhanced peripheral blood monocyte activity would seem to oppose the findings of others that chemotactic function of monocytes is depressed even in early malignant disease (5,8). There is no explanation for this though the two functions of monocytes, expression of Fc receptors and chemotaxis may be modulated independently. On the other hand both chemotaxis assays and the present studies detect a factor produced by tumours which inhibits monocyte function and which may therefore facilitate the growth of the tumour.

The present work demonstrates the similarity between the humoral inhibitors extracted from tumour and present in normal serum. Both factors have similar physical properties (molecular weight less than 25,000 daltons, heat stable at $56^{\circ}C$) though final confirmation of this must await more detailed analysis.

On the basis of these data we are tempted to conclude that the inhibitory factor from normal serum and tumours are the same. Therefore whereas systemic monocyte activation may be an appropriate response to the presence of carcinoma cells the tumour continues to grow because it is able to produce a normal physiological inhibitor of monocyte activation.

REFERENCES

1. Alexander, P., The functions of the macrophage in malignant disease. Ann. Rev. Med. 27, 207-224 (1976).

2. Currie, G., Immunological aspects of host resistance to the development of growth of cancer. Bioch. Biophys. Acta. 458, 135-165 (1976).

3. Carr, I., Macrophages in human cancer: a review, in "The macrophage and cancer". Eds. James, K., McBride, W. and Stuart, A. Edinburgh (1977).

4. Snyderman, R. and Pike, M. C., An inhibitor of macrophage chemotaxis produced by neoplasms. Science. 192, 370-372 (1976).

5. Hausman, M. S. and Brosman, S. A., Abnormal monocyte function in bladder cancer patients. J. Urol. 115, 537-541 (1976).

6. Rhodes, J., Macrophage heterogeneity in receptor activity: the activation of macrophage Fc receptor function in vivo and in vitro. J. Immunol. 114, 976-981 (1975).

7. Rhodes, J., Altered expression of human monocyte Fc receptors in malignant disease. Nature, 265, 253-255 (1977).

8. Boetcher, D. A. and Leonard, E. J., Abnormal monocyte chemotactic response in cancer patients. J. Natl. Cancer Inst. 52, 1091-1099 (1974).

T AND B LYMPHOCYTES IN PATIENTS WITH BLADDER TUMOURS

M HORŇAK

Department of Urology, Medical School

80946 Bratislava-Kramare, Czechoslovakia

In following up the cellular component of the immunity system in man, attention has been focused upon two cellular types: the subpopulation of T and B lymphocytes. Our work has aimed at following up the immunological reactivity in patients with bladder tumours and the correlation between immunological reactivity parameters and the clinical stage of the disease.

Thirty-five patients have been followed up. The patients were classified according to TNM. The control group was made up of 27 patients hospitalised for non-tumourous disease. T and B lymphocytes were identified by using a modification of the rosette method (Jondal et al, 1972).

TABLE I

T AND B LYMPHOCYTES IN PATIENTS WITH BLADDER CANCER

	No. of Patients	T	B
Control group	27	$64,65 \pm 5,66$	$25,73 \pm 3,42$
Bladder Cancer	35		
T1	15	$55,97 \pm 4,58$	$35,77 \pm 5,40$
T2	3	$55,17 \pm 0.76$	$34,83 \pm 2,02$
T3	11	$49,27 \pm 7,52$	$39,50 \pm 4,95$
T4	6	$48,58 \pm 4,18$	$42,92 \pm 3,36$

155

Table I shows the percentage of T and B lymphocytes in the control group and in patients with bladder tumours according to the clinical stage. In comparing the percentage values of T and B lymphocytes between the individual clinical stages the differences were not statistically significant.

REFERENCE

1.   Jondal, M., Holm, G. and Wigzell, H., Surface markers on human T and B lymphocytes. I. A large population of lymphocytes forming non-immune rosettes with sheep red blood cells. J. Exp. Med. 136, 207-215 (1972).

ABH-ANTIGENICITY IN T1 UROTHELIAL TUMOURS

G JAKSE and F HOFSTÄDTER

Department of Urology and Department of Pathology

University of Innsbruck, Innsbruck, Austria

The urothelial cells have, besides other surface antigens, also the isoantigens A, B and H which are identical with the blood group antigens.

The specific red cell adherence (SRCA) test, originally developed by Davidsohn et al, allows the disclosure of these antigens (3).

The blood group antigens can be demonstrated by a sandwich technique, where firstly the tissue is incubated with an isoantibody. Then the occurring antigen-antibody reaction can be visualised by adherence of the erythrocytes of the respective blood group.

In the course of dedifferentiation the urothelium will lose its antigenicity, as shown by Davidsohn (1). Benign urothelial hyperplasia reveals the same antigenicity as normal urothelium. With the occurrence of atypia there is a loss of antigens. As a rule negative tests were associated with atypical hyperplasia and carcinoma in situ which are areas of potential malignant and invasive tumours (2). The same could be demonstrated on cytological preparations and the results are in close correlation with the histological material from tumours.

The SRCA test was applied in a retrospective study of 36 patients with recurrent transitional cell carcinoma stage O/A, Grade 1-3 (Jewett and Strong, Broders). All these patients were initially treated by transurethral resection (TUR) only.

1. Positive tests. A positive result means that more than one half of the urothelium shows an antigen antibody reaction.

Twenty of the 36 patients had a positive SRCA test. None of these patients had a recurrence of higher stage or grade during the follow up, from 4-17 years.

2.   Negative tests.   In 16 of the 36 patients the test was negative. Of these, 10 failed to respond to conservative treatment and died of progressive cancer after a period between one year ten months and 13 years with an average of 3.5 years. In six patients with four to nine years of follow-up the test was negative but no invasive tumour has so far developed.

The recurrence for patients with positive and negative tests are shown in Table I.

No correlation has been established between the number of recurrences and the results. Those with negative tests have shown fewer recurrent tumours because of the shorter life span of these patients. Furthermore no correlation could be found between multi- plicity of tumours and negative test results. In the SRCA positive group there were significantly more multiple tumours (nine of 20) than in the negative group (three of 16).

In 15 patients with recurrent TCC we could correlate the SRCA test results with the DNA distribution of the same tumours. In the positive group every patient has a diploid DNA distribution (Table II). On the other hand there were three specimens with normal DNA content but negative SRCA test. One of these died from a progressive tumour (Table III).

TABLE I

RELATIONSHIP BETWEEN RECURRENCE OF TUMOUR AND SRCA TEST

Recurrences

SRCA	STAGE	1	2	3	4	5	6	7	8	9	10
Pos. Follow-up 4-17 yrs.	O	1	-	2	2	2	-	-	1	2	-
	A	-	3	1	2	1	1	-	1	-	1
Neg. Follow-up 2-13 yrs.	O	-	1	1+[2]	1+[2]	1+[2]	-	-	-	-	-
	A	-	[1]	1	1	[3]	-	-	-	-	-

[ ] - patients who have died with tumour

TABLE II

POSITIVE SRCA-TEST AND DNA-CONTENT IN EIGHT PATIENTS WITH
STAGE O/A BLADDER TUMOURS

Name	Survival (years)	Grade	DDQ[+)]	SQ[++)]	DNA-Dist.	SRCA-Test
W.B.	8	2	0.86	0.88	2c-4c	+++
K.H.	5	2	1.17	1.14	2c	+++
W.A.	5	2	1.13	1.06	2c-4c	+++
W.F.	4	2	1.31	1.06	2c-4c	+++
N.A.	7	1	1.12	1.05	2c-4c	++
W.J.	6	2	1.06	1.01	2c	++
K.M.	9	2	1.26	1.01	2c-4c	++

[+)]DDQ = Diploid deviation quotient=rel. DNA-Content $(\bar{x})$/2c-extinct.
(Leucocytes).

[++)]SQ = stem line quotient=rel. DNA-Content $(\bar{x})$/tumour stem line
$(\bar{x})$.

TABLE III

NEGATIVE SRCA-TEST AND DNA-CONTENT IN SEVEN PATIENTS WITH
STAGE O/A BLADDER TUMOURS

Name	Survival	Grade	DDQ[+)]	SQ[++)]	DNA-Dist.	SRCA-Test
K.E.	5	1	1.16	1.07	2c-4c	-
H.A.	9	1	1.28	1.00	2c-4c	-
E.J.	5 (+)	2	2,31	1.71	3,5c-7c	-
W.L.	2 (+)	2	1.19	1.01	2c-4c	-
B.R.	3 (+)	2	1.45	1.12	2,5c-5c	+
S.A.	3 (+)	3	1,84	1.43	3c-6c	-
B.J.	2 (+)	3	2,70	1.81	3,5c-7c	-

[+)]DDQ = Diploid deviation quotient=rel. DNA-Content (x)/2c-extinct.
(Leucocytes).

[++)]SQ = stem line quotient=rel. DNA-Content $(\bar{x})$/tumour stem line
$(\bar{x})$.

CONCLUSIONS

Urothelial metaplasia shows the same antigenicity as normal urothelium.

A differentiation into SRCA positive and negative tumours is also possible using cytological preparations.

A diploid DNA distribution can be associated with a negative test and does not exclude an aggressive, recurrent tumour. The ABH antigenicity enables a prognosis to be made in T1, G1-3 transitional cell carcinomas in that in our opinion an SRCA negative test means that a recurrent aggressive tumour is very likely, whilst an SRCA positive test makes a recurrent, aggressive tumour very unlikely.

REFERENCES

1.   Davidsohn, I., Immunopathological diagnosis of urinary bladder tumours. Proc. Inst. Med. Chgo. 30, 37-38 (1974).

2.   Jakse, G., Hofstadter, F., Further experiences with the Specific Red Cell Adherence Test in bladder cancer. Eur. Urol. 4, 356-360 (1978).

3.   Kovarik, S., Davidsohn, I., Stejskal, R., ABO antigens in cancer. Archs. Path. 86, 12-21 (1968).

HUMORAL AND CELLULAR IMMUNE RESPONSE IN PATIENTS WITH TRANSITIONAL CELL CARCINOMA OF THE URINARY BLADDER (TCC) AGAINST BLADDER CARCINOMA CELLS IN TISSUE CULTURE

S PAULI, M TROYE, Y HANSSON, M KARLSSON, H BLOMGREN and B JOHANSSON
Department of Immunology, University of Stockholm and
Department of Urology and Radiumhemmet, Karolinska
Hospital, Stockholm, Sweden

ABSTRACT

Non-irrádiated and irradiated patients with TCC of the urinary bladder as a group show disease related cytotoxicity. Moreover, our results strongly suggest that the effector cell(s) involved in these allogeneic reactions are of the K-cell type, ie. SIg- and FcR+ lymphocytes acting through antibodies. Furthermore, about 30% of the isolated IgG-fractions from patients sera had ADCC-inducing capacity. By means of using these antibodies in an insolubilised form we are presently trying to identify and characterise the tumour-associated antigens.

Highly purified peripheral blood lymphocytes (PBL) from five different groups of donors, each comprising approximately 30-40 individuals were tested in a 51Cr-release assay against a small panel of allogeneic target cells of established cell lines (7). The different groups of blood donors were: 1) untreated TCC-bladder patients; 2) TCC-bladder patients treated by local radiotherapy 1-12 years before testing; 3) age and sex matched clinical controls comprising mainly patients with cancer of the prostate also untreated for their disease; 4) age and sex matched patients with acute cystitis, and 5) healthy donors. The target cell panel consisted of five different cell lines: two being of TCC-bladder origin, distinct from each other in expressing different caryo-types and HLA antigens (unpublished observations); one derived from normal bladder epithelium; one from colon carcinoma and one from malignant melanoma. Percentage cytotoxicity was expressed by subtracting the percentage background in the lymphocyte-free medium controls from that in the lymphocyte containing experimental samples.

We found that as a group PBL from both non-irradiated and irradiated patients had significantly elevated mean cytotoxicity against TCC-bladder cell lines as compared to other cell lines. Furthermore, among the irradiated TCC group there was a close correlation between year of irradiation and disease related cyto- toxicity, ie. treatment just before testing generated either high non-specific reactivities or no reactivity, while patients treated 7-12 years prior to testing followed the pattern of the control groups. However, patients treated 1-6 years before testing showed strongly significant disease related cytotoxicity, a phenomenon not seen among the three control groups. Thus, PBL from these TCC- bladder patients had disease related cytotoxicity, while selectivity (ie. reactivity against some test target cells but of no particular histological type) was found among all five groups tested. Non- selective cytotoxicity, (ie. killing of all or most cells unrelated to the patients' histological type of cancer) was rare.

Furthermore, fractionation of the lymphocytes on various immune complex columns revealed that the effector cells involved were surface Ig-negative (SIg-) and Fc-receptor bearing (FcR+) lymphocytes (2,3). It is well established that antibody dependent cell-mediated cytotoxicity (ADCC) is dependent on SIg- and FcR+ killer (K) cells (1). The question whether antibodies were involved in our cyto- toxicity systems was solved by adding immunosorbent purified Fab- fragments of rabbit anti-human immunoglobulin to the incubation mixture (6). Thus, in almost all cases tested, addition of such fragments inhibited the cytotoxic reactions, strongly suggesting that antibody dependent mechanisms are mainly if not exclusively res- ponsible for the lysis of the allogeneic tumour target cells. More- over, we have isolated IgG-fractions from various sera by affinity chromatography on Protein A-Sepharose and tested these fractions for ADCC-inducing capacity against our target cell panel. About 30% of the isolated IgG-fractions were strongly reactive and antibodies from the TCC-bladder patients were significantly more reactive against tumour cells of TCC-bladder origin as compared to cells of other origins. The results from one single experiment are shown in Figure 1, where the IgG-fractions from three TCC-bladder patients and two healthy donors were tested against one cell line of TCC-bladder origin and one from colon carcinoma.

When ^{125}I-labeled plasma membranes from different cell types were analysed by Na-dodecylsulphate-polyacrylamide gel electro- phoresis (SDS-PAGE), followed by autoradiography, a characteristic pattern of membrane polypeptides was found for each of the cell lines. However, all bladder derived cells were highly similar (4,5). Experiments are now performed to establish whether or not differences in expression of certain polypeptides correlates with differences in cytotoxicity of TCC patients' lymphocytes against the various

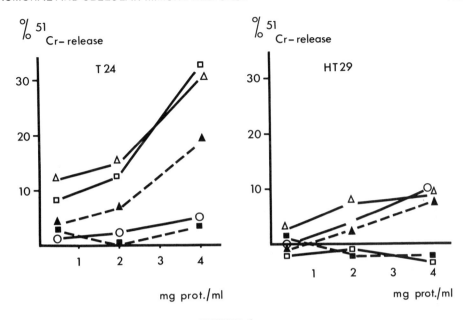

FIGURE 1

targets. For this purpose the ADCC-inducing antibodies found in
sera from patients and normal donors are insolublised by coupling
to Sepharose 4B or Protein A-Sepharose. By means of affinity
chromatography ^{125}I-labeled antigens are then purified from
detergent (NP-40)- or other plasma membrane extracts and then
analysed by SDS-PAGE followed by auto-radiography of the gels. By
means of this technique it will be possible to identify and
characterise the tumour-associated polypeptide specifically bound
by patients' antibodies.

REFERENCES

1.   Cerottini, J. C. H. and Brunner, T. K., Cell-mediated cyto-
     toxicity, allograft rejection and tumour immunity. Adv.
     Immunol. 18, 67-132 (1974).

2.   Pape, G. R., Troye, M. and Perlmann, P., Characterisation of
     cytolytic effector cells in peripheral blood of healthy in-
     dividuals and cancer patients. I. Surface markers and K-cell
     activity after separation of B-cells and lymphocytes with Fc-
     receptors by column fractionation. J. Immunol. 118, 1919-1924
     (1977).

3.   Pape, G. R., Troye, M. and Perlman, P., Characterisation of

cytolytic effector cells in peripheral blood of healthy individuals and cancer patients. II. Cytotoxicity to allogeneic
or autochtonous tumour cells in tissue culture. J. Immunol.
118, 1925-1930 (1977).

4.   Schneider, M. U., Troye, M., Pauli, S. and Perlmann, P., Plasma
      membrane associated antigens in transitional cell carcinoma of
      the urinary bladder. I. Immunological characterisation of plasma
      membrane antigens on intact human TCC-bladder and "normal"
      bladder cells in tissue culture. Int. J. Cancer. Submitted
      (1978).

5.   Schneider, M. U., Pauli, S., Troye, M. and Perlmann, P., Plasma
      membrane associated antigens in transitional cell carcinoma of
      the urinary bladder. II. Identification of plasma membrane
      associated antigens on cultured human TCC-bladder and "normal"
      bladder cells on the molecular level. Int. J. Cancer.
      Submitted (1978).

6.   Troye, M., Perlmann, P., Pape, G. R., Spiegelberg, H. L.,
      Naslund, I. and Gidlöf, A., The use of Fab-fragments of anti-
      human immunoglobulin in the spontaneous cytotoxicity to
      cultured tumour cells by lymphocytes from patients with bladder
      carcinoma and healthy donors. J. Immunol. 119, 1061-1067
      (1977).

7.   Troye, M., Pape, G. R., Perlmann, P., Pauli, S., Blomgren, H.,
      and Johansson, B., In vitro cytolytic lymphocytes in trans-
      itional cell carcinoma of the human urinary bladder. I. Post-
      treatment expression of disease-related cytotoxicity after local
      radiotherapy. Int. J. Cancer. Submitted (1978).

ACKNOWLEDGEMENT

     This work was supported by grant no. 365-B78-09XA and 1065-B78-
02R2 from the Swedish Cancer Society.

IMMUNOTHERAPY IN BLADDER CANCER

S BROSMAN

Department of Urology
Harbor General Hospital
University of California, Los Angeles, USA

INTRODUCTION

The realisation that the host-cancer relationship involved the
immune system led to the hope that assessment and manipulation of the
immune system in man could be beneficical. Work in animal tumour
systems provided important information and indicated that immune
modulation or immunotherapy could, in carefully controlled
conditions, completely eliminate an established cancer. These
successes led to numerous clinical trials in humans involving many
different tumours systems (1). In this report, I will relate our
experiences in patients with bladder cancer.

CLINICAL EXPERIENCE

Our initial clinical trials dealt with patients having
metastatic bladder cancer (2,3). These patients, as well as those
with lesser stages of disease, were selected on the basis of
several criteria.

1.   A histological diagnosis of bladder cancer.

2.   In those with metastatic cancer, the tumour could be
     confirmed and measured by x-ray, ultrasound, physical
     examination or cystoscopy.

3.   The patient had a performance status of three or better
     which meant that they were ambulatory, able to care for
     themselves and were able to receive outpatient therapy.

4.   The metastatic disease had been present for less than
      three months. Those with lesser stages of bladder cancer
      had completed treatment within three months.

5.   No other disease was present which would limit the
      patient's life expectancy.

6.   The patient was receiving no other cancer therapy.

Thirty-one patients with metastatic disease who satisfied these
criteria were randomised into two groups. There were 15 patients
who received eight weekly inoculations of Tice strain BCG (Bacillus
Calmette-Guerin). One ampoule was applied to different areas using
the scarification technique.

In order to maintain the same doctor-patient contact with the
control group, 16 patients were seen on a weekly basis for eight
weeks but received only symptomatic and supportive therapy. After
the eight week period, all the patients were seen monthly or sooner
if additional medical examinations and therapy were necessary.

Most patients receiving BCG had some toxic effects but these
were usually minor. Fever and malaise were common and lasted
several days following each treatment but patients did not consider
this to be severe. The skin lesions left by the scarification were
painful, healed slowly and were considered unsightly.

The data indicated that there was no difference in survival
between the two groups.(Figure 1). The mean survival time for the
BCG group was 26.4 weeks while the controls lived for a mean time
of 24.7 weeks. There were no instances of tumour regression in the
BCG treated or untreated groups. The study was terminated when
statistical analysis confirmed our clinical observations. Immune
response as measured by delayed cutaneous hypersensitivity,
cytotoxicity, and quantitation of T-cells and Fc receptor bearing
cells showed no differences between the two groups.

The next group of patients to be treated by immunotherapy were
those with invasive cancer, (stage B,C or P3NoMo, G3-4) and had been
treated with preoperative radiation, radical cystectomy and pelvic
lymphadenectomy. The patients were considered to be at high risk
for tumour recurrence. The immunotherapeutic agent in this trial
was Corynebacterium Parvum. Like BCG, it is a bacterium but
important differences exist. C. Parvum is a killed bacterium and
the dose can be quantitated. The protocol was designed to randomise
patients into a C. Parvum treated group and those who received no
immunotherapy. Neither group received additional anticancer therapy.
The C. Parvum was administered intravenously each week for a total
of six weeks. Although we had already used C. Parvum in patients
with metastatic disease and were familiar with the potential

toxicity, we were disturbed by the severity of the reactions in this group of patients. High fevers, rigors, nausea and malaise began within hours after the injection and lasted for several days. The patients and their private physicians as well as ourselves were concerned about these reactions and we halted the trial.

Additional studies related to the toxicity and immuno-pharmacology of C. Parvum indicated that the severity of the reaction would diminish after each successive treatment and that the adverse reactions could be eliminated by treating the patients with cortisone. The use of cortisone did not alter the immunostimulatory effects of C. Parvum. We noted that patients who were immuno-suppressed as indicated by their anergic state tended to have no adverse reactions to C. Parvum. Those who maintained some degree of immunocompetence were likely to have toxic effects and these could be greatly modified by the use of cortisone.

After knowing how to use this agent safely, we resumed the trial. However, referring physicians remembered the previous experience and patient entry into the study was slow and poor. Twenty-one patients were randomised into C. Parvum treated and no treatment groups. No difference in survival was found between the two groups although the C. Parvum group seemed to have tumour recurrences and died earlier than the non-treated group. The number of patients enrolled in this study were not large enough to make the results statistically valid. The difficulty in patient recruitment prompted us to terminate the study.

The third group of bladder cancer patients to be studied were those with superficial disease (Stage O.A; T1NxMo, G1-2). There tumours had been removed by transurethral resection. The patients were considered tumour free prior to entry into the protocol and were randomised into two groups. One group received the synthetic antihelminthic, Levamisole, while the other group received no anti-cancer therapy. This study was managed by my colleagues, Drs Jean de Kernion and Robert Smith. The object of this study was to determine if tumour recurrence could be diminished by the use of this agent. Levamisole is a synthetic immunostimulant which primarily affects monocyte and T-cell function. Suppressed activity can be returned to normal but normal function is not enhanced.

Levamisole was given orally by tablets and there were no significant adverse reactions. The 42 patients who had been randomised were followed for a minimum of one year or until a tumour recurrence was found. The data indicated that the frequency of recurrences was not influenced by the use of Levamisole.

Immune function was evaluated in each of these groups of patients by the use of skin testing, lymphocyte quantitation, lymphocyte cytotoxicity and in some instances, monocyte chemotaxis.

The cancer patients as a group differed from non-cancer controls but no significant or sustained changes could be seen between those receiving immunotherapy and other cancer patients.

DISCUSSION

The inability to achieve clinical success in controlling or decreasing the tumour burden should not be interpreted as a failure of immunotherapy. As our knowledge of the immune system has increased, we realise that the complex interactions between the various components will not easily yield to our naive attempts at immunotherapy. A brief review of some of the principles of immune response will help to explain our failures. Had this knowledge been available earlier, we could have predicted that our attempts at immunotherapy, particularly in patients with large tumour burdens, would be unsuccessful. Our efforts in immunotherapy have given us needed information about the host response to cancer as well as the behaviour of this disease (4).

One of the fundamental principles in cancer immunobiology is that the normal cell surface antigens are altered when the cell becomes neoplastic. Antigens can be demonstrated in cancer cells which are not usually found in normal adult tissue. The cell surface contains numerous antigenic structures which are modified, deleted or added to, when malignant transformation occurs. Unfortunately, the newly formed tumour associated antigens tend to lack specificity for any particular cancer and they vary greatly in their antigenic potency(5).

The host is able to mount an antigenic response against cancer cells. This response is mediated by the lymphoid cells and monocytes. The interactions of these cells are complex and are only beginning to be understood. Whereas we once considered only T-cells (thymus derived cells) and B-cells (bursa cell equivalents) as being important, we now recognise that there are a number of lymphocyte subsets which interact with each other and with monocytes. There are mechanisms to enhance and suppress lymphocyte functions and specific cells which carry out these activities. The monocyte is now considered to be an important effector cell in the immune response. These cells can detect changes in cell surface antigens, augment lymphocyte response and exert a specific cytotoxic reaction. In some human cancers and particularly in the early stages of cancer, we are often unsuccessful in being able to observe these subtle changes in the immune system because we do not have the proper assays and techniques.

The immune response lacks specificity in human tumours. The neoplastic process itself probably initiates the same or a similar type of immune response for all types of cancer. The vigor of the

response relates to the antigenicity of the cancer and to numerous
other factors. In animal systems, there does seem to be more
specificity, particularly when viral induced tumours are compared
to chemically induced tumours.

The concept of immunosurveillance had been questioned
particularly in regard to solid tumours (6). The ability of the
immune system to recognise and eliminate cancer at its earliest
stage may occur but this means of early detection and elimination
is either nonoperative or ineffective in most instances and has
never been proven in human cancer.

Currently, there is no single or group of tests which measure
immune competence. The tests which are available evaluate isolated,
complex functions of the immune system which have not been integrated
into the total sphere of immunocompetence. These various assays show
differences between groups of cancer and non-cancer patients but
various assays tend to lack specificity, reproducibility, and do not
serve to measure serial changes in a single individual. The assays
require large amounts of blood, are difficult to perform and require
extremely careful controls. Presently, all are useful only in the
research laboratory and are of no clinical value to the urologist.

Even though a number of immunotherapeutic agents have shown
beneficial effects in carefully controlled animal experiments, they
have yet to show benefits in human cancers. Non-specific immune
adjuvants such as BCG and C. Parvum represent a conglomeration of
antigenic substances and evoke a variety of host responses. There
is no way of determining all the effects upon the host immune system.
One fraction of the bacterial cell could stimulate while another
fraction could be suppressing immune response. We may determine that
the overall effect is stimulatory, but in some clinical instances,
immunosuppression has prevailed.

Recently, synthetic molecules have been developed which offer
the hope that specific components of the immune system can be
manipulated in an orchestrated manner (7). For example, the active
stimulatory principle in BCG is a substance known as MDP. This
agent activates macrophages, induces mitogenic activity, stimulates
lymphocyte activating factor, enhances the titer of circulating
antibodies, augments cell mediated cytotoxicity and shows no toxic
effects.

Other synthetic immunoadjuvants have structural analogies to
native substances. An example of these are the polynecleotides.
These serve to increase antibody synthesis, alter T-cell function
through their action on helper and suppressor lymphocytes, and
serve to stimulate cytotoxic cells.

In the years to come, improved immunotherapeutic agents will become available (8). The ability to use specific tumour cell vaccines will continue to have great interest. With these developments must also come improvements in the study of immunopharmacology and toxicology. Pharmacologic interactions, the effects of these agents individually and in combination upon cellular kinetics and their complications must all be carefully evaluated before clinical trials can be undertaken.

CONCLUSION

We have passed through the first phase of immunotherapy. Our early hopes were not fulfilled but our knowledge of the cancer process has been greatly increased. Manipulation of the immune system as an adjuvant in cancer therapy remains feasible. We must be patient and wait for our knowledge of cancer immunology to increase before we can expect any significant success with immunotherapy.

REFERENCES

1. Muggia, F. M., Cancer Immunol. Immunother. 3, 5-9 (1977).

2. Brosman, S. A., Neoplasm Immunity; Solid Tumour Therapy. Franklin Institute Press, Chicago, 97-107 (1977).

3. Brosman, S. A., Neoplasm Immunity; Solid Tumour Therapy. Franklin Institute Press, Chicago, 109-117 (1977).

4. Prager, M. D. Cancer Immunol. Immunother. 3, 157-161 (1978).

5. Weiss, D. M. Cancer Immunol. Immunother. 2, 11-19 (1977).

6. Allison, A. C. Cancer Immunol. Immunother. 2, 151-155 (1977).

7. Johnson, A. G., Audibert, F., Chedid, L. Cancer Immunol. Immunother. 3, 219-227 (1978).

8. Gutterman, J. U. Cancer Immunol. Immunother. 2, 1-9 (1977).

INTRAVESICAL BCG (BACILLUS CALMETTE-GUERIN) IN THE MANAGEMENT OF

T1 Nx Mx TRANSITIONAL CELL TUMOURS OF THE BLADDER: A TOXICITY STUDY

M R G ROBINSON, B RICHARDS, R ADIB, A AKDAS, C C RIGBY
and R C B PUGH
The Yorkshire Urological Cancer Research Group and
the Department of Pathology, Institute of Urology
London, England

ABSTRACT

In 10 patients with recurrent category T1 bladder carcinoma the
use of intravesical BCG was followed by complete or partial
regression in four patients. Toxicity was evident in three patients.

INTRODUCTION

The Urologist has a problem in the management of recurrent
category T1 (U.I.C.C. classification) bladder tumours which are not
controlled by repeated transurethral resection or coagulation
diathermy. If the lesions are confined to the epithelium of the
bladder the disease can be cured by total cystectomy. This
treatment, however, is very radical and traumatic for non-invasive
cancer. Many alternative ways of managing such tumours have been
advocated but none is entirely satisfactory.

Immunotherapy has not been fully assessed in this disease.
Recently there have been reports that a combination of intradermal
and intravesical BCG are effective in controlling category T1 bladder
cancer. Morales et al (1976) reported that the pattern of recurrences had been favourably altered in nine patients with recurrent
superficial tumours. Bladder biopsies from their patients
demonstrated marked inflammatory cell infiltration and macrophage
granulomas typical of a delayed hypersensitivity reaction to BCG.
Douville et al (1978) reported that four of six patients had a
complete regression of recurrent bladder papillomata. Two of their
patients, however, had major systemic complications of BCG therapy
which necessitated hospitalisation and antituberculous therapy.

This paper reports the preliminary experience of the Yorkshire Urological Cancer Research Group, using intravesical, without intra-dermal, BCG in the management of recurrent category T1 bladder tumours. The objectives of this study have been to determine:-

i.   Local and systemic toxicity due to BCG therapy.
ii.   The histological changes in the bladder following intra-vesical BCG with particular reference to tumour destruction.

SELECTION OF PATIENTS

Patients entered into this study have all had recurrent category T1 transitional cell bladder tumours. The protocol does not require extensive investigation for metastases but known clinical or radio-logical evidence of secondary deposits are criteria for exclusion. A careful history is taken to exclude conditions which may depress the immune response eg. eczema, infective dermatoses, hypergamma-globulinaemia, diseases of the lymph nodes, spleen and liver, and treatment with cytotoxic drugs or corticosteroids. All the patients are Mantoux tested (1:10,000, 1:1,000, 1:100). On entering the study each has an intravenous urogram to exclude upper urinary tract pathology. At the pre-treatment cystoscopy biopsies are taken of the tumour and normal bladder epithelium. The tumour is not resected at this stage.

TREATMENT

Glaxo freeze-dried BCG vaccine (1 ml diluted in 5 ml normal saline) is instilled into the bladder via a urethral catheter weekly for four weeks then monthly for 11 months. The patient retains the BCG until he next voids urine naturally. At each visit a history is taken of any symptoms due to local or systemic toxicity.

FOLLOW-UP

Follow-up is at one month and then three monthly. On each occasion a cystoscopy and bimanual examination are performed under general anaesthesia. Biopsies are taken of the tumour surface, tumour base, normal bladder mucosa and any bladder mucosa which appears abnormal. Residual bladder tumour is resected.

RESULTS

Eighteen patients have so far been entered into this study. Ten have completed one or more months treatment and are assessable.

Local toxicity has been manifested by frequency, dysuria and haematuria and systemic toxicity by pyrexia, rigors, malaise and abnormal liver function tests. Severe local toxicity has been observed in one patient and local and systemic toxicity in two patients (Table I).

Complete regression has been seen at one month in two patients and partial regression in four (Table II). Patients having a regression have shown inflammatory cell infiltration and macrophage granulomas in the lamina propria of the bladder adjacent to tumours.

DISCUSSION

This continuing study has already demonstrated that intravesical immunotherapy with BCG can result in complete or partial regression of recurrent category T1 bladder carcinoma. Toxicity, however, can be severe although intradermal BCG is not given concurrently. One patient required hospitalisation and antituberculous therapy with Rifampicin and Ethambutol. She did not respond to Isoniazid. Her tumours regressed completely during treatment. The other two patients with toxicity had a partial regression of their tumours.

Further evaluation of BCG immunotherapy for category T1 bladder carcinoma should be reserved for recurrent tumours which do not respond to resection and diathermy. None of the patients in this series had evidence of a depressed immune response before treatment.

Patients whose tumours have responded to BCG immunotherapy have had histological reaction in their bladders characterised by an inflammatory cell infiltration and macrophage granulomas. This reaction has been confined to the lamina propria and has not been observed so far within the malignant epithelium.

TABLE I

TOXICITY FOLLOWING INTRAVESICAL BCG IMMUNOTHERAPY

Type	No. of Patients	Remarks
Local	1	Responded by delaying further treatment for one day (partial tumour regression).
Local and Systemic	2	Both required hospitalisation. 1 patient responded to withdrawal of treatment (partial tumour regression). 1 patient required anti-tuberculous therapy with Rifampicin and Ethambutanol. She failed to respond to Isoniazid. (Complete tumour regression).

TABLE II

TUMOUR RESPONSE TO INTRAVESICAL BCG IMMUNOTHERAPY

Patients	10
Complete Regression	2
Partial Regression	4
No Change	2
Progression	2

REFERENCES

1. Union Internationale Contre le Cancer.   TNM classification of malignant tumours. 2nd Edition, Geneva 79-82 (1974).

2. Morales, A., Eidinger, D., Bruce, A. W., Intracavity Bacillus Calmette-Guerin in the Treatment of Superficial Tumours. J. Urol. 116, 180-183 (1976).

3. Douville, Y., Pelouse, G., Ray, R., Charrois, R., Kibrite, A., Martin, M., Dionne, L., Coulonoval, L., Robinson, J., Recurrent Bladder Papillomata Treated with Bacillus Calmette-Guerin: A Preliminary Report (Phase 1 Trial). Cancer Treatment Reports, 62, 551-552 (1978).

BCG VACCINE IN THE TREATMENT OF NON INFILTRATING PAPILLARY TUMOURS OF THE BLADDER

J A MARTINEZ-PIÑEIRO

Service of Urology, La Paz Clinic

Faculty of Medicine, Universidad Autonoma, Madrid

Papillary tumours of the urinary bladder are usually well differentiated, have little tendency to infiltrate and can be successfully treated by means of endoscopic resection in more than 80% of the cases. The major problem with this kind of tumour is the high recurrence rate. To prevent recurrences after TUR, or even after partial cystectomy, long term chemoprophylaxis has been recommended. Intravesical instillations with Thiotepa and Epodyl seem to be the most popular agents, capable of reducing the recurrence rate from around 60 to 25% (1-4,7). Encouraging results have been also reported with orally administered drugs, such as retinoic acid (5), SLA (6) and procarbazine (7), but the efficacy of these agents seems to be less than that of the intravesical agents.

Recent evidence indicating that tumour development and progress are, to some extent, controlled by the immune system (8,9) and that patients suffering from bladder tumours present immunological deficiencies, directly related with the stage of the disease (10,12) and the rate of recurrences (13,14), has led to new avenues of treatment implicating the modulation of the immune system by means of immunostimulation. Our group has been engaged since 1975 in a study to assess the value of BCG vaccine as an immunostimulant. The preliminary results (15) suggested that BCG could be effective both in the treatment and prevention of these types of tumours; when used with curative intention the initial results have shown a clear advantage of the intralesional injections over the systemic administration via dermal scarifications, but we found that the injections, besides being uncomfortable for the patients, were not free of risks, such as anaphylactic shock in sensitised patients.

Bloomberg et al (16) in 1975 investigated the effects of BCG instillations in the dog after experimental bladder injury, their findings suggesting that topical BCG induces a strong inflammatory reaction that would support the idea of immunotherapy via this route. Almost simultaneously Morales et al (17) reported the results of intravesical instillations of BCG combined with intradermal administration in tumour bearing patients; of four cases treated with curative intention, three showed complete tumour regression and the biopsies demonstrated the presence of necrosis and formation of granulomas; in nine patients the recurrence rate dropped dramatically. They argued that the easy accessibility of the bladder permits the delivery of a high local concentration of Calmette Guerin bacilli in close contact with the tumour cells, without concomitant systemic effects, and concluded that the intracavitary route met all the desirable criteria to be a successful immunotherapeutic procedure. Based on these studies we modified our BCG programmes, introducing a protocol which included intravesical instillation alone or in combination with scarification.

Herein we present our overall experience in the treatment and prophylaxis of papillary non infiltrating tumours with BCG since 1975, including the follow-up of the nine cases presented in a previous preliminary report (15).

PATIENTS AND METHODS

Thirty patients have entered four different studies (Table I); however one of them, assigned first to receive intra-tumoural injections, was included later on in the group receiving scarifications. Thus, for the evaluation of results, the total number of cases herein mentioned will sometimes be 31.

Eight patients had Tis (O-Jewett) tumours, 20 T1 (A-Jewett) and two T2 (B1); 16 were recurrent and 14 were primary tumours. Eleven were treated primarily with curative aim, but afterwards were also treated with prophylactic aim, raising the total number of cases in whom BCG treatments were given prophylactically to 29.

The therapeutic schedules have suffered slight changes with respect to those previously reported; in Group 1 and in seven patients of Group 2, BCG Pasteur vaccine (R) was used, while in the remaining patients Immuno BCG Pasteur vaccine (R) was employed, following the methodology specified in Table II.

Pretreatment studies included a complete history of the disease, physical examination, blood and urinalysis, IVP, chest x-ray, immunologic profile (skin tests), endoscopy and bimanual palpation under anesthesia and partial biopsy or complete transurethral resection.

TABLE I

Treatment Modality	Aim[x]	Stage	Grade	Recurrent Disease
Group 1 - Local Injection (2 cases)	C - 2	T1 - 2	G1 - 2	1
Group 2 - Cutaneous Scarification (10 cases)	C - 3 P - 10	T1 - 8[xx] T2 - 2	G1 - 5 G2 - 5	4
Group 3 - Vesical Instillation (12 cases)	C - 3 P - 12	Tis - 5 T1 - 7	G1 - 2 G2 - 10	5
Group 4 - Instillation & Scarification (7 cases)	C - 3 P - 7	Tis - 3 T1 - 4	G1 - 1 G2 - 6	6
Totals 31 cases (30 patients)	C - 11 P - 29	Tis - 8 T1 - 21[xx] T2 - 2	G1 - 10 G2 - 21	16 Tis - 4 T1 - 12 G1 - 4 G2 - 12

[x] C = Curative, P = Prophylactic

[xx] One of these cases was crossed-over from Group 1, and is therefore counted twice.

TABLE II

THERAPEUTIC SCHEDULES[x]

Direct injection into the tumour:

    37,5 mg BCG vaccine injected by means of an endoscopic needle into the tumour, once per month, during three to four months.

Cutaneous Scarification:

    150 mg BCG vaccine (2 ampoules of 75 mg each), applied over 10 scarifications of 5 cm length. Weekly for one month. Monthly for one year, and every three months for another year.

Intravesical Instillations:

    150 mg BCG vaccine (2 ampoules of 75 mg each), diluted in 50 ml saline instilled into the bladder. Weekly for one month and monthly for a minimum period of one year.

    In patients treated with a combination of instillations and scarifications, both were administered the same day.

[x] PPD negative patients must be converted to positive before the outset of treatment. This can be achieved by means of 1 mg BCG injected intradermally for three or four times at weekly intervals.

The follow-up included endoscopy, urinary cytology and immunological assessment at six and 12 weeks; thereafter every three months during the first year and every six months in subsequent years.

The average duration of follow-up in months has been 24,5 for Group 1 (range 13-36 months), 21 for Group 2 (range 9-42), 10, 9 for Group 3 (range 5-17) and 10,7 for Group 4 (range 6-17).

RESULTS

1. Tumour response to curative treatment

Eleven small tumours (less than 1 cc mass) were treated with this aim. Two tumours receiving local injections showed partial regression (15); five months after the start of treatment both were resected.

One of the patients did not receive any further treatment and developed a recurrence nine months later, being lost to follow-up afterwards. The other patient was crossed over to prophylaxis with scarifications and his tumour has not recurred in three years. He is still getting scarifications every three months.

Of three patients treated by means of cutaneous scarifications, one showed a rapid progression of the existing tumours and the appearance of new multiple tumours, as reported previously (15) (enhancement?), and underwent a radical cystourethrectomy; after the operation he continued receiving scarifications until one year later, when a papillary tumour was discovered in the left renal pelvis and inferior calyces. A left nephro-ureterectomy was performed, and the patient died of post-operative complications. In another patient the tumour progressed very slowly and was resected 11 months after start of therapy; he continued under treatment for a further one and a half years without any recurrence before being lost to follow-up. In the third patient, in whom at first no objective regression was seen (as reported previously (15)), a regression took place four months later and a TUR biopsy revealed only a urothelial dysplasia. He continued on treatment for another one and a half years, when he died of intercurrent illness, but without any recurrence.

Three tumours treated with instillations regressed completely, two after four instillations each, and one after nine instillations. The three patients are still receiving instillations one year after start of treatment and none has had recurrence; the actual cytology is IIIa in all of them.

Of three tumours treated with a combination of scarifications and instillations, one showed a complete regression after six instillations, and in spite of being a recurrent tumour (twice in two years), it has not recurred one year afterwards. The two remaining tumours did not respond to treatment; both were also recurrent many times (five in 11 years, 11 in eight years). After TUR the patients continued to receive BCG treatment; in one a recurrence was detected five months later and the other patient was lost to follow-up disease free six months afterwards (cytology II).

In Summary (Table III), five (45.4%) patients showed a complete tumour regression, three (27.2%) a partial regression and three (27.2%) did not respond. Four of seven recurrent tumours and all four primary tumours responded.

Of the five total responders, three were primary tumours and two were recurrent; of the three partial responders two were recurrent; the three non responders all had recurrent tumours. The most effective treatment modality was the intravesical instillation alone or with scarification, yielding four regressions in six patients (Table III).

TABLE III

RESULTS OF CURATIVE TREATMENT

Treatment and No. of patients		Progression		Complete Regression		Partial Regression	
Local Injection	2	-		-		2/2	(1R 1P)
Scarification	3	1	(R)	1	(P)	1	(R)
Instillations	3	-		3	(2R 1P)	-	
Instillations + Scarification	3	2	(R)	1	(P)	-	
Total		3/11 27.2% 3 (R)		5/11 45.4% (3P 2R)		3/11 27.2% (1P 2R)	

In brackets: R = Recurrent disease, P = Primary tumour.

BCG appeared to be most effective in Tis (O. Jewett) tumours, both of whom showed complete regression; in T1 tumours three of nine showed complete regression and another three partial regression. Similar figures were seen in G1 and G2 tumours in whom six of seven and two of four respectively showed regressions.

2. PROPHYLAXIS OF RECURRENCES

Of 29 cases treated prophylactically none of the 14 primary patients had recurrences, but six of the 15 recurrent patients (40%) developed further tumours whilst on treatment; of these, five had only one recurrence and the remaining patient had two recurrences.

The analysis of each treatment group is indicated in Table IV. From this table can be seen the recurrences, the follow-up and the recurrence rate before and after treatment. The recurrence rate in each treatment group was lower after treatment.

TABLE IV

RESULTS OF PROPHYLACTIC TREATMENT WITH BCG FOLLOWING TUR IN 15 PATIENTS WITH PREVIOUSLY RECURRENT BLADDER TUMOUR

	Scarification		Instillation		Scarif. + Instil.	
Patients Entered	4		5		6	
Recurrences Before and After Treatment	Before	After	Before	After	Before	After
	13	3	17	1	34	3
Months Follow-up	180	65	450	69	548	67
Recurrence Rate per 100 Patient/Months	7.22	4.41	4.78	1.45	6.2	4.48

NB. NONE of 14 additional patients treated with BCG after resection of a primary tumour showed a recurrence.

Analysis by the chi-square test revealed that the differences were not significant; nevertheless, the patients treated only with instillations had less frequent recurrences than patients with other regimes, although without reaching the necessary margin of confidence ($p = 0.09$). It is likely that the small size of the sample may account for the apparent lack of significance.

IMMUNOLOGICAL RESPONSE

Table V shows the results of the DNCB test both before and during therapy. It can be seen that before the treatment only five (16.6%) patients reacted normally, while after the treatment 23 (76.6%) presented a normal reactivity. In table VI each group of patients is analysed separately, and it can be seen that the improvement rates are similar for the different types of treatment.

The relation between immune response and the appearance of recurrences during treatment is presented in Table VII. Three (13.6%)
out of 22 patients with a normal reactivity had recurrences, while
three (42.8%) out of seven having an abnormal or a negative reactivity had recurrences, the difference being not significant, but
highly suggestive (p = 0.09).

TABLE V

CELL-MEDIATED IMMUNE RESPONSE (DNCB TEST) IN 30 PATIENTS

Immune Response	Normal	Abnormal	Anergy
Before BCG Therapy	5	2	23
3 Months after BCG start	24	3	3
At last follow-up	23	3	4

TABLE VI

IMMUNE RESPONSE BY TREATMENT

Treatment Modality No. of patients		Patients with normal DNCB Test	
		Before Treatment	After Treatment
Scarifications	10	0	7
Instillations	12	2	10
Instil. + Scarif.	7	3	5
Local Injection	2	0	1

The patients receiving only instillations seemed to be the best
responders, either from the point of view of immunologic response or
recurrences; eight out of 10 anergic patients reverted to normal
reactivity, and none of these eight, together with the two who had a
normal response prior to treatment, had recurrences; this zero rate
of recurrences in patients with normal immune response, in comparison
to 50% in patients with abnormal response, is significant
(p = 0.045).

TABLE VII

BCG IN PAPILLARY BLADDER TUMOURS

Relationship between Immune Response and Recurrences

Treatment	DNCB Test	
	Normal	Abnormal
Scarifications	2/7	1/3
Instillations	0/10	1/2
Instil. + Scarif.	1/5	1/2
Total	3/22 13.6%	3/7 42.8%

Numerator = Patients with recurrences.
Denominator = Patients at risk.

4. COMPLICATIONS

The treatment was tolerated remarkably well by the majority of the patients, minor local discomfort and/or fever during the following day being the most usual complaints. However, eight patients (26.6%) had complications attributable to BCG. One patient receiving instillation had a serious hypersensitivity reaction after the third injection and treatment was discontinued. One patient receiving scarifications presented an impressive growth of new tumours after the tenth series of scarifications, which might have been due to an immunological enhancement and later on presented with pulmonary TB. Among the 19 patients receiving instillations alone or in combination, six (31.5%) suffered cystitis, which was severe in two (after seven and nine instillations each), necessitating discontinuation of the intravesical treatment and cross over to scarification; one of these two patients had serious haematuria twice. The remaining four cases had only mild symptoms and are still getting instillations; in two of them cystoscopy revealed typical lesions of cystitis cystica which were confirmed by biopsy; this lesion was combined in one case with tuberculoid granulomas.

In one more patient, free of any bladder symptomatology, acid-alcohol-resistant bacilli were found once in a routine urinalysis.

DISCUSSION

The results from this study seem to confirm the effectiveness of nonspecific immunostimulation with BCG in non-infiltrating papillary bladder tumours, as previous preliminary reports (15,17,18) had suggested.

When used with curative aim 45.4% of the tumours were eradicated and a further 27.2% showed partial regressions. The most effective modality seems to be the intravesical application, either by means of direct injection into the tumour or by instillations, supporting the current feeling that BCG is most active when entering into close contact with the tumour cells. Recurrent Tis (0) tumours of low degree of malignancy responded better than T1 (A) and G2, and the same was true for primary tumours.

When used prophylactically 20.6% of the patients developed recurrences, a percentage which is markedly lower than the 36.3% yielded by Thiotepa or 62% by VM26 in the controlled clinical trial carried on by the EORTC Genito-Urinary Tract Cooperative Group (19). BCG yielded the best results in primary tumours, where the recurrence rate was nil.

The analysis of recurrences per 100 patient months of follow-up was zero for primary tumours.

The same analysis repeated for recurrent tumours separately showed that before prophylaxis the recurrence rate per 100 patient months was 5.43 versus 3.43 following treatment, and the partial rates revealed again that the groups receiving scarifications, and instillations plus scarifications respectively, showed poorer results than the group getting only instillations (4.41 and 4.48 versus 1.45).

The explanation of such differences may lie in the fact that the patients entered into the group receiving instillations only had, before the onset of prophylaxis, a lower recurrence rate per 100 patient months than the patients entered into the other two groups (3.78 versus 7.22 + 6.2).

From an immunological viewpoint, BCG on the one hand seemed to improve the response in 19 patients (63.3%), and on the other it was observed that patients with a normal immune response had 13.6% recurrences, while patients with a depressed response had 42.8%.

Of the four groups, the one receiving instillations alone showed the highest rate of favourable responses in both senses.

Side-effects were of minor importance in the majority of the cases, and only in four patients (13.3%) were serious enough either to discontinue the treatment in two (hypersensitivity and pulmonary TB), or to cross over to another modality of BCG treatment in another two (intense cystitis); four more patients also had mild cystitis, requiring symptomatic medication.

On the whole the incidence and severity of complications was
moaest, and it can be said that BCG immunostimulation is a safe
procedure, particularly when used by intravesical instillation.

Our findings suggest that the best method of administrating
BCG for non infiltrating bladder tumours is by topical instillation,
either for the treatment of small growths or for the prevention of
recurrences, and that its efficacy seems to be higher than that of
the cytotoxic drugs currently used.

SUMMARY

BCG vaccine has been used as non-specific immunostimulant in
30 patients with papillary bladder carcinomas, following four
different therapeutic schedules:- intralesional injection, dermal
scarifications, intravesical instillations and instillations plus
scarifications. In 11 cases the aim of treatment was curative.
Tumours disappeared in five (45.4%) and regressed partially in three
(27.2%). In 29 cases (10 of the group treated primarily with
curative purpose and 19 more treated after TUR) the aim of treatment
was the prevention of recurrences. Recurrences occurred in six
patients (20.6%) from a group of 15 with a previous history of
history of multiple recurrences; in 14 patients with primary tumour
no recurrences were detected during follow-ups ranging between five
and 42 months (mean 15.1). The most effective schedule was
intravesical instillation with 100% regressions and 8.3% recurrences.

REFERENCES

1. Pavone-Macaluso, M. Brit. J. Urol. 43, 701 (1971).

2. Martinez-Pineiro, J. A., Arocena, F., Hernandez Armero, A.,
    y Camacho, M. XVI Congrès de la Societé Internationale
    d'Urologie. Amsterdam. Ed. Doin, Paris, 2, 511 (1973).

3. Riddle, P. R. Brit. J. Urol. 45, 84 (1973).

4. Riddle, P. R. and Wallace, D. M. Brit. J. Urol. 43, 181 (1971).

5. Evard, J. P. and Ballag, W. Schweiz. Med. Wschr 102, 1880
    (1972).

6. Ichikawa, T., Akasaka, H., Ishikawa, M. J. Urol. 108, 571
    (1972).

7. Pavone-Macaluso, M. XVI Congrès de la Societé Internationale
    d'Urologie. Amsterdam. Ed. Doin, Paris. 1, 234 (1973).

8.   Burnet, M. Brit. Med. Bull. 20, 154 (1964).

9.   Klein, G. and Oettgen, H. F. Cancer Res. 29, 1741 (1969).

10. Catalona, W. J., Chretein, P. B. J. Urol. 110, 526 (1973).

11. McLauglin, A. P., III, Kessler, W. O., Triman, K. and
     Gittes, R. F. J. Urol. 111, 233 (1974).

12. O'Boyle, P. J., Cooper, E. J. and Williams, R. E. Brit. J.
     Urol. 46, 303 (1974).

13. Olsson, C. A., Chute, R. and Rao, C. N. J. Urol. 111, 173
     (1974).

14. Martinez-Pineiro, J. A., Muntanola, P. and Hidalgo, L. Eur.
     Urol. 3, 159 (1977).

15. Martinez-Pineiro, J. A. and Muntanola, P. Eur. Urol. 3, 11
     (1977).

16. Bloomberg, S. D., Brosman, S. A., Hausman, M. S., Cohen, A.
     and Battenberg, J. D. Invest. Urol. 12, 423 (1975).

17. Morales, A., Eidinger, D. and Bruce, A. W. J. Urol. 116,
     180 (1976).

18. Douville, Y., Pelouze, G., Roy, R., Charrois, R., Kibrite, A.,
     Martin, M., Dionne, L., Coulonval, L. and Robinson, J.
     Cancer Treat. Rep. 62, 551 (1978).

19. Schulman, C. C. and EORTC Urological Group. Recent Results in
     Cancer Research, Springer-Verlag, Berlin, Heidelberg. Ed.
     G Mathe. (In Press).

Editorial Note (F Corrado)   It is widely accepted that the
immune response plays some role in the control of the growth of a
bladder carcinoma.

Morphological studies show that the peritumoral lymphocytic
infiltration is associated with a specific stage of the neoplastic
disease. When infiltration is sparse the neoplasm is usually
aggressive. Furthermore, specific cytotoxic lymphocytes against
TCCB lines are present in TCCB patients and this reaction disappears
after a 'complete' surgical removal of the neoplasm; its reappearance
is apparently always related to recurrence.

Other studies seem to demonstrate that the cytotoxicity reflects
the presence of a tumour in the host, while its absence might signify
either the presence of a large tumour burden or complete cure.

The studies reported here and our own work stress the diagnostic
and the prognostic relevance of specific immunological tests which are
able to reveal the presence or absence of immune-reactivity of the
patients against their tumours. Cytotoxicity tests may, however,
present some problems in interpretation. The role of the 'natural
killer' lymphocytes (non-specific cytotoxic lymphocytes) should also
be noted.

TRANSURETHRAL SURGERY

S ROCCA ROSSETTI

Department of Urology

University of Trieste, Italy

INTRODUCTION

During the First Urological Course in Erice in 1976 Professor Martinez-Piñeiro very clearly described his own experience and views on this topic. Very little has changed since that time. To speak of a single therapy for bladder tumours is less relevant than years ago; alternative therapies are showing an increasing value, so that it would be wrong to neglect or to ignore them.

Secondly I think we must compare the results of the different kinds of treatment. Bladder tumours often only represent the local manifestation of a generalised disease of the urothelium and in theory transurethral resection (TUR) should be considered only if the bladder cancer is thought to be localised. However, the results of endoscopic treatment are satisfactory and this is a very good reason to consider it valid.

These results allow us to assume that many bladder tumours originate locally and take varying lengths of time to spread, invade and enlarge (Hendry, 1976; van der Werf-Messing, 1976). In fact it is the task of the urologist to utilise, when possible, this lapse of time for endoscopic treatment and moreover to establish with reasonable certainty if a given tumour is still resectable or not.

INDICATIONS

Endoscopy is compulsory in the treatment of bladder tumours for diagnosis in all patients, treatment in many and palliation in some.

a)   Diagnosis and Biopsy.   Experience has shown that accurate
staging and grading are essential for the rational treatment of
bladder tumours; this is possible only if the biopsy is carried out
correctly. The TUR begins with the removal of the whole of the
protruding tumour, preferably including also a piece of apparently
normal mucosa. If the tumour is too big to be completely resected,
it is necessary to take many samples from different areas.

The underlying wall must be separately resected, taking care
to retain a proper orientation of the samples and to identify their
inner aspect (the resected slice has a curved appearance, whose
concavity corresponds to the mucosa). The depth of the resection
depends on whether the tumour is papillary and superficial, or
solid and infiltrating. In the latter case the whole wall, including
some perivesical tissue must be removed, otherwise it is impossible
to determine the proper T category.

If necessary a bladder perforation is performed intentionally,
as recommended by Marberger (1972). Accidental perforation is most
likely to occur when performing biopsies of superficial tumours,
beneath which the bladder wall is thin and there is little or no
fibrous reaction.

It the tumour is very deep it must be remembered that the
thickness of the wall of the distended bladder corresponds to the
depth of the resectoscope loop from the surface of the mucosa. If
tumour is present beyond this depth it should be placed in category
T3 or T4.

During biopsy-resection coagulation must be avoided in order to
prevent the damage to samples. This is nearly impossible when
resecting very big, obviously well vascularised, papillary tumours.
In these cases, as the removed tissue is abundant, coagulation does
not impair the value of histological examination, as long as it is
avoided in the deep layers. All suspicious areas, such as swellings
or redness, away from the tumours must also be removed.

The cold biopsy forceps are still useful in non-respectable
areas or after resection of areas looking suspicious of ca in situ.
In these cases it is essential to perform many forceps-biopsies in
multiple zones.

Resection of the bladder neck is sometimes useful or necessary
to allow access to the lateral walls.

When the tumour appears benign, circumscribed and superficial,
an ample resection, including the deepest layers, not only
corresponds to a biopsy but becomes ipso facto, a curative treatment.

Since all future therapy depends on an exact diagnosis the

biopsy resection demands a competence which cannot be acquired
without long experience.

b)   Treatment.   TUR is the therapy of choice when there is
evidence that the tumour is localised; this holds true in the so-
called "benign papilloma" (T1 GO) and in category T1 transitional
cell carcinoma, grade G1-2 if papillary and G1 if solid. In these
cases lymphatic invasion and distant metastases are extremely
improbable and the 10 year survival is 70% as long as recurrences
are adequately treated.

Personally I do not consider that TUR is the treatment of
choice for ca in situ because of the absolute unpredictability of
the presence of undetected, invasive areas, or for adenocarcinoma.

c)   Alternative Treatment.   When the tumour is completely
resectable, but histology gives proof of muscular invasion or poor
cellular differentiation, regional lymphatic metastasis is
statistically probable. I do not consider that TUR is still a
rational therapy under such circumstances, and feel that radiotherapy
or cystectomy should be considered instead except when the patient
is of advanced age, refuses operation or is a poor surgical risk.
The results show that such an attitude is not illogical since five
year survival in these cases varies between 40% and more than 60%
(Martinez Pineiro, 1976). The view that a degree of anaplasia,
the presence of metaplasia and the involvement of lymphatic vessels
discourage one from performing a TUR is also shared by other authors
(Miller, 1969; Hendry, 1976).

During the last three years I have employed TUR more frequently
than in previous years due to the great epidemiological difference
between Cagliari, where I worked before, and Trieste, where I work
at present. In the patients of the first group ie. in Cagliari there
were 250 low stage - low grade papillary tumours as opposed to 46
invasive carcinomas, 29 of which were squamous. In this population
the highest incidence was from 50 to 65 years of age and the male -
female ratio was 7:1. In patients of the second group (Giarelli,
1978), out of 411 tumours only 119 were superficial and of low grade,
whereas 292 were frankly malignant; the male - female ratio was 4:1.
The highest incidence was found from 70-84 years of age for males
and from 70-79 for females. Only 1.6% were squamous.

The bladder tumour incidence in Trieste appears to be the
highest in Europe after Great Britain and it is surprising how low
the incidence is for the same tumours in adjacent Slovenia.

Therefore, I now perform TUR in T2 and T3 tumours more
frequently than I did in Cagliari because of the advanced age of
patients and the lower grade of tumours in Trieste.

In case of tumour recurrences the choice of the treatment depends on many factors, such as the frequency of recurrences, and their histological features, grade and stage.

d)   Palliative Treatment.   This can be a decision of necessity or of choice; results are not discouraging with 9% five year survival rate in T4 and 20% in T3 (Marberger, 1972; Haschek, 1978) and mostly depend on the elimination of local complications.

The main advantages of the TUR are:

a)   the correct staging of the tumour;
b)   the possibility of obtaining better identification and easier removal of suspicious areas than in open surgery;
c)   the low incidence of scar recurrences compared to open surgery (Martinez Piñeiro, 1976);
d)   low mortality and morbidity;
e)   short hospitalisation.

The main disadvantages are:

a)   the impossibility of detecting potentially curable lymphatic invasion.
b)   the possibility of causing either dissemination of neoplastic cells through open veins and exposed tissue or implantation of neoplastic cells in the traumatised vesical or urethral mucosa.

In addition TUR may be followed by complications such as undetected bladder perforation, urinary infection, sepsis and urethral strictures.

CONCLUSIONS

Eighty percent of bladder tumours can be treated endoscopically; when the tumour is still localised, TUR is the best treatment as long as it is technically possible and there is enough experience to prove that TUR is a better choice than conservative open bladder surgery.

However, TUR of tumours in the dome may be difficult and some urologists suggest that in such cases it should be performed as a multi-staged procedure, taking deeper bites at each subsequent session.

However, the good results of TUR even when the tumour is likely not to be localised and fully resectable (T2-T3) necessitate a critical reappraisal of the problem. A randomised study of TUR versus radical cystectomy may establish if TUR in these stages must be considered the best alternative treatment. At present, advanced age and low grade, small size, well circumscribed tumours are in favour of TUR as an alternative treatment in T2-T3 tumours.

Useful results can often be obtained with palliative TUR in T3-T4 cancer. The advantages are evident and noteworthy; the disadvantages are few and partly avoidable. The association of irradiation and chemotherapy may be valuable in achieving a control of occult lymph node metastases.

REFERENCES

1. Giarelli, L., Antonutto, G., Melato, M., Bologna., Osservazioni del patologo sui tumori epiteliali della vescica nell'anziano. Giorn. Geront. XXVI, 669 (1978).

2. Haschek, H. Personal communication.

3. Hendry, W. F., Bloom, H. J. G., Urothelial neoplasia: Present Postition and Prospect. In Recent Advances in Urology. Hendry, W. F. Churchill Livingstone, Edinburgh, London, New York (1976).

4. Marberger, H., Marberger, M., Decristoforo, A. The current status of transurethral resection in the diagnosis and therapy of carcinoma of urinary bladder. Int. Urol. and Nephr. 14, 35 (1972).

5. Martinez Piñeiro, J. A., Transurethral Treatment of Bladder Tumours. In The Tumours of the Genito-Urinary Apparatus. COFESE, Palermo 203 (1976).

6. Miller, A., Mitchell, J. P., Brown, N. J., The Bristol Bladder Tumour Registry. Brit. J. Urol. 41, suppl. 17 (1969).

7. Pugh, R. C. B., The pathology of the cancer of the bladder. Cancer, 32, 1267 (1973).

8. Van Der Werf-Messing, B., The experience of the Rotterdam Radiotheraphy Institute (RRTI) in the Treatment of Urological Tumour In The Tumours of Genito-Urinary Apparatus. COFESE, Palermo 93 (1976).

TRANSURETHRAL RESECTION OR CYSTECTOMY? AN ATTEMPT TO ANSWER THIS
QUESTION BY AN EVALUATION OF 688 PATIENTS WITH CARCINOMA OF THE
BLADDER (WITH SPECIAL REFERENCE TO AGE, SEX, STAGE AND THE PRESENCE
OF ASSOCIATED DISEASE)

G STUDLER and H HASCHEK

Urological Department
Allg. Poliklinik
Vienna, Austria

ABSTRACT

An analysis of age, sex, staging and medical risk of 688
patients with bladder tumours has been carried out. The collected
results are discussed with particular reference to the indications
for transurethral resection (TUR) and cystectomy. In a non-selected
group of patients it was found that approximately 75% should undergo
a transurethral operation and 10-15% a cystectomy. In a 25 year
follow-up of 331 patients over 70 years of age there has been a
marked increase in the use of TUR. The survival figures demonstrate
the success of this approach.

INTRODUCTION

The attitude of the various authors towards the treatment of
cancer of the bladder seems to depend greatly on the preference of
the surgical or the transurethral approach (TUR) and reminds us to a
certain extent of the present tendency to apply either one of these
operative methods as the treatment for adenoma of the prostate.

There seems to be no other reason why certain clinics treat 80%
or more of their bladder cancer patients with transurethral resection
(2,3) and why others tend to prefer the operative method (4,6).

As regards the approach, the problem is not really that of
partial resection of the bladder with and without ureteroneostomy
which in agreement with the literature is more and more limited to
the rather seldom found tumour localised on and near the dome.

The real question is whether to advise TUR or total cystectomy. It is unanimously agreed that localised tumours either without or with very little invasion (the so-called superficial bladder carcinoma A, B1 or T1, T2) are those most suited for TUR except for those tumours which are difficult to reach (on the anterior wall and dome) and in papillomatosis.

With this in mind the main question is whether deeply invasive bladder cancer (B2, C or T3) should be approached transurethrally or not. If so several sessions, sometimes including so-called controlled perforation, are necessary.

CLINICAL MATERIAL

The age distribution of our patients is in conformity with the literature; the peak incidence is between the seventh and eighth decade and 42.5% are older than 70.

74% of the patients are male and 26% female. Transurethral resection has been used in 38.1% of our patients. The staging of these patients is based on excretory urography, biopsy of the base and margin of the tumour and quite often on a repeated resection and bimanual palpation under anaesthetic. Bilateral pedal lymphangiography is seldom used.

The staging problem has often been discussed, (5,6) in particular the danger of understaging (1). Table I shows that superficial carcinoma of the bladder (A, B1 or T1, T2) was found in only 42% of patients, deeply invasive bladder carcinoma being present in 58%. Of these patients 91 (30%) were found to be stage D or T4 with metastatic tumours. A radical operation was therefore out of the question.

TABLE I

CLINICAL STAGING OF 688 PATIENTS
WITH BLADDER CANCER

STAGE		No. of Patients	%	
A	(T1)	136	19.8	
B1	(T2)	158	23.0	42.8
B2		124	18.0	
C	(T3)	179	26.0	57.2
D	(T4)	91	13.2	

This left 303 patients (44%) in stage B2, C or T3 possibly suitable for transurethral resection or cystectomy. Table II shows an analysis of the size and position of these tumours. At least two thirds were unsuitable for a radical transurethral resection and therefore a cystectomy was called for (Figure 1).

We believe that 51 (16.8%) patients of this group were suited for a radical transurethral resection probably with controlled perforation as the tumour was less than 3 cm in diameter and because of its localisation.

Of the remaining 252 patients, 105 were older than 70 - an age at which such a radical operation can only be performed under ideal circumstances.

The quantification of the medical risk in the remaining 147 patients shows that for 23 patients there was an absolute contra-indication for total cystectomy. Seventy two patients could have been operated on at an increased risk after medical treatment. Only 52 patients (7% of the total) were obviously suitable for a radical cystectomy.

We realise that there may be objection to such statistics but we also believe that in spite of all uncertainty, we are able to say how often, in an unselected group of patients, transurethral resection or cystectomy should be performed.

TABLE II

EVALUATION BY SIZE AND LOCALISATION OF 303 PATIENTS
STAGES B2, C or T3 WITH BLADDER CANCER

TUMOUR SIZE	No. of Patients	%
Up to 3 cm	60	19.8
Up to 5 cm	157	51.8
More than 5 cm	86	28.4
LOCALISATION		
Dome of the Bladder	28	9.2
Lateral/Posterior Wall	149	49.2
Base of the Bladder	96	31.7
Anterior Wall	10	3.3
Multiple	20	6.6

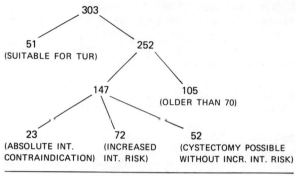

Urological Department, Allg. Poliklinik Vienna

FIGURE 1

EVALUATION OF 303 PATIENTS WITH BLADDER CANCER

AT STAGES B2, C OR T3

Of course there is the personal inclination towards the surgical procedure or transurethral resection, but it seems that in most cases of bladder cancer TUR is correctly chosen as the commonest method of treatment (approx. 75%). Radical cystectomy is the best treatment in perhaps 15% of cases. A partial resection could be performed successfully in about 5%.

It remains to be seen how far these statements may have to be corrected by the appropriate use of radiotherapy but one can imagine that in doubtful cases a combination of TUR and irradiation could be chosen with, if no response occurs after a relatively short period of observation, the removal of the bladder.

BLADDER CANCER IN THE ELDERLY PATIENT

During the past 25 years 331 patients with cancer of the bladder over 70 years of age came to the Urological Department of the Vienna Poliklinik for their first examination.

The staging of the tumours in these patients showed no significant difference from those under 70 years of age (Table III). The histological grading which has been carried out according to Mostofi since 1974 also did not differentiate between these two groups of patients (Table IV) nor was there any difference in the size and the localisation of the tumours.

During the past few years there has been a very marked increase in the use of transurethral resection at the expense of open surgery

TABLE III

COMPARISON OF STAGING IN PATIENTS OVER AND UNDER 70

(761 Patients with Bladder Cancer 1953-1977)

Clinical Stage		Pts. under 70 n=430		Pts. over 70 n=331	
		No.	%	No.	%
A	(T1)	96	22.3	60	18.1
B1	(T2)	108	25.1	78	23.6
B2	(T3)	79	18.4	54	16.3
C		96	22.3	93	28.1
D	(T4)	51	11.9	46	13.9

or symptomatic treatment. The reasons for preference of TUR are as follows:

1.   Even though 70 years of age is a random choice and correctly one should speak of the biological age, radical operations. such as cystectomy and urinary diversion are rarely suitable except in special cases.

2.   Arteriosclerotic and cerebral changes are frequently present and make urinary diversion extremely difficult for these patients to tolerate.

TABLE IV

HISTOLOGICAL GRADE OF TUMOUR

(321 Patients with Bladder Cancer 1974-1977)

Grade of Tumour	Pts. under 70 n=101	Pts. over 70 n=120
WHO I	32.7%	24.2%
WHO II	35.6%	41.7%
WHO III	27.7%	25.8%
WHO IV	4.0%	8.3%

3.   The short life expectancy of this group also makes the recommendation of such large operations questionable.

These considerations explain the resons for our preference for TUR. Table V shows that of the 186 patients over 70 years of age who were treated for bladder cancer in the last ten years, 84.9% were operated on transurethrally. Cystectomy and partical resection of the bladder was carried out only in 8.1%. Between 1953-1967 the percentage treated by TUR was only 10.3%.

TABLE V

CHANGE IN THE DISTRIBUTION OF THE METHODS OF TREATMENT

(331 Patients over 70 with Bladder Cancer)

Method of Treatment	1953-1967		1968-1977	
	No.	%	No.	%
TUR	15	10.3	158	84.9
Partial Cystectomy	54	37.3	14	7.5
Irradiation	35	24.1	2	1.2
Symptomatic Therapy	40	27.6	11	5.9
Total Cystectomy	1	0.7	1	0.6

We almost always operate under epidural anaesthetic. As a result respiratory complications hardly ever occur and the patients can readily be ambulated after the operation. Even with wide indication for operative treatment, the post-operative mortality rate was only 0.5% in this group of patients.

Whilst the use of transurethral resection is generally recognised - except for certain tumours of the anterior wall of the bladder and in papillomatosis - in stage A and B1 (T1 and T2) TUR is more problematical in stages B2 - D (T3/T4). We believe that it is possible to operate histologically radically by resection, some-times with controlled perforation on a significant percentage of the circumscribed tumours, especially in stage B2. Should the radical removal of the tumour by TUR not be possible, tumour reduction often makes irradiation more successful. By the correct use of irradiation, that is on localised tumours of not more than 3-4 cm in diameter, and with the new techniques of radiotherapy, it is possible to avoid the once dreaded complication of radiocystitis with all its consequences.

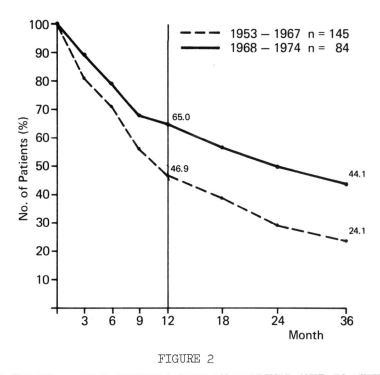

FIGURE 2

ALL STAGES, 3 YEAR SURVIVAL RATE IN PATIENTS OVER 70 WITH

BLADDER CANCER (Comparison 1953-1967 and 1968-1974)

Figure 1 shows the comparison of the results from 1953-1967 and from 1968-1974 of 229 patients over 70. Even though we only show the three year survival rate, we believe that comparison of the survival rate with the group of patients treated before 1968 clearly points out the correctness of our method of treatment.

REFERENCES

1. Cox, C. E., Cass, A. S., Boyce, W. H., Bladder cancer; A 26 year review. J. Urol. 100, 550-558 (1969).

2. Marberger, H., Marberger, M., Decristoforo, A., Die Stellung der transurethralen Elektroresektion in Diagnostik und Therapie des Blasencarcinoma. Int. Urol. a. Nephrol. 4, 35-44 (1972).

3. Mauermayer, W., Tauber, R., Die Tumoren der Harn-Blase-Indikation, Technik und Ergebnisse der transurethralen Therapie Urologe A 16, 185-189 (1977).

4.   Mayor, G., Zur Therapie des Blasencarcinoms.   Urologe A 16,
     175-176 (1977).

5.   Whitmore, W. F., Vortrag anlaBlich des 10.   Internationalen
     Krebskongresses in Houston 1970 Referat : G. Lunglmayr,
     Urologe 10, 95 (1971).

6.   Zoedler, D., Hoffmeister, R., Wienhower, R., Uber die
     Indikation zur operativen Blasen-Tumor-Therapie (anhand einer
     10-Jahres-Statistik).   Urologe A 16, 177-179 (1977).

PARTIAL CYSTECTOMY

E J ZINGG, Th ZELTNER

Department of Urology, Inselspital

University of Berne, Berne Switzerland

From a purely operative point of view partial resection of the urinary bladder is a perfectly logical method for the removal of a bladder tumour without impairing the integrity of the vesical function.

Well into the fifties the segmental resection was a procedure widely used for non infiltrating and infiltrating carcinomas (4,6). You all are very familiar with the operative procedure, described in every textbook of operative urology. The procedure has been improved. Hemicystectomy with subtotal prostatectomy and the trigonal cystectomies are described.

Haschek (1976), reported 40% partial resections of the bladder and 10% transurethral resections for bladder tumours in one year. Esch (1973), mentioned that, by reviewing the literature, between 20% and 48% of all bladder tumour cases are suitable for a partial resection. The operation is rarely carried out these days.

In 1972 10% of our bladder tumour patients in Bern underwent a partial cystectomy; last year (1977) we did not perform this operation at all.

Quite a few papers have been published on this subject in recent years (Table I). The analysis of these papers yields the following results: the five year survival rate for tumours of stage O and A treated with partial cystectomy varies between 50 and 70%, in stage B between 30 and 50%, in stage C between 10 and 30%. The average postoperative mortality is close to 5%.

Why then is this simple operation with apparently good results

TABLE I

FIVE YEAR SURVIVAL AFTER PARTIAL CYSTECTOMY FOR BLADDER CARCINOMA ACCORDING TO STAGE

	No. Cases	STAGE O-A %	STAGE B %	STAGE C %	STAGE D %	OPERATIVE MORTALITY %
MARSHALL AND ASSOCIATES 1956[10]	115	63 →	X	22	—	6.5
RESNICK AND O'CONNOR 1973[13]	102	59	45	22	20	2
EVANS AND TEXTER 1975[5]	47	69	31	0	0	0
UTZ AND ASSOCIATES 1973[15]	187	68	44	29	0	3
MASINA 1965[11]	72	82	50	38	0	8.5
MAGRI 1962[9]	104	80	38.4	26.3	0	9.6
LONG AND ASSOCIATES 1972[8]	42	73	33	9	0	7
RICHES 1960[14]	88	58	36	0	0	6.7
COX AND ASSOCIATES 1969[2]	59	61	27	17	0	-
JEWETT AND ASSOCIATES 1964[7]	133	58	30	16	0	-
NOVICK AND ASSOCIATES 1976[12]	50	67	53	17	25	0
BRANNAN AND ASSOCIATES 1978[1]	45	84.4	58.5	33.3	-	-

not used more often? There may be several reasons for this:-

    1.   With the decrease in the number of segmental resections
performed there has been a marked increase in transurethral
resection of bladder tumours. Due to better and more sophisticated
instruments and greater experience of the urologists the efficiency
of transurethral resection of bladder tumours has improved.

    2.   Transitional cell carcinoma of the bladder is a manifest-
ation of a disease of the entire vesical mucosa. As well as the
macroscopically visible tumour we can often find other changes in the
mucosa ranging from the common hyperplasia and cystic dysplasia to
actual carcinoma in situ. Even though each case is different
in the extent to which these mucosal changes are present, the
fact remains that apart from endoscopically visible tumour other
pre-cancerous and truely cancerous changes of the mucosa may exist
which cannot be recognised by means of the endoscope. Even by
performing a resection with a large margin and by obtaining frozen
sections of the margin we may not resect all cancerous lesions.
Esch and Rummelhardt (1973), reported that they found in 30% of
partial resections cancer infiltration in the margin of the specimen.
Therefore, these operations were not radical.

    3.   The attempt to compare the papers reporting partial
cystectomy and to analyse the cumulative results is of doubtful
value. The only two characteristics that all these patients have in
common are that they have had a partial cystectomy and that they have
been followed over a period of five years. Their pre- and postoperative treatment is not uniform with regard to the type and
number of operations as well as the addition of chemotherapy or
radiotherapy.

    4.   The multi-centric growth of the tumour in the bladder
results in the high recurrence rate amounting to 50 to 75% in all
series. Most of these recurrences were later on treated by one or
several transurethral resections.

    5.   The danger of tumour spread was considered an essential
shortcoming of the partial cystectomy. Many authors, therefore,
recommend a preoperative transurethral resection which should be
as radical as possible. Moreover some argue that a preoperative
radiotherapy of at least 3,000 rads delivered to the tumour is
necessary to avoid metastasis within the wound. The results seem
to be improved by this preceding radiotherapy (van der Werf-Messing,
1978). However, there are no prospective randomised studies.

    6.   The efficacy of postoperative irradiation or split dosage
irradiation has not been clearly defined. Even a precise unbiased
analysis of the results of partial cystectomy published during the
last twenty years does not give objective guide-lines concerning the

indication for pre- and postoperative radiotherapy. The decision
is largely subjective and remains up to each individual urologist.

CONCLUSIONS

Our indications for partial cystectomy are:

1.   Solitary lesions
2.   Tumour localised to the bladder dome (Urachal tumour) or
posterior bladder wall (mobile part of the bladder).
3.   Inaccessibility to adequate transurethral resection.
4.   Infiltration (UICC) T1 or T2.
5.   Multiple biopsies of the macroscopically normal mucosa
must be negative.
6.   Special indication is a tumour in a vesical diverticulum.

Contraindications for partial cystectomy are prior irradiation
of the bladder, multiple tumours, inability to obtain adequate
margins, incolvement of the vesical neck, evidence of extravesical
extension of the tumour, or regional lymphnode metastasis, carcinoma
in situ and the presence of microscopic tumour foci in multiple
biopsies of the macroscopically normal mucosa. On rare occasions
we have to rely on the segmental resection when the patient refuses
a total cystectomy.

With regard to operative technique, we are in agreement with
Brannan (1978), prior to the segmental resection most parts of the
tumour should be resected transurethrally. Before segmental
resection we perform extravesical dissection including perivesical
fat, peritoneum and lymphnodes. The cystostomy is done
asymmetrically well away from the tumour. As much as possible frozen
sections of the margins should be obtained. If uretero cystoneostomy
is necessary, an antireflux procedure is not mandatory. To decrease
potential cellular implantation we suggest preoperative flash
radiotherapy.

REFERENCES

1.   Brannan, W., Ochsner, M. G., Fuselier, H. R. and Landry, G. R.
     J. Urol. 119, 213 (1978).

2.   Cox, C. E., Cass, A. S. and Boyce, W. H. J. Urol. 101, 550
     (1969).

3.   Deweerd, J. H. and Colby, M. Y. J. Urol. 109, 391 (1973).

4.   Esch, W., Rummelhardt, S. Helv. Chir. Acta, 40, 459 (1973).

5.   Evans, R. A. and Texter, J. H.   J. Urol. 114, 391 (1975).

6.   Haschek, H., Schimatzek, A. and Vedrilla, D.   Helv. Chir. Acta
     40, 453 (1973).

7.   Jewett, H. J., King, I. R. and Shelley, W. M.   J. Urol. 92, 668
     (1964).

8.   Long, R. T. L., Grummon, R. A. and Spratt, J. S.   Cancer, 29,
     98 (1972).

9.   Magri, J.   Brit. J. Urol. 34, 74 (1962).

10. Marshall, V., Holden, J. and Ma, K. T.   Cancer, 9, 568 (1956).

11. Masina, F.   Brit. J. Surg. 52, 279 (1962).

12. Novick, A. C. and Stewart, B. H.   J. Urol. 116, 570 (1976).

13. Resnick, M. I. and O'Connor, V. J.   J. Urol. 109, 1007 (1973).

14. Riches, E.   J. Urol. 84, 472 (1960).

15. Utz, D. C. and Schmitz, St. E.   Cancer, 32, 1075 (1973).

16. van der Werf-Messing, B.   Report to the International School
     of Urology, Erice 1978.

AUTOLOGOUS HUMAN SKIN FLAPS IN PARTIAL REPLACEMENT OF THE BLADDER WALL

A ROST

Department of Urology, Klinikum Steglitz
Free University of Berlin
Germany

INTRODUCTION

Different materials, eg. muscular fascia, intestine, peritoneum and synthetic products, have been used with varying degrees of success as partial replacement for the wall of the bladder (1-5,7,8). For several years now, our hospital has also been dealing with the problem of partial replacement of the bladder. Lyophilized dura and skin have been tested and applied in animal experiments and clinically (3,5).

After the good results achieved with full-skin flaps in the cat experiments we have performed partial bladder replacement with an autologous skin flap in five patients.

SURGICAL TECHNIQUE

An oval-shaped piece of skin with subcutaneous tissue, 15 cm long and 8 cm wide, is taken from the lateral region of the patient's abdomen, and the wound is closed after mobilisation of the edges. The epidermis of the skin flap is scraped off with the scalpel, then the subcutaneous fatty tissue is removed (6).

After resecting the lesion with a 2 cm margin of healthy mucosa the graft is inserted into the defect by an overlapping technique using atraumatic 2-0 chromic catgut U-sutures stitched vertically and knotted at the exterior surface. Between the U-sutures, interrupted stitches are applied between the edge of the skin flap and the bladder wall (Fig. 1).

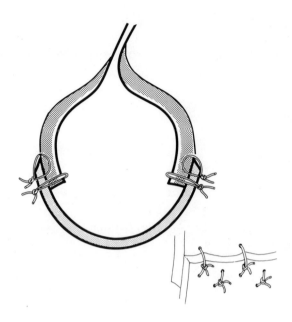

Fig. 1

Waterproof overlapping suture technique between bladder wall and
skin flap.

        Fig. 2 shows the graft in situ. With this technique it is
possible to achieve a waterproof closure of the bladder. Transurethral and suprapubic catheters are inserted. The space of
Retzius is drained by a 4 x 6 mm latex drain. Eight days after
surgery, an IVP is performed to demonstrate the absence of extravasation, after which the suprapubic catheter is removed. On the
fourteenth post-operative day the transurethral catheter is also
removed.

                              RESULTS

        In four patients the post-operative course was without
complications. In one, extravasation of contrast medium persisted
for four weeks. One patient showed a late extrusion of fragments
from the graft without further complications.

        After an observation period of six months the patients were
able to empty their bladders without residual urine and to hold
urine for at least three hours. In all patients the normal preoperative bladder capacity was regained. The result of this
operation is demonstrated in a cystogram (Fig. 3).

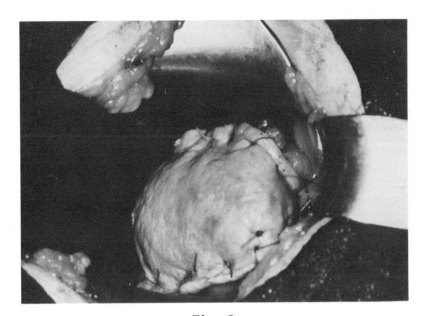

Fig. 2

Operation sites after completion of replacement of the bladder wall.

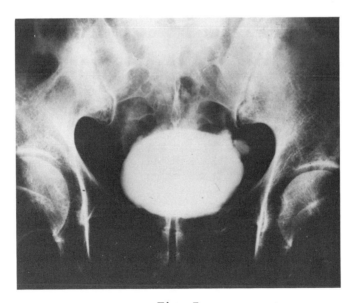

Fig. 3

Patient: female, 62 years old, post-operative cystogram

CONCLUSIONS

This preliminary report demonstrates that the application of
an autologous skin flap is a simple method for replacing even
extensive areas of the bladder wall. This material can be also
used for increasing the capacity of contracted bladders. Skin is
always available and can be used easily. It is elastic and adapts
itself to the wound edges, allowing a waterproof closure to be
easily achieved. Our experience shows that in selected cases the
replacement of the bladder wall with an untreated full thickness
skin graft is a good and technically simple method.

REFERENCES

1.   Bandhauer, K., Frick, J. and Födisch, H.J., Die Homotrans-
      plantation tiefgekühlter Blasenanteile im Tierversuch.
      Verh. Ber. Dtsch. Ges. Urol. 22, 214-220 (1969).

2.   Hradec, E.A., Bladder Substitution: Indications and Results in
      114 Operations. J. Urol. 94, 406-417 (1965).

3.   Kelâmi, A., Duraplasty of the Urinary Bladder - Results after
      two to six years. Eur. Urol. I, 178-181 (1975).

4.   Kolle, P., Wiederherstellung und Ersatz der Harnblase.
      Münch. med. Wschr. 115, 265-270 (1973).

5.   Pust, R., Butz, M., Riedel, B. and Rost, A., Replacement of
      urinary bladder wall in the cat by autologous X-ray treated
      full thickness skin graft. Urol. Res. 3, 139-143 (1975).

6.   Rehn, E., Das Kutane und subkutane Bindegewebe als plastisches
      Material. Münch. med. Wschr. 61, 118-121 (1914).

7.   Simons, E. and Pieritz, E., Defektdeckung der Blase durch
      homoiologe und heterologe Transplantate. Verh. Ber. Dtsch.
      Ges. Urol. 22, 225-229 (1969).

8.   Tsuji, J., Ishida, H. and Fujieda, J., Experimental cysto-
      plasty using preserved bladder graft. J. Urol. 85,
      42-44 (1961).

INDICATIONS FOR CYSTECTOMY

S ROCCA ROSSETTI

Department of Urology

University of Trieste, Italy

INTRODUCTION

There are three main indications for radical cystectomy:

a) to cure tumours localised to the bladder or with a single involved regional node,
b) the minimal possibility of curing tumours no longer localised to the bladder but still confined to the anterior pelvic space,
c) the necessity to relieve symptoms due to the tumour or arising following previous treatment or associated neoplasms.

The increasing use of alternative therapy may markedly modify the indications especially since the results of cystectomy have not been very encouraging in the past. One may consider the indications under the categories of compulsory and of optional and alternative treatments.

COMPULSORY INDICATIONS

In certain situations it is impossible to use any other kind of therapy for theoretical or practical reasons:

a) when the tumour actually or potentially affects all the bladder and/or the urethral mucosa, as in true diffuse papillomatosis, ca in situ with multiple foci and in patients whose tumours show rapid recurrences in different zones especially if presenting a higher stage or grade.

Another indication for cystectomy for T2 tumours is that at this
stage it is still possible to avoid preoperative radiotherapy. A
rectal bladder with intrasphincteric sigmoidostomy or with colostomy
can be performed safely if the pelvis has not been irradiated. It
should be noted that this is the only method of diversion which some
patients accept.

Cystectomy is only one step in the treatment of T3 tumours. If
possible, it should be preceded by radiotherapy. This indication is
often due to ureteral obstruction.

The quality of life one can offer a patient is in my opinion a
factor which determines the indication. In some patients the
residual bladder makes life unbearable; in these cases cystectomy
must be performed for humanitarian reasons.

Moreover, urologists know that if after cystectomy a patient
has metastasis he rarely suffers. The contrary is often true in
patients whose bladder is not removed and who undergoes other
treatments.

OPTIONAL OR ALTERNATIVE INDICATIONS

They are those in which other kinds of less aggressive therapies
are possible.

In this group we find category T4a, tumours downstaged T3
lesions and patients with multiple repeated recurrences, tumour in a
small or congenitally abnormal bladder, a neurogenic bladder or
associated with severe urethral stenosis.

Another indication arises due to the aversion of some urologists
to partial cystectomy, which can never be considered as radical
treatment from the oncological point of view.

All these indications are alternative because of the possibility
of other more conservative, associated therapies whose results cannot
at present be fully evaluated.

The opinions of various authors concerning the therapy of
purulent cystitis after urinary diversion are also of interest and
are contrasting. Personally, I believe that this severe, painful
situation must be avoided by cystectomy.

CONCLUSIONS

The indication for cystectomy for bladder tumours derives
essentially from a doctrinal point of view:

b) when there are associated urological tumours such as lesions
of the renal pelvis and ureter, or prostatic cancer;

c) when TUR is technically impossible or inappropriate (tumours
of the anterior wall, the dome and in diverticula);

d) when high grade or stage gives a higher suspicion of
initial invasion of the lymphatic channels in the bladder wall;

e) when, independently of the staging, there is ureteral
obstruction, which needs a complicated urinary diversion; in
these cases cystectomy does not add much to the surgical trauma;

f) when complications due to previous treatment of the tumours
have rendered life unacceptable (eg. haemorrhage and pain);

g) when the patient does not accept or cannot undergo the
endoscopic check-ups required.

Some points must be emphasised: ca in situ, ie. non-papillary
and non-invasive intraepithelial tumour, is so dangerous as to
merit careful and expert follow-up. The fact that different patterns
of superficial and of deep infiltration can be found in unsuspected
areas of bladder removed for ca in situ convince me that cystectomy
is the aggressive answer to an extremely aggressive tumour.

In six of 21 cystectomy specimens, I found multiple areas
of carcinoma of the apparently normal prostate (latent or occult
carcinoma); this association between adenocarcinoma of the prostate
and transitional cell carcinoma of the bladder probably merits
greater interest and in my opinion is one of the indications for
radical cystectomy.

Category T2 and T3 tumours undoubtedly represent the crucial
point of the discussion; T2 because they are often resectable
endoscopically, T3 because 10 year survival rates are very disappointing. In favour of cystectomy for T2 tumours there are the
following considerations:

a) radical cystectomy is curative in T2 No Mo Lo Vo and may be
so also in T2 N1 Mo if there is only one positive regional lymph
node;

b) an error of staging is possible and not rare (27%).

c) associated areas of ca in situ are found in 20% of cases
(Van der Werf-Messing, 1969) as well as high grade areas (27%)
or unhomogeneous histological features in the tumour itself
(22%) (Hendry, 1976). Only a thorough randomised study will
permit us to reach a more selective indication for cystectomy

a) cystectomy can cure tumours localised to the bladder or in the anterior pelvic space;

b) cystectomy is the only means of avoiding in some conditions extreme discomfort or danger for the patient.

In either situation cystectomy must always be preceded by endoscopic resection, if possible complete, of the tumour.

However, the potentially favourable results of other therapies, oblige us to keep the indications for cystectomy under continuous critical revision, through which increasingly highly selective indications will emerge. Randomised studies are indispensable for this aim.

REFERENCES

1. Baker, R., The accuracy of clinical versus surgical staging. J.A.M.A. 206, 1770 (1968).

2. Dretler, S. P., Ragsdale, B. D., Leadbetter, W. F., The value of pelvic lymphadenectomy and the surgical treatment of bladder cancer. J. Urol. 109, 414 (1973).

3. Hendry, W. F., Bloom, H. J. G., Urothelial Neoplasia. Present position and prospect in recent advances in urology. Churchill Livingstone, Edinburgh, London, New York (1976).

4. Jewett, H. J., King, L. I. R., Shelley, W. M., A study of 365 cases of infiltrating bladder cancer: relation of certain pathological characteristics to prognosis after extirpation. J. Urol. 92, 668 (1964).

5. Melicow, M. M., Tumours of the bladder: a multifaceted problem. J. Urol. 112, 467 (1974).

6. Miller, L. S., Bladder Cancer: Superiority of Preoperative Irradiation and Cystectomy in Clinical Stages B2 and C. Cancer, 39, 973 (1977).

7. Young, H. H., The value of lymphadenectomy in the surgical treatment of bladder tumours. "The tumours of Genito-Urinary Apparatus. COFESE, Palermo 237 (1976).

THE RESULTS OF TOTAL CYSTECTOMY FOR CARCINOMA OF THE BLADDER

R E WILLIAMS, P B CLARK AND P H SMITH

The General Infirmary and St James's University

Hospital, Leeds

ABSTRACT

This paper reviews 68 cases of radical cystectomy done for
bladder cancer with a five year follow-up. Radical cystectomy is
associated with a higher operative mortality and morbidity than
simple cystectomy, especially in the presence of previous high
energy radiation. It offers the possibility of a five year cure
in a few patients who have lymph node metastases in the pelvis.

INTRODUCTION

Between January, 1967 and October, 1978 164 total cystectomies
for bladder carcinoma were carried out in the Urological Services
of Leeds. The present survey covers a period from 1967 until
October, 1973 and thus allows for a possible five years' survival.
During this period 68 radical cystectomies were done and 11 simple
cystectomies; the latter number is too small for analysis but does
provide some interesting data for comparison. The radical
cystectomies comprise 54 men and 14 women, most of whom were over
55 years of age and about 20% were over 70 years of age. In 30
patients the cystectomy was an elective procedure, the commonest
indication being invasive tumour. Salvage cystectomy following
failure of radiotherapy to control tumour growth was performed on
38 patients and on 24 of these the operation was precipitated by
persistent and sometimes uncontrolled bleeding.

SURGICAL TREATMENT

Cystectomy was a one-stage procedure and was accompanied by urinary diversion usually with an ileal conduit, though six of the earlier cases had a ureterosigmoidostomy and one had a rectal bladder. In women, cystectomy was included in an anterior exenteration procedure while for men the seminal vesicles and prostate were removed with the bladder in both simple and radical cystectomy. When radical cystectomy was done, the dissection was extended to include the lymph node chains from the bifurcation of the common iliac artery to the inguinal ligaments along with the peri-vesical fat and pelvic fascia in continuity with the bladder.

RESULTS

Simple cystectomy had no operative mortality but that for radical cystectomy was 16%. Salvage cystectomy following failed radiotherapy was associated with a higher operative mortality (22%) than when radical cystectomy was done as an elective procedure (7%).

Post-operative complications included urinary fistula, faecal fistula, abdominal dehiscence and osteitis pubis. Late complications included stomal stenosis, uretero-ileal stenosis and electrolyte imbalance associated with ureterosigmoidostomy. The later development of urethral carcinoma required urethrectomy in four patients while four other patients developed transitional cell carcinoma in the renal pelvis or ureter. Pitting oedema occurred in 10% of patients after radical cystectomy and non-pitting oedema in 15%. On some occasions lymphoedema was due to pelvic tumour but on other occasions it persisted for many years in the absence of recurrent tumour and was presumably due to damage to lymphatic drainage.

Carcinomatosis was the commonest cause of death within five years following radical cystectomy. The five year survival is 54% after simple cystectomy and 31% after radical cystectomy. When the radical cystectomies are broken down into elective and salvage procedures, values of 23% and 35% respectively are obtained. These differences can be explained by the different operative mortalities and the proportion of category P1 tumours in the various groups. When the values are corrected for post-operative deaths, the difference between the five year survival after simple and radical cystectomy becomes 54% and 38% respectively, whereas the difference between elective and salvage radical cystectomy becomes greater - 25% and 47% respectively. In addition, there was a high percentage of P1 cases in the radical cystectomy group due to the large number of salvage cases which showed no evidence of muscle invasion on the cystectomy specimen.

In 14 patients lymph node metastases were found on histological examination of the cystectomy specimen and three of these patients survived for five years. In all of these patients elective radical cystectomy had been done and none had received radiotherapy.

DISCUSSION

In this series, radical cystectomy has a greater operative mortality than simple cystectomy. However, Whitmore and Marshall (1962) and Richie et al (1976) compared operative mortality in simple cystectomy, radical cystectomy and radical cystectomy with node dissection and found no significant difference. The number of simple cystectomies in this series is too small for analysis and probably the value of 5% operative mortality reported by Cordonnier (1968) is a realistic figure for this operation. The dangers of cystectomy after high energy radiation were pointed out by Higgins et al (1966) and this factor contributes to the high operative mortality of 16% for radical cystectomy in this series. Probably an operative mortality of 10% would be reasonable for radical cystectomy in the absence of high energy radiation.

The significance of lymph node metastasis has been debated in the past. Whitmore and Marshall (1962) reported survival of two patients out of 13 who had one or two positive lymph nodes but only 4% survival of all their patients with lymph node involvement. Dretler et al (1973) recorded a 33% five year survival for those with only one or two nodes involved. Laplante and Brice (1973) considered that a few positive nodes within the pelvis did not appear to render radical cystectomy any less effective and pointed our that while radical cystectomy might offer the possibility of cure for a few of these patients, there was no report of any patient surviving with proved nodal spread beyond five years without surgical treatment.

In a personal series, Clark (1978) reported three patients out of 12 with lymph node involvement who survived for five years or more after cystectomy.

Radical cystectomy offers the possibility of cure to a few patients with lymph node invasion but this must be balanced against the higher operative mortality and morbidity. The results in this paper suggest that simple cystectomy should be performed for patients with papillomatosis, carcinoma-in-situ and as a salvage procedure, for these patients have a low incidence of lymph node metastasis. Radical cystectomy, on the other hand, should be reserved for elective cases of invasive tumour of the bladder as these are known to have a high incidence of lymph node metastasis and for these patients in whom metastatic iliac node metastasis are found at operation.

REFERENCES

1. Clark, P. B. Brit. J. Urol. 50, 492-495 (1978).

2. Cordonnier, J. J. J. Urol. 99, 172-173 (1968).

3. Dretler, S. P., Ragsdale, B. D. and Leadbetter, W. F. J. Urol. 109, 414-416 (1973).

4. Higgins, P. M., Hamilton, R. W. and Hope-Stone, H. F. Brit. J. Urol. 38, 311-318 (1966).

5. Richie, J. P., Skinner, D. G. and Kaufman, J. J. J. Urol. 113, 186 (1976).

6. Whitmore, W. F. and Marshall, V. F. J. Urol. 87, 853 (1962).

RADICAL CYSTECTOMY IN ADVANCED BLADDER TUMOURS

F PUTTI

Department of Urology
Ist. Regina Elena
Rome, Italy

The Department of Urology of the Institute Regina Elena in
Rome has seen about 300 cases of advanced bladder tumours between
1970 and the end of 1977, of which only 120 were treated surgically.
Some were primary transitional bladder cancer, others were secondary
tumours of neighbouring structures invading the bladder wall.

The clinical study was undertaken to check the value of
aggressive operations, often added to chemotherapy and radiotherapy,
and to see if such agressive surgical management is justified or not.
In all we performed 44 urinary diversions and 76 total cystectomies.
Herein we will report only the results concerning patients undergoing total cystectomy.

Of these, 26 were for primary bladder tumours and 50 for
secondary tumours. All the patients suffering from transitional
cell tumours had T3 growths, often with involvement of some regional
lymph nodes, but with no evidence of distant metastases. The
secondary tumours were recurrences of previous neoplastic disease
affecting other adjacent organs and were therefore T4 growths.

We have nearly always performed a radical cystectomy with
urinary diversion according to the methods described by Mauclaire,
Gersuny and Heitz Boyer, but in the cases needing a total or partial
exenteration the Bricker method of urinary diversion was used.

The mortality within one month of operation was 15% (11 of 76
patients), 35 patients of the 65 survivors lived for a mean period
of 16 months and 13 patients were lost to follow up. Seventeen
patients (23%) are presently alive and free of disease, seven of

them having been followed for periods ranging from three to eight years after the operation. In all these cases the tumour category was P3 - P4 N1+ N2+, as confirmed by histo-pathologic post-operative study.

The main conclusion to be drawn from our experience is that, if it is possible to obtain 23% long term survival in patients already "condemned to death", such aggressive operations are worthwhile. Even in the patients who did not survive for more than one year, we feel that the operation was justified by the palliation of the terrible end stage symptoms of this disease; these patients usually die of metastases but free of local suffering.

Moreover, it is possible by cystectomy to give to Chemotherapists and to Radiotherapists the opportunity to help these patients, since the reduction of tumour burden by surgery permits other adjunctive treatments to be effective.

Because of all these considerations we believe that radical cystectomy still has a place in the treatment of the very advanced bladder tumours, whether primary or secondary.

CANCER OF THE URETHRA FOLLOWING CYSTECTOMY

S COLLEN and A EK

Department of Urology

University Hospital of Lund, Lund, Sweden

Several authors have called attention to the risk of recurrence of malignancy in the urethra left at cystectomy and recommend routine prophylactic cystourethrectomy (2,3,6). Others reserve this procedure for patients with bladder tumours which encroach upon the bladder neck and/or have cancer in situ involving the proximal urethra (4,5).

We have found "secondary" cancer of the urethra in nine out of 800 patients treated for cancer of the bladder in 1966-1973, ie. approximately 1%. However, seven of these recurrent urethral tumours occurred among 63 cystectomised patients. That makes a frequency of "secondary" urethral cancer in cystectomised patients of almost 11%. All except one were diagnosed within two years of the cystectomy.

TABLE 1

INCIDENCE OF SECONDARY URETHRAL CARCINOMA FOLLOWING
CYSTECTOMY FOR BLADDER CANCER

Number of Patients	Histological Grade	Secondary Cancer of the Urethra
0	I	0
12	II	1
44	III	6
7	Undifferentiated	0

In five cases the urethral tumour was diagnosed because of local symptoms such as palpable tumour, pain or urethral bleeding. All these died of cancer in spite of aggressive surgery and radiotherapy. In one patient a tumour of the penile urethra was found four years after cystectomy for multiple, well-differentiated bladder cancer without muscular or urethral invasion. The urethrectomy specimen showed a highly malignant urethral tumour with possible invasion of the corpora cavernosa. One month later a total peno-scrotal amputation was performed followed by radiotherapy. However, this patient soon developed cutaneous and skeletal metastases and died five months later.

Two patients without local symptoms were diagnosed by cytological examination of urethral saline-lavage. In one no tumour was seen at urethroscopy but because of a consistent cytologic finding a secondary urethrectomy was performed. In the specimen a very small tumour was found, invading the corpus spongiosum of the urethra. After the urethrectomy he had radiotherapy, but is now in poor condition with pulmonary metastases. The other case of "secondary" urethral cancer diagnosed by cytology had a small, superficial, moderately differentiated tumour and carcinoma in situ. He is without recurrence after three years observation.

In our small series no obvious factors predisposing to secondary urethral malignancy could be found. However, Table 1 could indicate a higher risk for patients with grade III cancer, though the differences are not significant.

Previous authors (2,6) have found a higher incidence of secondary urethral cancer in patients with multiple bladder tumours compared to patients with solitary tumours. We found no difference in this respect. Two of the 16 patients with multiple and five of the 47 patients with solitary bladder tumours developed "secondary" urethral cancer.

The urethral tumour in the cystectomised patients may be an expression of multicentric carcinogenesis, but the high frequency may also imply that tumour cells could be implanted or spread through urethral lymphatic or venous plexuses due to bladder squeezing during the cystectomy. As carcinoma in a retained urethra has a dismal prognosis we now routinely perform cystourethrectomy en bloc instead of simple cystectomy. Simultaneous urethrectomy performed by the assistant is a simple procedure with a negligible complication rate and probably no undesirable future consequences for the patient (7). Urethras left behind for various reasons may be removed or monitored by cytological examination of urethral lavage.

REFERENCES

1. Baird, B., Bush, L. and Livingstone, G., Urethrectomy subsequent to total cystectomy for papillary carcinoma of the bladder: case reports. J. Urol. 74, 621-625 (1955).

2. Cordonnier, J. J. and Spjut, H. Jr., Urethral occurrence of bladder carcinoma following cystectomy. J. Urol. 87, 398-403 (1962).

3. Goning, N. F. C., Urethral carcinoma associated with cancer of the bladder. Brit. J. Urol. 32, 428-438 (1960).

4. Johnsson, D. E. and Guinn, G. A., Surgical management of urethral carcinoma occurring after cystectomy. J. Urol. 103, 314-316 (1970).

5. Raz, S., McLorie, G., Johnsson, S. and Skinner, D., Management of the urethra in patients undergoing radical cystectomy for bladder carcinoma. J. Urol. 120, 298-300 (1978).

6. Stams, U. K., Gursel, E. O. and Veenema, R. J., Prophylactic urethrectomy in male patients with bladder cancer. J. Urol. 111, 177-179 (1974).

7. Whitmore, W. F. and Mount, B. M., A technique of urethrectomy in the male. Surg. Gynec. & Obstet. 31, 303-305 (1970).

SUPRAVESICAL URINARY DIVERSION

E J ZINGG, K VENETZ, and D BERCHTOLD

Urological Department, University Hospital, Inselspital

CH-Berne, Switzerland

In recent years interest has become focussed once more on the controversy concerning the best method of supravesical urinary diversion. Indeed, it has become almost impossible to remain familiar with the abundant literature on the subject. In this paper it is unnecessary to deal with the individual basic principles underlying the different types of urinary diversion, since it can be assumed that the members of this audience are already familiar with the concepts involved.

Let us start by summarising the characteristics of an ideal supravesical urinary diversion (28).

1. Free drainage of the urine from the upper urinary tract.

2. Absence of stenosis at anastomoses between ureter and intestine, ureter and skin, or intestine and skin.

3. Low-pressure reflux of the urine.

4. Absence of ascending infection.

5. Absence of electrolyte imbalance.

6. Urinary continence.

The types of supravesical urinary diversion which are currently feasible are summarised in the following table:

- Direct drainage of the urinary tract to the exterior

    - cutaneous ureterostomy

- cutaneous transureteroureterostomy

- lateral ureteric fistula

- nephrostomy

- Drainage to the exterior via an isolated intestinal segment

   - ileal conduit

   - colonic conduit

   - cecal conduit

   - jejunal conduit

- Drainage into the non-isolated intestine

   - ureterosigmoidostomy

- Drainage into an isolated segment of the large intestine with transanal pull-through of the colon

   - rectal bladder according to Heitz-Boyer-Hovelaque

   - rectal bladder according to Gersuny

ILEAL CONDUIT

The principle of this method lies in the isolation of a 15-25 cm long segment of the terminal ileum. The ureters are divided and anastomosed to the ileal segment, and the distal end of the ileum is fashioned into a cutaneous ileostomy.

Pathophysiology

In a discussion of the pathophysiology of this type of urinary diversion a number of problems need to be examined particularly closely (Table I).

TABLE I

PATHOPHYSIOLOGICAL PROBLEMS

1. Resorption of Vitamin B12 and Bile Acids
2. Hyperchloremic Acidosis
3. Peristalsis in the Ileal segment
4. Change in the Ileal Mucosa

Hyperchloremic Acidosis. The small intestine has a number of important endocrine, excretory, resorptive, and mechanical functions. It produces a secretion which has a pH of 6.9-7.6 and which is isotonic with blood plasma. The pH is largely determined by the secretion of bicarbonate into the lumen in exchange for chloride ions. The resorption of chloride and the secretion of bicarbonate involve active transport processes. When the ileum is used as a conduit the resorption of chloride is of functional importance. Hyperchloremic acidosis rarely occurs in the presence of normal renal function. If the renal function is compromised owing to impairment of the regulatory function of the distal tubule by pyelonephritis or back-pressure, construction of a conduit is followed at an early stage by hyperchloremic acidosis in approximately 60% of cases (8). The incidence of late hyperchloremic acidosis reported in the international literature lies between 2% and 10%.

Resorption of Vitamin B12 and Bile Acids. The specific functions of the ileum include the resorption of vitamin B12 and bile acids. This function cannot be assumed by any other part of the intestine. If the construction of an ileal conduit involves isolation of a long segment from the intestinal flow the resorption of B12 may be diminished. Since the organs possess very large reserves of this vitamin which suffice to supply their needs for several years it takes some time for the vitamin B12 deficiency to become manifest.

Following extensive ileal resections (30-100 cm) or ileocecal resections the resorption of bile acids decreases. Thus larger amounts of these acids enter the colon and may cause diarrhoea (37). The loss of bile acids is usually compensated for by increased hepatic synthesis. The resorption of fat is not affected.

Peristalsis. According to Boyarsky, (5) the contractile patterns in the ileal conduit vary from hyperactivity to little more than slow writhing. All forms of peristaltic activity are compatible with satisfactory function of the conduit. Campbell (6) and Minton (30) obtained similar results. Only in 40-56% of cases does one find spiking contractile patterns of activity associated with peristaltic waves. A particularly noticeable feature is the total lack of coordination of any kind whatsoever between the contractions of the ureters and those of the ileum. The pressures in the ileal conduit lie between 10-20 mm Hg. The conduit contains little or no residual urine. It does not act as a reservoir (23).

Changes in the Mucosa. A certain flattening and widening of the villi of the ileal mucosa is already evident four weeks after construction of a conduit. After one year the changes are very marked. In addition, extensive inflammatory infiltration is seen. However, the intestinal epithelium does not actually lose its characteristic features. Neither in ileal conduits nor in colonic conduits does adaptive metaplasia occur, even after a period of years (17,20,22).

As Tapper (52) showed recently, marked lymphoid depression is seen in the ileal segments. At the same time reactive hyperplasia of the lymph nodes in the mesentery of the intestinal loop occurs. The cause of these changes is not known. Does urine contain a lymphocyte suppression factor? The lymphoid depression could explain not only the late mid-loop strictures but also the recurrent infections and the progressive renal deterioration.

With regard to the physiology of an ileal conduit, we would like to stress the following points: 1) An ileal conduit is a low pressure system, 2) the transport time of the urine in the system is important, 3) loopograms are unphysiological examinations.

Surgical Technique

The surgical technique has largely been standardised. Following isolation of the ileal segment the continuity of the small intestine can be restored with one or two layers of sutures. The ureter is usually joined to the ileum in the Bricker fashion with a single-layer end-to-side anastomosis and without attempting anti-reflux plasty. The anastomosis should be retroperitonealised. The distal end of the conduit is brought directly forwards to the anterior abdominal wall rather than retroperitoneally, eg. behind the cecum. A full-thickness cylinder is excised from the abdominal wall. The use of intracutaneous Dexon[R] or Vicryl[R] sutures to ensure perfectly contiguous union between the skin and mucous membrane has been found to be a worthwhile measure for the prevention of stenosis of the stoma. The mesentery of the distal part of the loop should not be shortened excessively, since this might compromise the blood supply to the stoma.

Postoperative Mortality

The postoperative mortality following construction of an ileal conduit is currently 2-12% in the case of adults with malignant disease and 0-4% in children suffering from benign conditions.

Early Complications

The most important early complications are wound dehiscence, mechanical or paralytic ileus, urinary leakage, and acute pyelonephritis. The frequencies of these complications vary from 1-10% (11,13,29,38,56).

The morbidity in the ureteroileal diversion after prior radiation therapy is higher (wound infection, urinary leakage, paralytic ileus), the average postoperative hospital stay is longer (23,30).

Long-Term Results

Nowadays the interest in all types of urinary diversion is focussed on the long-term results, ie. the results after five, 10 or 15 years (11,12,13,32,40). The success of a given type of procedure cannot be judged until the true long-term results are known. The first long-term survival statistics to become available are the five and 10 year figures which are now being reported in the field of pediatric urology. The survival of patients with malignant disease tends to be shortened by the malignancy itself. For this reason there are relatively few adults with carcinoma of the bladder who have been followed up over a long period after supravesical diversion.

The most important late complications are: ascending infection and pyelonephritis, impairment of renal function, urolithiasis, stenosis of the ileo-ureteric anastomosis, mid-loop stenosis, and stenosis of the stoma (9,26).

Infection. The normal flora of the ileum is of a mixed oral and fecal type, and anerobic organisms usually predominate. The bacterial count amounts to 10^4/ml or more. The conduit flora differs qualitatively from that of the healthy ileum and usually comprises a mixture of gram negative bacteria. Earlier bacteriological investigations showed significant colonisation of the ileal conduit with gram negative organisms in 60-100%. It was only when Durham-Smith (12), and Gracey (20) carried out their investigations with a suitable double-catheter technique that it became apparent that the bacterial counts in urine taken from the depths of the conduit under sterile conditions are below 10^4ml in the majority of cases. These results have been confirmed by Spence (49), Stromenger (50) and ourselves (Table II). This explained the discrepancy, which had been known for years, between the permanently infected state of the conduit and the normal conditions in the upper urinary tract. The stomal end of the conduit is always infected; at the proximal end in the vicinity of the ureteral ostia, on the other hand, there is some bacterial colonisation (in the range of 10^2-10^4/ml) in the majority of patients with normal upper urinary tracts. The significance of this is still in question.

Pyelonephritis. The published data on pyelonephritis as a complication of conduit diversion is difficult to interpret. The frequency of pyelonephritis - which, for the majority of the authors, means the clinically unequivocal form of the disease - lies between

TABLE II

BACTERIURIA IN INTESTINAL CONDUIT IN URINARY DIVERSION

		%
Rickham	1964	50
Campbell	1965	70
Retik	1967	15
Holland	1968	56
Engel	1969	100
Needham	1970	72
Spence	1971	82
Graley	1971	91

WITH USE OF DOUBLE CATHETER

Spence	1972	59
Strohmenger	1976	23
Bishop	1972	0
Zingg	1977	7

10 and 20%. Subtle pyelonephritic changes in the urogram are un-accompanied by clinical signs or symptoms are certainly more frequently encountered and occur in approximately 30% (38).

Urolithiasis. Secondary stones in the upper urinary tract form in approximately 5-15% of the patients. Stone formation is influenced by urinary tract infection, the length of the ileal loop, the intestinal peristalsis, and outflow obstruction due to stomal stenosis. In our experience stone formation increases greatly with the duration of the urinary diversion.

Stenoses. The areas which are susceptible to stenosis are the ileal stoma, the ileo-ureteric anastomosis, and the ileal segment itself. In children stomal stenoses occur in 30-40% and are at the head of the table of late complications. In adults changes in the stoma rarely occur if a suitable technique is used.

The stricture rate is not influenced by the ileo-ureteral anastomosis technique. The frequencies of stenosis associated with the original Bricker technique and with the Wallace modification are identical (14). It should be noted that stenoses can occur at this site years after the operation. It is extremely important that patients with urinary diversions be followed up at regular intervals.

Hardy (23) recently reported 15 stenoses of the loop itself. This complication, too, occurs at a late stage and is clinically

often latent. The suggested causes include inflammatory changes,
lymphocyte depletion, and abnormal and compromised local defence
mechanisms.

State of the Kidneys. A decisive measure of the success of a
urinary diversion is the subsequent state of the kidneys. According
to Gregory, pyelographic changes provide the earliest and most
reliable evidence of postoperative improvement or worsening of the
renal situation.

Long-term follow-up of children with ileal conduits revealed
an alarming rate of renal deterioration in persons in whom the
upper urinary tract had previously been normal. Schwarz (43)
followed up 96 children with conduits for an average period of 11
years and found renal deterioration in 56%. A similarly disappointing result in children was reported by Shapiro (45); during
an average follow-up period of 11.2 years late complications occurred
in not less than 69.7%. The results in terms of renal function
were somewhat better than those published by Schwarz; in 70% of the
cases with previously normal uretero-renal units there was no
deterioration following urinary diversion. Long-term data of this
type in adults is not yet available. According to Gregory (21),
Schmidt (42) and Engel (13) urographic follow-up over periods of
two to eight years reveals no changes in 70-80% of the cases with
normal preoperative urograms (Table III). Our own results also
point in this direction.

Conclusion

The ileal conduit has been used for urinary diversion for
approximately 28 years. The results published to date are not yet
uniform. An extremely high complication rate is found in children
who are followed-up for 10-15 years, and some pediatric surgeons

TABLE III

ILEAL CONDUIT : COMPARISON PREOPERATIVE AND POSTOPERATIVE
UROGRAPHIC FINDINGS COMPILED FROM THE LITERATURE

	Preop. Normal Postop. No Change	Preop. Abnormal Postop. Improved
	%	%
Delgado, Muecke 1973	69	65.8
Schmidt 1973	72	70.7
Gregory 1974	71	17
Remigailo 1976	76	17

(Hendren, Hohenfellner (25)) now prefer the colonic conduit to the
ileal conduit. In adults, particularly those with preoperatively
normal upper urinary tracts, the results are not as alarming. In
the majority of the latter cases the upper urinary tract is still
normal after three to eight years.

We agree with Remigailo (38) that the ileal conduit operation
is not a difficult procedure but one which requires very great
attention to detail. The greater the proportion of cases which are
operated on by experienced staff members who possess the appropriate
surgical skill, the greater is the success rate. The ileal conduit
still has an indisputable place in the treatment of adults with
malignant disease and in our department, is the method of choice
for urinary diversion (Table IV).

TABLE IV

SUPRAVESICAL URINARY DIVERSION

Department of Urology, Inselspital, University of Bern
July 1971 - Oct. 1978

Intestinal conduits		116
Ileum	101	
Jejunum	5	
Colon	4	
Coeco-Ileal	6	
Uretero-Sigmoidostomy		49
Cutaneous Ureterostomy		20
Trans-Uretero-Ureterostomy		11
TOTAL		196

JEJUNAL CONDUIT

In cases in which the ileum has been damaged by radiation the
ileal conduit is associated with an excessively high complication
rate. Under these circumstances Morales and his co-workers (33)
recommend use of a jejunal conduit, whilst Hohenfellner (25) and
Schmidt (41) prefer the transverse colonic conduit.

The transport characteristics of the jejunum are basically
different from those of the ileum and colon. Sodium is first
actively resorbed, mainly as bicarbonate which disappears completely
from the lumen. The permeability of the jejunum is such that the

movement of water through its wall is almost totally determined by
osmotically active concentration gradients. This results in loss
of water, sodium chloride and bicarbonate, and in a considerable
reduction in extracellular volume (53). According to Clark (7) and
Morales (33) episodes of severe pre-renal uremia and hyperkalemia
have occurred in approximately 50% of patients with a jejunal
conduit. Thus hyperchloremic acidosis does not result but these is
loss of sodium, chloride, and bicarbonate. The syndrome simulates
water intoxication, a salt-losing nephritis, and adrenal failure.

In five of our own cases we were able to prevent severe
electrolyte disturbances by regular postoperative follow-up The
jejunal conduit operation does not present any difficulties from
the technical point of view. It can be used for urinary diversion
in exceptional cases, but the colonic conduit is preferable.

COLON CONDUIT

Uebelhör (54) in 1952, was the first to describe the use of an
isolated segment of the large intestine for urinary diversion in
cases of malignancy of the female genital organs. The procedure
was resurrected by Mogg (31,32) and the same author reported the
first large series of cases. On the Continent it is mainly
Hohenfellner who has advocated use of the colonic conduit (1,2).

Surgical Technique

The surgical technique is now largely standardised. A colon
segment approximately 15 cm in length is isolated and the proximal
end is closed with two layers of sutures. The segment is opened
along the antimesenteric teniae. The ureters are pulled through
the mesentery into the intestine, with excision of a small piece of
muscularis in order to prevent stenosis. The ureter is anastomosed
to the intestine with a reflux plasty in the form of a submucous
tunnel. The intestinal continuity is restored by anastomosis with
two layers of sutures.

Pathophysiology

From the pathophysiological point of view the pressures are
approximately the same as those in an ileal conduit or, at most,
10% higher. The contents of the colonic segment are propelled
through the conduit by longitudinal contractions. The residual
urine volumes are less than 15 ml.

Postoperative Mortality

The overall postoperative mortality corresponds to that
following construction of an ileal conduit and is shown in
Table V.

Early Complications

The early complications do not differ in type or frequency from
those associated with the ileal conduit.

The procedure is definitely contraindicated in the presence of
marked changes in the large intestine such as diverticulitis or
radiation damage, or in patients with ureters which are excessively
short or, above all, distally damaged.

Long-Term Results

Here again, the long-term results are assessed in terms of
renal function and the long term course. The incidence of calculi,
stenosis and stomal stenosis between ureter and colon in children and
in adults is of the order of 2-7% (1,28,32,51) whilst the incidence
of pyelonephritis varies from 6-35% (28,32,51). According to
Altwein (2) in children only 17% of the preoperatively normal uretero-
renal units subsequently show urographic signs of pyelonephritis.
Dilation of the ureters proximal to a colonic conduit is hardly
ever seen in children and is rare (5%) in adults. Despite the
reflux plasty reflux is found in 10-15% of patients. In children
stenosis of the stoma of a colonic conduit is less common than that
of an ileal conduit.

The large intestinal conduit has the following advantages
when compared with its small intestinal counterpart:

- The contents of the large intestine are propelled in one direction

TABLE V

COLON CONDUIT : POSTOPERATIVE MORTALITY

| | No. of Patients | | Mortality % |
	Adults	Children	
Altwein 1977	-	64	1.5
Lindenauer 1974	45		2.2
Mogg 1969	75		0

by longitudinal contraction; true peristalsis is absent.

- The colon has a rich blood supply which allows the isolation of very short intestinal segments.

- The ureter can be anastomosed with the intestine in such a way as to prevent reflux.

- Stomal problems are very rare.

- Because stomal stenosis is rare and the conduit segment is usually short metabolic disturbances hardly ever occur.

Conclusion

The results obtained to date with the colonic conduit, particularly those in children, are very promising. Because of the effective protection against reflux the colonic conduit is particularly suitable for cases in which the urinary diversion is subsequently undiverted.

In an adult the situation is more complex. Until now no long-term data have been available. It is precisely in the elderly patient with malignant disease that one is faced with a short sigmoid mesentery with large amounts of adipose tissue and changes in the sigmoid colon such as diverticulosis and diverticulitis. In our experience the technical difficulties associated with the colonic conduit are more serious than those which accompany ileal loop diversion. We therefore feel that, in the adult, the colonic conduit is not a significantly better alternative to the ileal conduit.

URINARY DIVERSION WITH CONTINENT UROSTOMY

The possibility of diverting the urine through a continent stoma has occupied numerous surgeons for many years. Since 1949 several trials, including those of Pearl (36), Kock (27) and Gilchrist (18) have been described. The procedures currently in use are still at the stage of clinical trial and include Kock (27) and Leisinger's ileal pouch with a continent stoma, our method with a continent ileocecal pouch, and Ashken's (3) ileocecal conduit.

A basically different technique is embodied in Feustel (15) and Sigel's (46) continent diversion with a magnetic closure.

None of the procedures described are in widespread clinical use yet. It is too early at this stage to make a final assessment of their worth.

URINARY DIVERSION BY DIRECT CUTANEOUS URETEROSTOMY

Terminal cutaneous ureterostomy or the creation of a lateral ureteral fistula are procedures which are seldom used for urinary diversion in the treatment of carcinoma of the bladder.

In our experience transureteral cutaneous ureterostomy is justifiable for cases in which terminally damaged ureters and the poor general condition of the patient rule out an ileal conduit, and in which one of the ureters is so dilated that it can be used to bridge the gap between the non-ectatic ureter and the skin. In eight of our own cases the rate of fistula formation was very high but, on the other hand, the operation placed little stress on the patients.

IMPLANTATION OF THE URETER INTO THE INTESTINE (URETEROSIGMOIDOSTOMY)

Uretero-intestinal anastomosis is the oldest type of urinary diversion. In 1852 it was carried out for the first time by Simon (47) in London. It is one of the few operations which, with the changes in technique, indication, and biochemical insight over the last few decades, has been both fervently acclaimed and heartily condemned.

Since 1967, however, ureterosigmoidostomy has recovered some of its popularity. Due to more careful selection of the cases and improvements in technique including, in particular, anti-reflux anastomosis of the ureter, the range of indications for this procedure has widened. In 1967 Williams (55) recommended restriction of the operation to a carefully chosen group of indications, meticulous postoperative chemotherapy, specific and carefully monitored replacement of potassium and alkali losses, and urographic follow-up. Spence (49) also advocates ureterosigmoidostomy, as did Rettmer (39), in publications in the seventies, Noszkei (35) and Batke (4). Since 1975 ureterosigmoidostomy has been undergoing a veritable renaissance, with reports by Zincke (57), Spence (49), Segura (44) and Hohenfellner (25).

Optimum selection of the patients is decisive, and the following considerations should be borne in mind:

- The procedure is contraindicated if the kidneys have been damaged by urinary back-pressure or pyelonephritis.

- If the intestine shows inflammatory changes at the time of the operation these is a danger of subsequent stenosis.

- The question of postoperative radiotherapy is still open.

There have been no conclusive publications on this topic and
uretero-intestinal implantation might therefore be risky for the
treatment of bladder malignancy if the urinary diversion was to be
followed by radiation therapy. However, all of our few cases of
uretero-intestinal implantation have tolerated postoperative high-
voltage radiation therapy well.

- Fecal continence is, of course, a prerequisite.

Surgical Technique

We use the transcolic procedure of Goodwin (19). The ureters
are divided far distally near their junction with the bladder. The
sigmoid colon is opened along the antimesenteric tenia and the ureter
is pulled through the sigmoid mesentery and anastomosed with the
intestine via a submucosal tunnel.

Important features of the operation are: the retroperitoneal
course of the ureters throughout their lengths; excision of a small
segment of bowel mucosa to avoid ureteral stenosis; and creation of
a submucosal tunnel to prevent reflux.

The immediate postoperative mortality is in the region of 9%.
Early complications such as obstructive ileus, urinary extravasation
pyonephrosis, and wound dehiscence occur in 2-8% of cases, and are
significantly more frequent in adults with malignant disease than
in children.

TABLE VI

URETERO - SIGMOIDOSTOMY : LATE COMPLICATIONS

	No. of Pts.	PYE %	C %	H A %	U-S S %
Harvard and Thompson 1951	144	70	10	40	
Spence 1966	31	71	13		
Zincke and Segura 1975	173	20	3		
Lindenauer 1974	45	20	6.6	2.2	4.4
Hohenfellner 1976	24		8.3	8.3	8.3

PYE = Pyelonephritis; C = Calculi; H A = Hyperchloremic Acidosis;
U-S S = Uretero-Sigmoid Stenosis.

Long-Term Results

The long-term results (10) are evaluated in terms of complications such as uretero-intestinal stenosis, urolithiasis, obstruction to urinary flow, and pyelonephritis (Table 6). Additional criteria include the postoperative acid-base and electrolyte balance, the frequency of defecation, and the degree of fecal continence.

In adults 16% of the uretero-renal units show subsequent urographic signs of pyelonephritis. Seventeen percent of the children and 40% of the adults with preoperatively normal ureters show evidence of slight dilatation caused by obstruction to urinary flow following the operation.

Acid-base and electrolyte distrubances do not present problems if the renal function is intact. A base excess of more than -5 mmol/l is seen in only approximately 5-7%.

The anti-reflux anastomosis is of decisive importance. Uretero-intestinal implantation is followed by late complications in 70% of cases in which no anti-reflux procedure was performed (24) and in 11.8% of those which included an anti-reflux procedure (7).

Meticulous follow-up is of paramount importance to the success of any urinary diversion. Surgeons and surgical units should never undertake urinary diversion procedures unless they are prepared to follow the patients up regularly and, if necessary, perform any further surgery which may subsequently become necessary. It is generally considered that the follow-up examinations should include abbreviated urograms at six monthly intervals, together with regular measurements of the serum electrolytes and blood gas analyses. If there are signs of renal failure it is advisable to determine the split clearances with iodohippurate sodium I-131. If a postoperative dilatation does not regress within six months reoperation is necessary.

When evaluating the results of a diversion procedure one should also take into account the patients' postoperative quality of life. Excessively frequent defecation or fecal incontinence are very serious problems which greatly impede the social reintegration of the patient. Of our patients who were followed up more than one year after ureterointestinal implantation, 16% reported a bad functional result with defecation at one to two hourly intervals, 50% reported a good result with defecation every two to four hours, and in only 34% had an optimum result been achieved with bowel motions every four to six hours. All the 50 patients were fecally continent.

URINARY DIVERSION BY CONSTRUCTION OF A RECTAL BLADDER

Urinary diversion by construction of a rectal bladder using the technique of Gersuny or Heitz-Boyer Hovelacque is a topic which I do not intend to deal with in detail. In our opinion these types of diversion following total radical extended cystectomy for carcinoma of the bladder and, if applicable, postoperative irradiation, are never indicated. I am, of course, fully aware that many members of the audience will not be prepared to share this opinion, especially here in Italy.

CONCLUSIONS

This survey is not intended to be exhaustive. The topics which one chooses and the emphasis which one places on them are always determined to a marked degree by subjective influences. However, I hope that this paper will provide some interesting insights into current trends and developments, and that some of the points may stimulate further discussion.

REFERENCES

1. Altwein, J. E., Hohenfellner, R. Surg. Gyn. Obst. 104, 33 (1975).

2. Altwein, J. E., Jonas, U., Hohenfellner, R. J. Urol. 118, 832 (1977).

3. Ashken, M. H. Brit. J. Urol. 46, 631 (1974).

4. Batke: Zit. Lutzeyer, W., In Zingg, E., Tscholl, R: Supra-vesikale Harnableitung, H. Huber, Bern (1977).

5. Boyarski, S., Kaplan, N., Martinez, J., Elkin, M. J. Urol. 88, 325 (1962).

6. Campbell, J. W., Oliver, J. A., Mekay, D. E. Radiology, 85 338 (1965).

7. Clark, B. G., Leadbetter, W. F. J. Urol. 73, 999 (1955).

8. Chisholm, J. In Zingg, E., Tscholl, R: Supravesikale Harnableitung, H. Huber, Bern (1977).

9. Clark, S. S. J. Urol. 112, 42 (1974).

10. Corbett, C. R. R., Lloyd-Daves, R. W. Eur. Urol. 2, 221 (1976).

11.   Delgado, G. E., Muecke, E. C.   J. Urol. 109, 311 (1973).

12.   Durham-Smith, E.   J. Ped. Surg. 7, 1 (1972).

13.   Engel, R. M.   J. Urol. 101, 508 (1969).

14.   Esho, J. O., Vitke, R., Ireland, G., Cass, A.   J. Urol. 111,
      600 (1974).

15.   Feustel, H., Henning, G.   Dtsch. Med. Wschr. 100, 1063 (1975).

16.   Flanigan, R. C., Nursh, E. D., Persky, L.   Amer. J. Surg.
      130, 535 (1975).

17.   Garner, J. W., Goldstein, A. M. B., Cosgrove, M. D.   J. Urol.
      114, 845 (1975).

18.   Gilchrist, R. K., Merricks, J. W., Hamlin, H. H., Rieger,
      J. L.   Surg. Gyn. Obst. 90, 752 (1950).

19.   Goodwin, W. E., Harris, A. P., Kaufman, J. J., Beal, J. M.
      Surg. Gyn. Obst. 97, 295 (1953).

20.   Gracey, M., May, E., Bishop, R. F., Durham-Smith, E.,
      Anderson, C. M.   Invest. Urol. 8, 596 (1971).

21.   Gregory, J. G., Gerrsahani, M., Schoenberg, H. W.   J. Urol.
      112, 327 (1974).

22.   Guerrero, M., Gonzales, A., Ortiz, F.   J. Urol. 104, 406
      (1970).

23.   Hardy, B. E., Leibowitz, R. L., Baez, A., Colodny, A. H.
      J. Urol. 117, 358 (1970).

24.   Harvard, B. M., Thompson, G. J., J. Urol. 65, 223 (1951).

25.   Hohenfellner, R., Marberger, M.   In: Zingg, E., Tscholl, R.
      Supravesikale Harnableitun, H. Huber, Bern, 210 (1977).

26.   Kafetsioulis, A., Swinney, J. Brit. J. Urol. 42, 33 (1970).

27.   Kock, N. G.   Progr. Surg. Vol. 12, Karger, Basel (1973).

28.   Lindenauer, S. M., Cerny, J. C., Morley, G. W.   Surgery, 75
      705 (1974).

29.   Malgieri, J. J., Persky, L.   J. Urol. 120, 32 (1978).

30.   Minton, J. P., Kiser, W. S., Ketcham, A. S.   Surg. Gyn. Obst.
      119, 541 (1964).

31. Mogg, R. A. Brit. J. Urol. 39, 687 (1967).

32. Mogg, R. A., Syme, R. R. A. Brit. J. Urol. 41, 434 (1969).

33. Morales, P. A., Whitehead, E. D. Urology, 1, 426 (1973).

34. Nichols, W. K., Krause, A. H., Donegan, W. L. Amer. J. Surg.
     124, 311 (1972).

35. Noszkei: Zit. Lutzeyer, W: In Zingg, E., Tscholl, R. Supra-
     vesikale Harnableitung, H. Huber, Bern (1977).

36. Pearl, J. I. Surgery, 25, 217 (1949).

37. Rangel, D. M., Yakeishi, Y., Stevens, G. H., Fonkalsrud, E. W.
     Surg. Gyn. Obst. 129, 1189 (1969).

38. Remigailo, R. V., Lewis, E. L., Woodard, J. R., Walton, K. N.
     Urology, 7, 343 (1976).

39. Rettmer: Zit. Lutzeyer, W: In Zingg, E., Tscholl, T. Supra-
     vesikale Harnableitung, H. Huber, Bern (1977).

40. Richie, J. P. J. Urol. 111, 687 (1974).

41. Schmidt, J. P., Hodgson, N. B. J. Urol. 112, 536 (1974).

42. Schmidt, J. D., Hawtrey, C. E., Buchsbaum, H. J. J. Urol.
     113, 308 (1975).

43. Schwarz, G. R., Jeff, R. D. J. Urol. 114, 285 (1975).

44. Segura, J. W., Kelalis, P. P. J. Urol. 114, 138 (1975).

45. Shapiro, S. R., Lebowitz, R., Colodny, A. H. J. Urol. 114
     289 (1975).

46. Sigel, A., Henning, G., Wilhelm, E., Hager, Th. In Zingg, E.,
     Tscholl, R. Supravesicale Harnableitung, H. Huber, Bern
     (1977).

47. Simon, J. Lancet, 2, 568-570 (1852).

48. Spence, B., Esho, J., Case, A. J. Urol. 108, 712 (1972).

49. Spence, H. M., Hoffman, W. W., Pate, V. A. J. Urol. 114, 133,
     pp 21 idem (1975).

50. Strohmenger, P. Acta Urol. Belg. 43, 424 (1975).

51. Symmonds, R. E., Gibbs, C. P. Surg. Gyn. Obst. 131, 687
     (1970).

52. Tapper, S., Folkman, J. J. Ped. Surg. 11, 871 (1976).

53. Truniger, B. In: Zingg, E., Tscholl, R. Supravesikale
     Harnableitung, H. Huber, Bern (1977).

54. Uebelhör, R. Langenbecks Anh. Klin. Chir. 271, 202 (1952).

55. Williams, R. E., Davenport, T. J., Burkinshaw, L., Hughes, D.
     Brit. J. Urol. 39, 676 (1967).

56. Zingg, E., Mayor, G. 4. Jenaer Harnsteinsymposium, pp 215,
     (1975).

57. Zinke, H., Segura, J. J. Urol. 113, 324 (1975).

TREATMENT OF THE CANCER OF THE BLADDER BY IRRADIATION, CYSTOPROSTATECTOMY AND ILEOCYSTOPLASTY

M CAMEY AND A LE DUC

Department of Urology

CMC Foch, 92151 Suresnes, France

The replacement of the bladder by a segment of ileum described by Couvelaire and which we have used for 20 years is the only procedure to maintain micturition through the urethra and to avoid the feeling of mutilation often caused by urinary diversion.

Among 245 patients who underwent cystoprostatectomy in our department after irradiation by telecobalt (3,500 rads 3 weeks or 1,200 rads flash), 87 received a new ileal bladder, the ileal loop being anastomosed by the top of the U to the membranous urethra, the surgeon carefully preserving the external sphincter.

It is a very long, and difficult operation that must be done perfectly on a carefully selected patient. Indeed the conditions required are very strict in order to achieve safety in the post-operative period an expectation of long survival and a good functional result:

The criteria for selection are:-

- physiological age $<$ 70 years,
- no significant obesity diabetes or pulmonary insufficiency,
- T $<$ 4 and no invasion of the neck of the bladder,
- perfect urethra and external sphincter,
- a well informed and willing patient able to understand and to accept the requisite reeducation hoping intensively to return to normal life is very important for the recovery of continence.

In these conditions the post-operative risk is not very high ($<$ 6% mortality) and the survival rate for patients without invaded

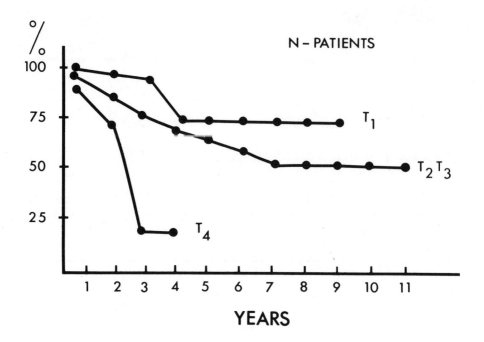

FIGURE 1

SURVIVAL RATE (ACTUARIAL)

INCLUDING FIVE PATIENTS WHO DIED IN THE POST-OPERATIVE PERIOD

nodes is 52% for T2 T3 and 76% for T1 at seven years (Figure 1).

The survival rate is rather better than that usually seen after cystectomy probably because this report is concerned with selected patients in particularly good general condition.

Following this operation the kidneys are frequently involved by reflux (mainly on the right because of the peristalsis of the ileum) but damage is rarely serious because this reflux occurs at low pressures and often with a sterile urine. The five renal failures that we observed must be avoided in the future by the new technique of antireflux implantation of the ureters that we have used for the last two years and which we proved effective by retrograde cystography.

In our opinion when operating upon the cancer of the bladder we must consider not only the length of the survival but also the quality of it.

In regard to the question of continence (and I think this is the

most important question) contrary to the classic concepts our
experience has demonstrated that continence was far better after
anastomosing the ileal bladder to the membranous urethra than by
preserving the tip of the prostate.

When the conditions required are respected, continence is normal
during the day, the patient voiding his new bladder every two or
three hours. The sensation of a full bladder which is effective
during the day, is generally insufficient to awake the patient who
must train himself to wake up twice or thrice a night. By this
means 70% of the patients prevent enuresis.

After the first four weeks or months these patients can do
everything they want including swimming and have so normal a life
that after some years they forget their disease.

A TYPE OF RECTAL POUCH FOR URINARY DIVERSION AFTER CYSTECTOMY

G S BARLAS

Admiral Bristol Hospital
Istanbul, Turkey

In our country, urinary diversion with devices such as urinary bags is very difficult for our patients to accept. The problem lies in finding good devices which can easily be managed by the patients. For this reason we have been performing uretero-sigmoidostomies. As is well known, after any kind of uretero-sigmoidostomy there are complications such as hyperchloremic acidosis and ascending infections (1,3,4).

While we were performing uretero-sigmoidostomies, we tried to find a method of diversion which did not need a bag or other device and which had fewer complications. In 1964 we read of the work of Dr. Modelski who reported a blind pouch (2). The main part of this procedure is to develop a rectal pouch and to anastomose the ureters and the sigmoid to this pouch far apart from each other. In this method there is less pressure in the pouch and the stool does not pass near the ureters.

After studying Dr. Modelski's work, we did several dog experiments and found only 25 cm. water pressure in the pouch, which was unexpectedly low due to the fact that peristalsis was arrested at the anastomosis site.

We have performed this type of anastomosis on seven patients. The surgical technique is shown in Figure 1.

After isolation of the ureters, cystectomy is performed and the sigmoid colon is resected at the rectosigmoid junction. The rectum is closed at this point and the ureters are implanted very proximally into the pouch. The sigmoid is then anastomosed to the pouch end to side as distally as possible. We operated on seven male patients.

247

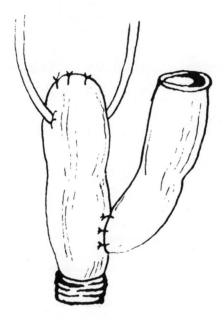

FIGURE 1

Diagram to show Rectal Pouch

Six of them were between 58 and 74 years old and had bladder cancer.
One, who was 19 years old, had a urinary fistula in the gluteus. He
had been operated on five times without any success and when we
decided to carry out urinary diversion we did not find any bladder
wall at all.

From the technical point of view there were no problems at
operation but one patient died on the ninth day following operation
from myocardial infarction, one other patient died on the eleventh
day of pulmonary embolism and a third patient on the 55th day after
discharge from hospital. At autopsy distant metastases to the brain
were found. The other four patients are well and have no electrolyte
imbalance. They are also free from kidney infection and urograms
show good kidney function. After barium enema, no reflux to the
ureters was observed (Figure 2 and 3).

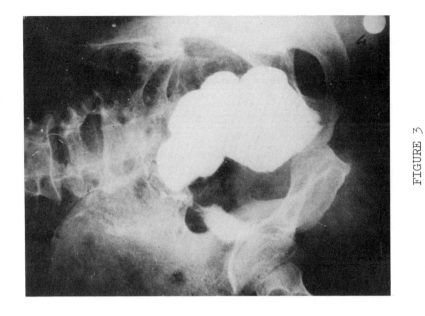

FIGURE 3

Ba enema following diversion by rectal pouch.

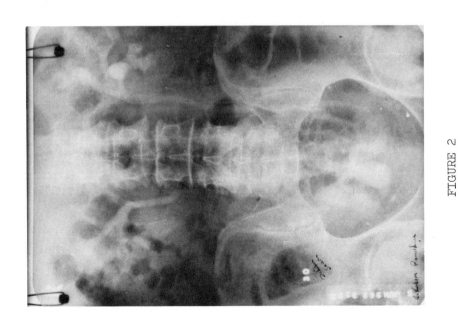

FIGURE 2

IVP following diversion by rectal pouch.

SUMMARY

We have used a Modelski type of urinary diversion in seven patients. This is a rectal pouch in which the ureters are anastomosed proximally and the sigmoid colon distally. Because of low pressure in this pouch neither kidney infection nor electrolyte imbalance were found.

REFERENCES

1. Hinman, Weyrauch, H. M., A critical study of different principles of surgery which have been used in uretero intestinal implantation. Trans. Amer. Ass. Genitourin Surg. 29, 156 (1936).

2. Modelski, W., Transplantation of the ureters into the partially excluded rectum. J. Urol. 87, 122 (1962).

3. Nesbit, R. M., Ureter-sigmoidostomy. J. Urol. 6, 726 (1949).

4. Turnbull, R. B., Higgins, C. C., Ileal valve pouch for urinary tract diversions, preliminary report of eight cases. Cleveland Clinical Quarterly, 24 187 (1957).

COMPARISON OF BRICKER AND WALLACE METHODS OF URETEROILEAL ANASTOMOSIS IN URINARY DIVERSION

J O ESHO

Unit of Urology, Department of Surgery

College of Medicine, Lagos University, Lagos, Nigeria

INTRODUCTION

Urinary diversion, as described by Bricker in 1950 was for use in adults who required pelvic exenteration for cancer. In this procedure, a 10 to 20 cm length of terminal ileum is isolated from the intestinal tract, and the continuity of the bowel re-established by open end-to-end anastomosis. The appendix is removed. The proximal end of the detached segment of ileum is closed. The ureters are divided from the bladder and anastomosed to the ileal segment, near its blind end through openings in the ileal wall cut to the exact size of each ureter. The distal end of the ileal segment is brought out to the surface of the abdomen in the right lower quadrant through a circular opening cut through skin, fascia, muscle and peritoneum and sutured to the skin to form a slightly protuberant ileal stoma. The various complications encountered with this procedure have prompted the introduction of several modifications. The Wallace method of ureteroileal anastomosis (1966) consists of splaying the distal ureters longitudinally. The medial edges are sutured together with a continuous 5-zero chromic catgut suture. The conjoined ureters are then sutured to the proximal ileal segment with a 4-zero chromic catgut suture at the apex of each ureter to the ileum and a continuous 5-zero chromic suture along the lateral edges. The entire anastomosis is retro-peritonealised. The ileal conduit is brought through the peritoneal cavity to the anterior abdominal wall where a stoma is constructed.

This report is based on comparison of 33 patients who had the Bricker method of diversion, with 33 patients who had the Wallace method. They were followed up for two years.

RESULTS

The results are shown in Table I.

TABLE I

		Diversion	
		Bricker	Wallace
Patients	Adults	11	11
	Children	22	22
Mean Operating Time		5 hr 56 min	4 hr 38 min
Post Op Deaths		1	0
Renal Stone Formation		2	2
% Upper Tract Dilatation at two years		7	11

CONCLUSIONS

A comparison was made of 33 consecutive patients having ileal diversions done by the Bricker method and an equal number of consecutive patients who underwent the Wallace method of conjoined end to end ureterointestinal anastomosis.

While the Wallace method had some technical advantages and resulted in shorter operating time, there was no significant difference between the methods at the end of two years.

The full text of this paper has already been published in the Journal of Urology, 111, 600-602 (1974).

LYMPHADENECTOMY IN BLADDER CANCER

J AUVERT and H BOTTO

Hospital Henri Mondor

94010 Creteil, France

INTRODUCTION

Lymphadenectomy is a valuable technique for the accurate staging
and grading of bladder cancer. It is performed in association with
every partial and total cystectomy which is intended to be curative
rather than palliative. We also recommended it as part of the
surgical technique during interstitial irradiation. Nevertheless,
it is debatable whether it has any therapeutic advantages.

TECHNIQUE AND PROGNOSTIC VALUE OF LYMPHADENECTOMY

Lymphadenectomy is bilateral when combined with total cystectomy
and unilateral when performed with partial cystectomy. It should
include the external and internal iliac nodes and the obturator
nodes and does not increase the operative mortality. An "en bloc"
technique is used if the bladder tumour is not too large. With
large tumours we remove the bladder first then perform careful
supplementary lymphadenectomy. Multiple clips are placed on lymphatic vessels to prevent lymph leakage. Frozen section of the nodes
at the time of surgery is of little value. More important is the
ability to resect the nodes. This is easier if only one or two
nodes are involved (N1 category) and more difficult in N2, N3 and
N4 categories.

THE RELEVANCE OF LYMPHOGRAPHY

The T N M classification does not pay enough attention to the
histological grading of malignant deposits in lymph nodes. It is

TABLE I

NODE INVOLVEMENT AND PATHOLOGICAL CATEGORY

PATHOLOGICAL CATEGORY

	P1	P2	P3	P4
% N₁	8	54	29	40

important to appreciate if the malignant cells are:-

a.   Restricted to the sub-capsular region.
b.   Invading the whole node.
c.   Involving the lymph node vessels.
d.   Infiltrating the surrounding fat.

These observations should be included in a more sophisticated histological description of lymph node involvement and related to prognosis. Resection of N3 category nodes which are fixed to the iliac veins and arteries is difficult and dangerous. Juxta regional nodes (N4 category) should be considered as distant metastases.

We have studied the relationship between the invasion of regional lymph nodes by bladder cancer and the pathological category of the primary tumour (Table I). There is also a good correlation between the invasion of lymph nodes and distant metastases (Table II).

Patient survival after total cystectomy correlates with the presence or absence of lymph node involvement. We divide our cases

TABLE II

CORRELATION BETWEEN NODE INVOLVEMENT (N+) AND METASTASES (M1)

	T CATEGORY		
	T1	T2	T3
Patients Treated by Lymphadenectomy	12	13	24
Patients with Positive Nodes (N+)	1	7	8
N+ Patients Developing Metastatses (M1)	0	3	5

TABLE III

RELATIONSHIP BETWEEN N CATEGORY AND SURVIVAL

	No. of Cases	Average Survival (mths)	Average Age (yrs)
N1	7	>12	48
N2	10	6	59

into N1 and N2 categories and see that even in a small series average survival for N1 disease is over a year but for N2 it is only six months (Table III).

These observations have led us to avoid total cystectomy in N3 category disease. Perhaps this policy should be adopted also for N2 disease. In such cases only palliative partial cystectomy or selective arterial embolisation should be done if the patient has severe bleeding or strangury.

CONCLUSION

Lymph node invasion occurs in 30-50% of T2/T3 category bladder tumours. Half of these patients develop metastases. The average survival in N2 cases is only six months. Radical cystectomy is an inappropriate operation for N2 and N3 category bladder cancer.

Editorial Note (J P Blandy)

Pansadoro (Rome) referred to advantages of Marberger's "controlled" perforation as adjunct to TUR giving useful information as to staging of tumours suspected of going deep into bladder wall. No morbidity arising.

Rost (Berlin) described a technique based on Newman's patch technique for enlarging bladder after partial cystectomy which seemed successful in a small number of cases though Blandy (London) questioned its originality and relevance to bladder cancer and Auvert (Paris) pointed out that it did not provide information about the extent of nodal invasion.

Brosman (Los Angeles) had analysed the results of survival of bladder cancer for UCLA and somewhat to everybody's surprise, showed no significant deterioration in survival in patients treated by partial cystectomy on a previous occasion. Furthermore, there was no difference in survival whether or not lymph nodes were invaded as evaluated by radical lymphadenectomy.

Against the advocates of TUR for the superficial tumour Auvert contended that the up to 25% involvement in T1 tumours meant that TUR alone was illogical and incomplete. However, de Voogt questioned whether the extra morbidity of radical operation was justified, since the outlook was so poor when the lymph nodes were involved. Auvert replied that morbidity was largely due to lymph leakage and could be avoided by meticulous closure of lymphatic channels at the time of operation: however, he agreed that lymphadenectomy was not worth attempting in N3 cases.

de Voogt asked Zingg where he was doing the "mapping" of the mucosa.

Bercovich pointed out also that partial cystectomy was in theory more extensive and radical than TUR and if found to be more extensive in the specimen, radiotherapy could be given afterwards.

Van der Werf-Messing was unclear whether TUR was for "diagnosis" or "cure", but Manthopoulos pointed out that radiotherapy was much less difficult for the patient when done after TUR than after partial cystectomy and Studler (Vienna) agreed that radiotherapy after TUR gave good results so long as only a relatively small area < 3 cm diameter was involved and special attention was paid to avoiding infection.

Pansadoro asked whether one or two stage operations were done for salvage cystectomy, to which Williams replied that he preferred a one stage operation.

Edsmyr, Chisholm and Hall were all concerned at the mix of
T - G stages in the material reported by Williams who agreed that in
many of the "salvage" cases, no tumour was found in the specimen.
As for the N stage, Van der Werf-Messing pointed out the value of
pre-operative cytological aspiration of the lymph nodes to give
some assessment of the N category without increasing the hazards
of lymphadenectomy.

Denis (Antwerp) praised the use of parenteral feeding to
avoid some of the postoperative morbidity.

Following radiotherapy Pansadoro reported that very often the
lymph nodes had been sterilised by radiotherapy and so questioned
the need for any such radical operation, however, all cystectomies
were facilitated by a synchronous perineal dissection.

Putti (Rome) drew attention to the fact that the mortality of
cystectomy was still high both in Rome and in Leeds. Smith
observed that the figures were similar to those quoted by Hodges
(J. Urol. 119, 216, 1978). Brosman advised that survival following
cystectomy was better if the duration of symptoms and of previous
treatment was minimal; also that the outlook for the patient with
a papillary tumour was better than if the tumour was solid.

In discussion of the paper on bladder replacement Camey
(Suresnes) stated that he had seen three urethral recurrences and
had never needed to remove the pubis. He also agreed that the
operation should be restricted to male patients. Pavone (Palermo)
commented that the original operation described by Couvelaire
involved retention of the apex of the prostate gland which may
increase the risk of urethral recurrence and supported the concept
of removing all the prostate gland.

EFFECTS OF INTRAVESICAL FORMALDEHYDE-INSTILLATION (EXPERIMENTAL AND CLINICAL RESULTS)

R PUST, Department of Urology, Klinikum Giessen
J. L.-University Giessen

A ROST, Department of Urology, Klinikum Steglitz
Free University of Berlin

ABSTRACT

Changes in the urinary bladder wall following intravesical instillation of 5 - 25% formalin were studied in 25 healthy female cats. The contact period varied from one to 20 minutes. With a 20% solution and one minute contact time the bladder urothelium proteins quickly precipitated without necrosis of sub-epithelial layers. Complete re-epithelialisation and normal bladder dynamics (x-ray control) were seen after three to four weeks.

No signs of formaldehyde intoxication were observed. In four of five patients with intractable bleeding of the bladder the intravesical formaldehyde therapy was effective.

INTRODUCTION

Conservative treatment of intractable bladder haemorrage has been attempted using various chemical agents (9,10,14).

Formaldehyde solution seems to be effective in animals and in clinical application (2,5,12,13,15) It can stop bleeding by coagulation necrosis of the whole bladder mucosa. Our purpose was to study the time-dependent effect of various formaldehyde concentrations on the epithelium of the bladder of the cat, as the structure is similar to that of the human urinary bladder (1).

MATERIAL AND METHODS

Laparotomy was performed in 25 adult female domestic cats under Nembutal anaesthesia. The bladder was emptied by needle puncture and 10 cc of formaldehyde solution were instilled. From the commercial aqueous formaldehyde solution dilutions to 5, 7.5, 10, 15, 20 and 25% were obtained and buffered with $NaHCO_3$ solution (pH 7). Contact times of between one and 20 minutes were used. The solution was completely aspirated and the bladder washed out several times with physiological saline.

X-ray controls (IVP) and histological examinations were performed.

RESULTS

No signs of general intoxication such as lacrimation, broncho-spasm, vomiting, tachypnoea or tachycardia were observed.

The histological examination of the whole bladder 10 days after formaldehyde instillation revealed the following results:

5% solution, five minutes contact time:
The transitional cell epithelium looks almost normal and is not demarcated from its base. Slight subepithelial oedema and leucocytic infiltration occurred. Similar alterations can be seen in the interstitial layers of the tunica muscularis.

5% solution, 20 minutes contact time:
Complete necrosis of the epithelium is achieved. Necrosis includes the submucosal and parts of the muscular layers (Figure 1).

7.5% solution, five minutes contact time:
The transitional epithelium is damaged to various degrees with loosening and detachment of cells. The submucosa is oedematous, with cellular infiltration and scattered haemorrhage. The deep muscular layers show loosening of the connective tissue.

10% solution, five minutes contact time:
Complete necrosis of the epithelium including parts of the submucosa is achieved. The oedema extends into the muscular layers. The whole bladder wall shows slight infiltration.

15% solution, five minutes contact time:
The destruction of the epithelium is similar to the 10% solution, but within the submucosa a small homogenous layer of necrotic tissue can be seen. The adjacent inner submucosa shows loosened collagenous connective tissue. The muscular interstitium is infiltrated by oedema, the muscle itself seems not to be affected.

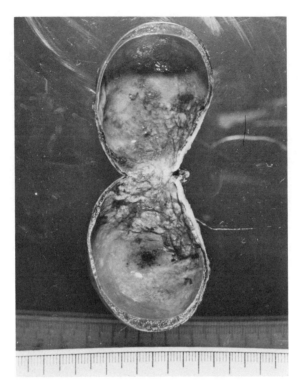

FIGURE 1

(5%, 20 minutes) Five days post op. Toxic effect. Complete necrosis of epithelium, submucosal and mucosal layers.

20% solution, one minute contact time:
The whole transitional epithelium is destroyed and transformed into a thin homogenous, condensed layer, equivalent to coagulated cellular proteins. The submucosal layer is oedematous without cellular infiltration. The muscular layer remains unaltered (Figures 2 and 3).

25% solution, one minute contact time:
The protein coagulation zone is deeper than in the case of the 20% solution and extends to the submucosal layers which are haemorrhagic. The muscular fibres look normal, the interstitium is extensively dilated by oedema.

The excretory urography (IVP), one to four weeks post-operatively, in cases treated with 20% formaldehyde solution and one minute contact time, shows no ureteral obstruction and a gradual normalisation of bladder capacity without residual urine.

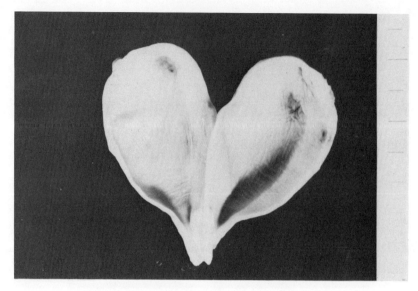

FIGURE 2

(20%, one minute) Eight days post op. Typical so called greyish-
white appearance of the bladder mucosa.

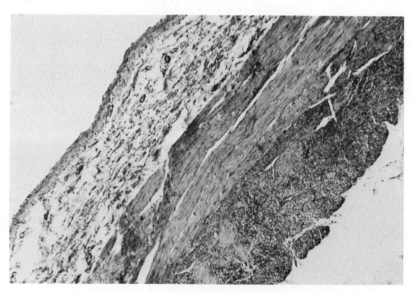

FIGURE 3

(20%, 1 minute) Eight days post op. Superficial protein precipitation of the epithelium, oedema of the submucosa.
V. Gieson stain (100 x).

FURTHER OBSERVATIONS

Depending on the degree of subepithelial destruction and the time-dependent demarcation of the necrotic material, regeneration of new transitional epithelium is obtained. In the group treated with 5% formalin concentration for a 20 minute period (for example), 75% mortality due to severe haemorrhagic cystitis was observed.

CLINICAL APPLICATION

In five patients with bleeding from bladder carcinomas that persisted after ligation or embolisation of the iliac artery, we tried the intravesical instillation of formaldehyde solution (50 cc, 20%, one minute contact time). Vesico-ureteric reflux had been excluded by cystography. In four cases it was possible to stop the bleeding by this therapy.

CONCLUSIONS

Intravesical formalin instillation can produce a precipitation of cellular proteins of all layers of the bladder, whose intensity depends on the formaldehyde concentration and the time of exposure (4).

Using 20% solution for one minute a superficial dense film of the bladder mucosa only results. The coagulated zone and the underlying reactive oedema prevent the formaldehyde from penetrating into the submucosal and the muscular layers. In this way it is possible to stop intractable bladder haemorrhage in humans (5, 15).

The re-epithelisation depends on the depth and extent of the necrosis. It can be speculated that this regeneration originates from the trigonal and the urethral regions (11).

Ureteral lesions in the cat were never observed when filling the bladder directly with formaldehyde solution. Reflex contraction of the trigone probably protects the cat's ureteral orifices. In man, the possibility of vesico-ureteric reflux must be excluded by prior high-pressure cystography before using intravesical formalin.

As a treatment of last resort in intractable bladder bleeding, intravesical formaldehyde instillation is often effective.

When using chemical agents, possible vesical reabsorption must be considered. A small dose of formaldehyde can be quickly oxidised to formic acid, which is an irreversible process. Formic acid is quickly eliminated as CO_2 (6,7,8).

REFERENCES

1. Albertini, V., A. Histologische Geschwulstdiagnostik. Stuttgard, G. Thieme Verlag (1955).

2. Brown, R. B. Med. J. Aus. 1, 23 (1969).

3. Fall, M., Peterson, S. Scand. J. Urol. Nephrol. Suppl. 33, 19 (1976).

4. French, D., Edall, J. T. Advances in Protein Chemistry, 2, 277 (1945).

5. Kumar, S., Rosen, P., Gragstald, H. J. Urol. 114, 540 (1975).

6. Malorny, G. Naunyn-Schmiedeberg's Archiv für experimentelle Pathologie und Pharmakologie, 255, 42 (1966).

7. Malorny, G., Rietbrock, N., Schneider, M. Naunyn-Schmiedeberg's Archiv für experimentelle Pathologie und Pharmakologie, 250, 419 (1965).

8. Malorny, G., Rietbrock, N., Schneider, M. Naunyn-Schmiedeberg's Archiv für experimentelle Pathologie und Pharmakologie, 247, 381 (1964).

9. Persky, L., Austen, G. Jr. J. Urol. 70, 724 (1953).

10. Pool, T. L. Surg. Clin. N. Amer. 39, 947 (1959).

11. Pust, R., Butz, M., Tost, A., Ogbuihi, S. and Riedel, B. Urol. Res. 4, 51 (1976).

12. Shah, B. G., Albert, D. J. J. Urol. 110, 519 (1973).

13. Whittaker, J. R., Freed, S. Z. J. Urol. 114, 866 (1975).

14. Wojewski, A., Roessler, R. Bull. Pol. Med. Sci. Hist. 8, 100 (1965).

15. Zechlin, H. H., Attobrah, F. Urologe B, 18, 106 (1978).

HYDROSTATIC PRESSURE TECHNIQUE AND INTRAVESICAL INSTILLATION OF

FORMALIN: METHODS FOR THE CONTROL OF SEVERE BLEEDING FROM THE BLADDER

M HORŇAK

Department of Urology

Medical School, Bratislava, Czechoslovakia

ABSTRACT

Bladder haemorrage in patients with widespread advanced tumours or haemorrhagic cystitis secondary to radiation therapy is frequently very resistant to treatment and presents a serious problem. In this group of patients we applied the hydrostatic pressure technique and also used intravesical instillation of formalin into the urinary bladder.

HYDROSTATIC PRESSURE TECHNIQUE

The hydrostatic pressure technique was originally described by Helmstein in 1972. The procedure is based on the decrease of the blood supply produced by increased intravesical pressure followed by hypoxia of the bladder wall and the tumour itself. In spite of some favourable records from the literature on tumour treatment, we have had no remarkable success with the treatment of the tumour itself and we have used the method only in patients with intractable haemorrhage from the bladder.

The technique is well known. We have used it in 12 patients in an attempt to stop persistent haemorrhage. In 10 the bleeding stopped, but in three this effect was only temporary and after several days, haemorrhage recurred. No complications related to the pressure treatment have been observed.

INTRAVESICAL INSTILLATION OF FORMALIN

Formalin was first used by Brown (1969), who instilled a 10% solution for 10 minutes.

Adequate pretreatment evaluation of patients for formalin therapy includes a cystogram. It extravasation and vesicoureteral reflux are demonstrated, we consider formalin instillation to be contraindicated. Before instilling formalin it is necessary to evacuate bladder clots under general or regional anaesthesia. Then, a Foley catheter is introduced and the urinary bladder filled with 100 to 150 mls of a formalin solution. Formalin that is 37.8% formaldehyde - is diluted to a 5% solution in sterile water. The Foley catheter is clamped for 30 minutes. When the solution is let out, the bladder is rinsed with 10% alcohol and subsequently with physiological saline. An indwelling catheter is maintained for 24 to 48 hours.

We have treated 34 patients with haemorrhage from the bladder by intravesical formalin instillation. In 27 patients bleeding stopped. In two patients haemorrhage recurred after seven and ten days, respectively. In two patients, the general condition improved to an extent which allowed us to proceed with radical cystectomy later.

The effect of formalin instillation has been explained by protein precipitation on the surface of the bladder mucosa. The histological investigation of the bladder wall following the instillation of formalin shows damage to the urothelium. Beneath the urothelium there is an inflammatory reaction with the deposition of amorphous and cellular substances. The inflammatory reaction and oedema involve the superficial muscle.

We have seen only one complication:- acute pyelonephritis which can be explained by vesicoureteral reflux. At that time we did not use cystography.

In conclusion, we have adopted the following policy for patients with troublesome bleeding from the bladder. For patients in whom vesicoureteral reflux is seen on cystography, we use the pressure treatment, otherwise we advocate the intravesical instillation of formalin.

REFERENCES

1. Helmstein, K. Brit. J. Urol. 44, 434-450 (1972).

2. Brown, R. B. Med. J. Austral. 1, 23-24 (1969).

INTRAVESICAL HYPERTHERMIA FOR TRANSITIONAL CELL CARCINOMA OF THE BLADDER

R R HALL

Department of Urology
Newcastle General Hospital
Newcastle-upon-Tyne, England

INTRODUCTION

It is more than four years since we presented our initial observations concerning the use of local hyperthermia in the treatment of bladder carcinoma. I now wish to present the results of our continued use of this treatment modality.

METHOD

Treatment involved the irrigation of the bladder with isotonic saline at a temperature of 42-45°C for three hours daily for five to fourteen days.

RESULTS

Tumour Necrosis

Prior to 1975, 52 patients with multiple stage T1 tumours were treated in nine of whom total tumour necrosis occurred and a further 23 showed more than 50% necrosis of the tumours within the bladder. Eight patients with stage T3 disease were also treated, three of whom showed superficial tumour necrosis but no evidence of deep tumour destruction (Table 1).

From 1975 to 1977 a further 24 patients were treated for extensive multiple superficial stage T1 disease. The results were not as good as previously, only six out of twenty four showing

TABLE 1

INTRAVESICAL HYPERTHERMIA FOR BLADDER CARCINOMA

RESULTS

Tumour Stage	No. of Treatment	Tumour Necrosis			
		100%	>50%	<50%	Nil
T1 (O.A)	52	9	23	10	10
T3 (B2,C)	8	0	3	1	4

worthwhile tumour necrosis (Table 2). I think the reason for the poor results during this period was that all patients undergoing hyperthermia were selected by myself and only patients with very extensive multiple superficial tumours were included in the study. By this I mean patients who had tumours covering at least 60% of the bladder surface, in many of them the bladder mucosa being almost completely replaced by tumour. On closer examination, it is clear that prior to 1975 although all patients had had multiple tumours, these were frequently small, the majority of patients having between 10 and 20 tumours, each a few millimetres in diameter.

In the past we have received criticism of our treatment on the basis that we did not guarantee complete bladder distension during treatment so that some tumours might not be thoroughly irrigated. In the final 7 patients of our study, the bladder was distended with a minimum of 300 mls of saline throughout treatment. Of these 7 patients only 1 showed worthwhile tumour necrosis (Table 3).

TABLE 2

INTRAVESICAL HYPERTHERMIA FOR BLADDER CARCINOMA

RESULTS (1975 - 77)

Tumour Stage	No. of Treatments	Tumour Necrosis			
		100%	>50%	<50%	Nil
T1 (O.A)	24	2	4	3	15

TABLE 3

INTRAVESICAL HYPERTHERMIA FOR BLADDER CARCINOMA
WITH BLADDER DISTENSION

RESULTS

Tumour Stage	No. of Treatments	Tumour Necrosis 100%	> 50%	< 50%	Nil
T1 (O.A)	7	1	0	1	5

These figures are included in Table 2.

Long Term Follow-up

No patient developed bladder contracture, invasive tumour or any other acute or long term complication referable to hyperthermia treatment.

The recurrence of tumours in patients treated by hyperthermia was studied in 40 patients where data was available 1 year following initial hyperthermia (Table 4). Thirty-two of 40 patients had developed recurrences in the bladder within 1 year. Of the 11 patients where total tumour necrosis was achieved initially by hyperthermia only 1 patient is known to be tumour free.

TABLE 4

INTRAVESICAL HYPERTHERMIA FOR BLADDER CARCINOMA
RECURRENCE OF BLADDER TUMOURS

Overall recurrence rate within 1 year 32/40

Recurrence rate in patients with total
   tumour necrosis initially

   recurred within 1 year 6/11

   recurred after $3\frac{1}{2}$ years 1/11

   lost to follow-up 3/11

   tumour free 1/11

CONCLUSIONS

1.   As a primary form of therapy in patients with very extensive multiple superficial stage T1 bladder carcinoma, hyperthermic irrigation of the bladder by the method I have described, does not provide a worthwhile form of therapy. While significant tumour necrosis may be achieved in patients with less extensive disease these are easily treated endoscopically with the modern resectoscopes currently available.

2.   Hyperthermic irrigation of the bladder does not prevent subsequent recurrence of tumour in these high risk patients.

3.   It has been suggested that continuous irrigation of the bladder for a minimum of 15 hours might prove more effective than the repeated short treatments that we employed. This has not yet been evaluated.

HYPERTHERMIA AND BLADDER CANCER

G D CHISHOLM and J R HINDMARSH

Department of Urology, Western General Hospital
Edinburgh and Department of Surgery
University of Edinburgh

INTRODUCTION

The use of hyperthermia in the management of patients with
malignant disease has generally been regarded with suspicion by the
medical profession. Over 100 years ago it was suggested that heat
might have a role in killing malignant cells. 'Coley's toxin' had
a vogue and various methods have been used to produce a fever
(Nauts et al, 1953). More recently Crile (1961) and Henderson and
Pettigrew (1971) have re-examined the possible role for this form
of tumour control. Interest has focussed on a properly controlled
form of hyperthermia using both local and total body techniques.

There is an experimental basis for this interest in hyperthermia. Cancer cells, both in vitro and in vivo are more
susceptible to heat than the normal tissues. A temperature above
40°C is necessary, but the optimum temperature and its duration for
bladder tumours remains uncertain. Ludgate (1977) has attempted to
determine the optimum conditions for the use of local hyperthermia
and has shown using thymidine uptake studies in vitro incubating
at 44°C for four hours, that transitional cell tumours are more
sensitive than normal transitional cell epithelium to hyperthermic
stress. Tumour necrosis consisted of loss of intracellular
constituents and lysis of lysosomes.

Heat causes an inhibition of nucleic acid synthesis at 41°C
and irreparable damage above 43°C. Tumour cells will show a 50%
reduction in DNA after heating for one hour. The effect on the cell
cycle is variable and in vitro cell cycle arrest occurs at 40-41°C
but some cells are thermostable and can pass on this quality to
subsequent generations (Overgaard and Overgaard, 1972). It appears

271

that even a change of 0.5°C temperature significantly influences the results.   Inhibition of repair occurs at 42°C and is irreversible when combined with radiotherapy (Ben-Hur and Elkind, 1975) or chemotherapy (Palzer and Heidelberger, 1973) at 42°C for 1.5 hours. The rate of cell death is approximately proportional to the heat gradient and there is a 12% cell death per degree above 40°C.   Thus, both tumour and normal cells are killed at 48°C.

The duration of exposure of heat at 44°C has been assessed in relation to (bladder) tumour effect.   Ludgate (1977) showed that there was no tumour effect until after two hours at 44°C; three to four hours seem to be optimum.

The single exposure to heat was regarded as optimal as fractionated heat was found not to summate.

The immediate macroscopic changes in bladder tumours have also been studied.   After one hour at 44°C there is no change but after three to four hours at 44°C there is patchy damage to the tumour which appears white with ghost-like villi.   Macroscopic appearances after three days show that with heat for four hours at 44°C the necrosis is so advanced that it is difficult to recognise the tumour.

The histological changes after four hours of heat at 44°C show nuclear vacuolation, pyknosis with vacuolation of cytoplasm and a reduction in epithelial adhesiveness.   The depth of damage is directly related to the duration of heat.   There is a cellular infiltration, particularly eosinophils, similar to any thermal injury.

CLINICAL EXPERIENCE

Clinical experience with hyperthermia may be considered under four headings:-

1.   Local hyperthermia for tumour control a) primary treatment, b) recurrent tumour after radiotherapy.

2.   Local hyperthermia for bleeding a) bleeding alone or b) tumour recurrence plus bleeding.

3.   Local hyperthermia for enhancement of a) radiotherapy or b) chemotherapy.

4.   Total body hyperthermia for advanced (metastatic) disease.

1.   Local Hyperthermia for Tumour Control

a)   <u>Primary Treatment</u>.   In 1974, Hall et al. reported their experience with 32 patients: 30 had T1 tumours and two had T3 tumours. The bladder was irrigated through a 20 FG 3-way Foley catheter using normal saline at 2 1/hour with an outflow temperature of 45°C. Most patients received 12 daily treatments for three hours.

Four patients had no tumour after completing the course. Most of the others showed partial regression but five showed no effect. Both of the patients with invasive carcinoma underwent necrosis of the visible tumour mass.

Although the long-term result in one patient was encouraging, the results using hyperthermia for primary treatment, using different regimes, have been unsatisfactory and it is no longer recommended (Hall, 1978 - this volume).

b)   <u>Recurrent tumour</u>. The effect of hyperthermia in the management of patients with recurrent tumour after radiotherapy has been reported by Ludgate et al (1976). The technique differed from that used by Hall: the aim was to distend the bladder during treatment and therefore required continuous epidural anaesthesia. The bladder was perfused with normal saline using an outflow gradient of 15-20 cm above the symphysis pubis. The outflow temperature was 43°C in three patients and 44°C in the other 10 patients. Duration of perfusion ranged from one to four hours.

Gross haematuria was arrested in all cases. After three hours at 44°C there was obvious tumour necrosis; the grey-white slough took up to two months to separate.

After four hours perfusion at 44°C the patients developed frequency and contraction of the bladder with capacities of 50-70 ml. Some of these patients required a urinary diversion because of intolerable urinary frequency rather than because of the recurrent tumour.

It was concluded that overall tumour control was poor and that the problems due to bladder contraction greatly restricted any value from this type of treatment.

2.   Local Hyperthermia for Bleeding

Since there was some measure of control of bleeding in the series reported by Ludgate, the technique has continued to be used in the Urological Department, Western General Hospital, Edinburgh, for those patients with intractable bleeding after radiotherapy either with or without recurrent tumour.

Twelve patients have been treated, in 11 the bleeding was due to recurrent tumour, the other being due to radiation telangectasia. The two hourly treatments at 44°C produced urinary frequency which generally settled down after two weeks. Five patients were treated twice, one was treated three times and six patients had one treatment.

In eight patients, haematuria was arrested for six weeks to six months after which time the tumour cases had recurrent haematuria. The patient with post-radiation haematuria only, has remained free of bleeding. Thus, two-thirds of the patients have had a useful period without bleeding.

In a recent series of six patients using one hour at 45°C treatment, three were successful but side-effects of frequency and dysuria were marked.

3.   Local Hyperthermia and Enhancement

a)   <u>With Radiotherapy</u>. In 1967 Cockett et al.reported an experimental study wherein the exposed (normal) dog bladder was heated to 42-44°C and then irradiated (1,500 rad). This produced destruction of the epithelium; the mucosa was swollen and vacuolation of cells was seen. Late effects were thrombosis of blood vessels and the development of granulation tissue.

These authors reported their experiments with this form of palliation in seven elderly patients. Using the combination of 43°C and 4,500-5,000 rad there was good reduction in the size of the tumour mass but no other details were given.

b)   <u>With Chemotherapy</u>. Shingleton (1962) found using the VX-2 rabbit carcinoma that the effect of radioactivity during nitrogen mustard administration was greater when the tumours were heated than when cooled. He used an inductive electromagnetic heating unit raising the temperature to 42°C. In vivo studies on bladder tumours using intravesical thiotepa (Lunglmayr, 1973) showed that pre-heating of the bladder to 44°C before instillation produced a complete or partial response in 50% of cases. This was a higher response rate than achieved by normothermic instillations. Unfortunately the enhanced absorption rate of thiotepa produced a high incidence of side-effects, so limiting its usefulness.

4.   Whole Body Hyperthermia in Advanced Malignancy

Pettigrew et al (1974) have used molten wax at 50°C to produce a body temperature of 41.8°C. In a study of 38 patients the most sensitive tumours were those of the gastrointestinal tract and sarcomas. The results with two urological patients, one with a transitional cell tumour and the other with a nephroblastoma were not encouraging.

In their series, four deaths occurred within 48 hours of treatment and all but one were associated with extensive tumour necrosis. In addition, there were no cures and few complete clinical remissions. In general, the patients responding to treatment experienced a remarkable sense of well-being during the period of remission, with relief of tumour pain. This quality of life was felt to be the main justification for this procedure.

It was noted that following treatment at 42°C there was a rise in serum enzymes and a period of jaundice. This did not occur when the temperature was 41.8°C. Also in this series there appeared to be an enhanced effect when hyperthermia was combined with chemotherapy.

SUMMARY

Local hyperthermia in the treatment of bladder cancer may be considered under three headings:-

1. Therapy of primary or recurrent tumours after radiotherapy or other forms of treatment. The results have been unsatisfactory.

2. Control of bleeding. Gross haematuria is usually arrested but severe symptoms and even bladder contraction may develop

3. Enhancement of radiotherapy or chemotherapy. The association with radiotherapy was reported to be useful, but the experience is limited. The association with chemotherapy seems to produce both a higher control rate and a greater toxicity from absorption.

REFERENCES

1. Ben-Hur, E. and Elkind, M. M., Mechanism for enhanced radiation induced cell killing in hyperthermic mammalian cells. Proceeding of the 1st International Symposium on Cancer Therapy by Hyperthermia and Radiation. Washington D.C. April 28-30th 34-41 (1975).

2. Cockett, A. T. K., Kazmin, M., Nakamura, R., Fingerhutt, A. and Stein, J. J., Enhancement of regional bladder megavoltage irradiation in bladder cancer using local bladder hyperthermia. J. Urol. 97, 1034-1039 (1967).

3.   Crile, G. Jr., Heat as an adjunct to the treatment of cancer:
      Experimental studies. Cleveland Clinical Quarterly, 28, 75
      (1961).

4.   Hall, R. R., Schade, R. O. K. and Swinney, J., Effects of
      hyperthermia on bladder cancer. B.M.J. 3, 593-594 (1974).

5.   Henderson, M. A. and Pettigrew, R. T., Induction of controlled
      hyperthermia in treatment of cancer. Lancet, 1, 1275-1277
      (1971).

6.   Ludgate, C. M., The effect of induced hyperthermia in advanced
      malignant disease. M.D. Thesis University of Edinburgh.
      p 204 and 219-220 (1977).

7.   Ludgate, C. M., McLean, N., Carswell, G. F., Newsam, J. E.,
      Pettigrew, R. T. and Tullock, W. S. Hyperthermic perfusion of
      the distended urinary bladder in the management of recurrent
      transitional cell carcinoma. Brit. J. Urol. 47, 841-848
      (1976).

8.   Lunglmayr, G., Czech, K., Zekert, F. and Kellner, G. Bladder
      hyperthermia in the treatment of vesical papillomatosis. Int.
      Urol. and Neph. 5, 75-84 (1973).

9.   Moritz, A. R. Studies of thermal injury. III. The pathology
      and pathogenesis of cutaneous burn, an experimental study.
      Am. J. Path. 23, 915-934 (1947).

10.   Nauts, H. C., Fowler, E. A. and Bogatko, F. H. A review of
      the influence of bacterial infections and of bacterial products
      (Coley's toxin) on malignant tumours in man. Acta. Med. Scand.
      145, Supplement 276 (1953).

11.   Overgaard, K. and Overgaard, J. Investigations on the
      possibility of a thermic tumour therapy. I: Short-wave
      treatment of a transplanted isologous mouse mammary carcinoma
      Eur. J. Cancer, 8, 65-78 (1972).

12.   Palzer, R. J. and Heidelberger, C. Influence of drugs and
      synchrony on the hyperthermic killing of Hela cells. Cancer
      Res. 33, 422-427 (1973).

13.   Pettigrew, R. T., Galt, J. M., Ludgate, C. M. and Smith, A. N.,
      Clinical effects of whole body hyperthermia in advanced
      malignancy. B.M.J. 4, 679-682 (1974).

14.   Shingleton, W. W., Selective heating and cooling of the tissue
      in cancer chemotherapy. Ann. Surg. 156, 408 (1966).

Editorial Note (PHS)   Attitudes to intravesical Formalin
varied. Camey had used 3% Formalin for 30 minutes without good
results. Blandy used 10% solution of conventional Formalin and
England (London) suggested that Formalin was preferable to the
Helmstein method as it was much simpler from the patient. Hall
(Newcastle) had used 10% Formalin and had noted anuria for 48 hours.
Attention was also drawn to the possible use of DMSO in controlling
the symptoms of post irradiation cystitis.

RADIOTHERAPY IN THE MANAGEMENT OF BLADDER CARCINOMA

F EDSMYR, P-L ESPOSTI and L ANDERSSON

The Radiumhemmet and the Department of Urology

Karolinska Hospital, Stockholm, Sweden

INTRODUCTION

At the Karolinska Hospital in Stockholm in the fifties a surgically treated series of patients with category T3 tumours showed a five year survival rate of 6%. Because of the disappointing results of surgery in treatment of patients with advanced bladder carcinoma, radiation therapy was introduced at the Radiumhemmet in Stockholm in 1957. This report covers a total number of 598 patients treated with full irradiation between 1957 and 1970, analysed and followed for at least five years or to death.

All tumours were histo-pathologically verified as carcinomas. The patients were clinically free of metastases at first diagnosis and have been categorized by the TNM system recommended by UICC in 1974.

In category T2 tumours, all the poorly differentiated and the largest of the highly differentiated types were selected for irradiation. All patients admitted without clinical metastases in categories T3 and T4 received irradiation.

TREATMENT METHODS

Radiotherapy consisted of external irradiation of either Cobalt-60 gamma rays in 1957 - 1968 or 6 MV X-rays in 1969 - 1970. The patients have in general been treated throughout with a calculated mean tumour dose of 6000 - 7000 rads over 7 - 8 weeks. The weekly tumour dose was 900 - 1000 rads given in five days. An individual irradiation plan was worked out for each case based on

the anatomical outlines of the patient in a horizontal section
through the centre of the treatment region. The regional lymph
node chains were considered to have been included in the irradiated
area defined as 75% of the average tumour dose.

RESULTS

Our results indicate that patients with transitional cell
carcinoma of the bladder treated by a full course of irradiation
have a significantly worse prognosis if the tumour is of higher
grade or T-category. The differences in survival rate at five and
ten years are high and significantly related to grades and
T-categories, whether assessed together or separately. The deaths
are mainly due to cancer (Table 1).

The complication rate after full dose irradiation is low.
Surgical intervention for complication has been necessary within
three years after therapy in only 1.2% (7 cases).

The quality of life seems to be good both at five and ten
years after irradiation when the patients are free of tumour.

Cystectomy with Bricker diversion was performed in 47 patients
six months to five years after irradiation. 36 of these patients
died of cancer and four of intercurrent disease. The remaining
seven lived more than five years after cystectomy and had superficial
tumour in the cystectomy specimen. The patients who died with
cancer all had tumour infiltrating deeply into the muscle layer of
the bladder wall.

The full details of this study are to be published in
Urological Research 1979.

TABLE 1

PERCENTAGE SURVIVAL AT FIVE AND TEN YEARS

FOLLOWING RADIOTHERAPY

Survival	Category			Grade	
	T2	T3	T4	G2	G3
5 YRS	31	20	10	26	18
10 YRS	22	14	4	19	13

CARCINOMA OF THE BLADDER CATEGORY T3 NX, 0-4 MO TREATED BY PRE-
OPERATIVE IRRADIATION FOLLOWED BY CYSTECTOMY AT THE ROTTERDAM
RADIOTHERAPY INSTITUTE

B   VAN DER WERF-MESSING

Rotterdam Radiotherapy Institute
Groene Hilledijk 297
Rotterdam, The Netherlands

SUMMARY

141 Patients with carcinoma of the bladder category T3 MO
were treated by preoperative irradiation (4000 rad in 4 weeks)
followed by simple cystectomy   Up to 1973 the preoperative
irradiation was applied to the true pelvis. After that period the
field was extended so as to include the region of lumbar 5. Surgery
was performed as soon as possible (preferably within a week after
finishing radiotherapy) but due to various circumstances it was
delayed in some cases up to 40 days.

The most important preoperative prognostic factors were age,
degree of differentiation, urographic findings and field size. The
prognosis worsened with increasing grade, urinary tract dilatation
and with the large field of radiotherapy, especially in older
patients.

Of the factors assessed after cystectomy, which influenced
prognosis significantly, the most important was T-reduction,
i.e. the diminishing of the depth of infiltration due to the preoperative irradiation. Less important but still influencing
prognosis were again age, degree of differentiation of the growth,
urological findings, the size of the irradiation field and the
interval between the end of irradiation and the cystectomy.

The most important postoperative factor, T-reduction, apparently
reflected the influence of irradiation on involved lymph nodes (no
lymphadenectomy was done) as in patients with T-reduction death with
involved lymph nodes was significantly lower than in cases without
T-reduction (7% and 40% respectively).

So far no reliable criterion has been found to predict
T-reduction but it can be stated that T-reduction is not due to
clinical staging error. In cases with T-reduction survival was
identical whether or not there was carcinoma in the biopsy specimen.
This biopsy was not always taken with the intent to include muscle.
A multifactorial analysis allows one to predict prognosis by preoperative factors and by postoperative factors.

The complete publication of this presentation will appear as
the del Regato lecture in Radiation Oncology Biology Physics.

SURGICAL TREATMENT OF 81 DEEP INFILTRATING BLADDER TUMOURS AFTER

PREOPERATIVE IRRADIATION

D TJABBES

Wassenaarseweg 93

Gravenhage, The Netherlands

Since 1964 deep infiltrating bladder tumours (category T3) have
been treated in our hospital with a combination of preoperative
irradiation and cystectomy. From 1964-1968 the patients received
6,000 rads followed after three months by cystectomy. Since 1968
irradiation has been restricted to 4,500 rads rotating telecobalt,
immediately followed by a subradical or total cystectomy. This
includes the prostate, uterus and vaginal wall but not radical
removal of the regional nodes. Urethrectomy was not performed unless
there was a history of frequent recurrences. With this technique
we are able to preserve and restore the pelvic peritoneum which
prevents some of the complications. We consider this preferable to
radical lymph node removal, as the small advantage of radicality in
case of a solitary lymphatic metastasis is more than outweighed by
the increase of complications. The results demonstrate the benefit

TABLE I

SUBRADICAL SURGERY OF DEEP INFILTRATING BLADDER TUMOURS (T3 No Mo)

Patients	Preoperative Irradiation	Operation	5 year Actuarial Survival
17	None	Cystectomy	20%
14	6,000 rads	Cystectomy	27%
48	4,500 rads	Cystectomy	45%

TABLE II

RESULTS OF SUBRADICAL CYSTECTOMY AFTER 4,500 RADS PREOPERATIVE
IRRADIATION OF DEEP INFILTRATING BLADDER TUMOURS T3 No Mo
(48 PATIENTS)

Living Without Tumour	48%	Tumour Cured	64%
Dead without Tumour	16%		
Operative Mortality	8%	Failed Treatment	32%
Dead with Tumour	24%		
Lost to Follow-up	4%		

of the combination of radiotherapy with cystectomy and show clear
differences in survival between the two radiotherapy regimes. In
addition, two patients who at operation were found to have a
positive node and who were treated by radical cystectomy died within
a year (Table I).

Real tumour cure rate is even better, as most patients are in
the age group over 65, and 16% died of unrelated causes without
evidence of tumour. The real tumour cure rate was 64%, with failure
of treatment in 32% (Table II).

The complications were acceptable: 7% died within one month
after operation; the causes were not related to the preoperative
irradiation. In 7% there were nonfatal postoperative complications,
which were probably related to the irradiation (Table III). No
wound ruptures were seen as we use a Pfannenstiel incision with
interchanging layers.

Late complications were seen in 18%. Rectal fistula and
osteitis pubis were probably caused by the combined treatment of
surgery and irradiation. All cases of osteitis recovered without
surgical intervention.

From the figures it would seem that limitation of the
extension of the fields of irradiation and of the radicality of
the operation do not reduce the survival rate.

TABLE III

COMPLICATIONS OF CYSTECTOMY AFTER PREOPERATIVE IRRADIATION WITH

4,500 RADS (48 PATIENTS)

EARLY COMPLICATIONS

Operative Mortality 7%

Cardiac	1 patient
Urosepsis	1 patient
Stress Ulcer	1 patient

Operative Morbidity 7%

Rectal Tear	1 patient
Ileus	1 patient
Faecal Fistula	1 patient

LATE COMPLICATIONS 18%

Renal Stones	2 Patients
Ureteral Stenosis	2 Patients
Rectal Fistula	1 Patient
Osteitis Pubis	3 Patients

CONCLUSIONS

From 1968 to 1978 48 patients were treated with total cystectomy immediately after rotating telecobalt irradiation with 4,500 rads. The results (45% 5-year survival) are at least as good as after radical cystectomy and there are fewer complications.

CYSTECTOMY FOLLOWING FULL COURSE IRRADIATION

F LUND

University Hospital

Copenhagen, Denmark

INTRODUCTION

Few surgeons - if any - deliberately embark on an apparently hazardous course of action, and yet situations do arise where circumstances force the reluctant surgeon to take on the task and run the risk. Performing a total cystectomy on a patient previously exposed to a full course of radiotherapy to the bladder implies increased complication rates, but it may nevertheless be strongly indicated to relieve the patient of severe and painful symptoms.

The following report deals with a series of patients where cystectomy has been the ultimate solution to their problems.

CLINICAL MATERIAL

From 1968 to 1970 a total of 429 patients with carcinoma of the bladder received radiotherapy totalling 6000 rad in five to six weeks given by a linear accelerator of 6 MeV (Walbom, 1972). The indications for treatment were histologically proven tumours (i) classified as T3 or T4, or with a histological malignancy grades III or IV regardless of the clinical classification, (ii) tumours not suitable for surgical treatment because of advanced age or poor general condition and (iii) tumours which had been treated by non radical surgical procedures. The three years survival rate for T3 tumours was 30%.

During the years of follow up some of the patients developed bladder symptoms of such an extent and severity that additional treatment was forced upon us.

TABLE I

TUMOUR CLASSIFICATION (UICC) IN 101 PATIENTS

UNDERGOING SECONDARY CYSTECTOMY

To	Tis	T1	T2	T3	T4	Not Known
3	8	31	8	40	10	1

Roughly 5% of the patients developed contracted bladders with frequency and urgency, often combined with haematuria caused by the radiotherapy. A similar number of patients developed recurrent tumours with symptoms severe enough to demand operation.

Despite the fact that secondary surgery has been considered hazardous by Higgins et al. (1966) and Edsmyr et al. (1971), a total of 101 patients were treated by cystectomy. The interval between the termination of radiotherapy and the surgical procedure averaged one year (5 months to 5 years). The classification of the tumours at the time of operation is shown in Table I, the majority being classified as T3 grade III tumours.

The cystectomy generally included prostatectomy in the males, and the urinary diversion was performed as a cutaneous uretero-ileostomy according to Bricker (1950) with 5-0 Dexon sutures. Perivesical fibrosis was always present to a varying degree, creating difficulty in dissecting the bladder. Lymph nodes were never seen or palpated after the irradiation! Many patients showed irradiation changes in the small bowel, and we rapidly learned to stay away from the field of irradiation.

The cumulative survival is shown in Figure 1. Apart from seven patients who died due to postoperative complications (gangrene of the ileal loop, anastomotic leakage, severe infection and cerebro-vascular catastrophies), a further 44 patients died during the first 12 months. These were almost exclusively those who had recurrent or residual tumour growth in the bladder at the time of the operation.

The patients with a contracted, bleeding bladder without tumour fared much better and following the first year of survival they approached the standard survival curve for corresponding age groups.

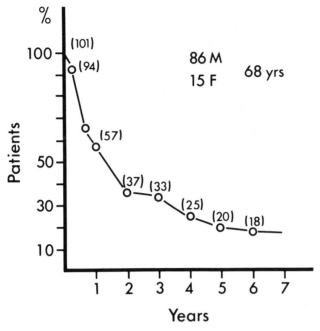

FIGURE 1

CONCLUSIONS

Total cystectomy following a full course of radiotherapy can be undertaken at an acceptable risk in terms of the complication rate. However secondary surgery (salvage surgery) as an attempt to cure the patient after failure of radiotherapy has given disappointing and unfavourable results and in our view radical surgery should be restricted to those cases in which operation is indicated because of intolerable symptoms such as contracted bladder or severe bleeding. Here the results and the survival rate seem to justify the surgical intervention.

REFERENCES

1. Bricker, E.M. Surg. Clin. N. Am. 30, 1511 (1950).

2. Edsmyr, F. et al. Scand. J. Urol. Nephrol. 5, 215 (1971).

3. Higgins, P. M. et al. Brit. J. Urol. 38, 311 (1966).

4. Walbom-Jørgensen, S. Scand. J. Urol. Nephrol. 6, suppl. 15, 113 (1972).

COMPLICATIONS OF IRRADIATION OF UROLOGICAL TUMOURS

F EDSMYR, C LAGERGREN and R WALSTAM

The Radiumhemmet, the Roentgendiagnostic Department and
the Institute of Radiophysics, Karolinska Sjukhuset
Stockholm, Sweden

INTRODUCTION

Using irradiation at the doses needed for destruction of
malignant tissue the borderline of tolerance in the normal tissues
is narrow and a systematic investigation of urological tumours to
investigate complications after radiotherapy is being undertaken in
Stockholm. The investigation of 598 patients with bladder
carcinomas, some followed over 15 years, has been completed and is
now continuing with over 400 testicular tumours, some followed over
30 years, and kidney tumours after pre- or postoperative irradiation.
This report concentrates on the patients with bladder carcinoma
treated with different models of irradiation.

TREATMENT

Treatment in all patients has been individually planned. The
tumour area includes the whole bladder with a wide margin in all
categories. The first lymph node station will be circumscribed at
the 75% isodose curve. The mean calculated dose is 6400 rads in
7 - 8 weeks using the three-field technique with cobalt-60 unit,
irradiating only one field daily without a rest period. The
regional lymph nodes and sigmoid bowel receive a calculated dose of
5500 rads.

COMPLICATIONS

1. Complications in the Bowel

From 1957 to 1970, 598 patients were treated with full irradiation. 130 have been examined by barium enema, before and after therapy. The observation time is over five years after the therapy.

Patients with a shorter interval than four months between investigations are excluded, since when the irradiation is completed oedema occurs, giving pseudostricture and thickening of presacral soft tissue. The X-ray picture returns to normal when the oedema disappears.

A. Complications not requiring surgical intervention
(a) Reduced capability of distension. A certain degree of reduced distensibility is often noticed at the recto-sigmoid junction. This is usually asymptomatic, but pain can occur with constipation. The reduced distensibility remains for many years. (b) Rectal irritation. In addition to reduced capability of distension, more frequent haustration in the distal part of sigmoid occurs as an expression of irritation. (c) Diverticulitis together with a strong irritability with frequent haustration in the distal part of sigmoid is often observed. In Scandinavia, diverticulitis of the sigmoid region is very common, increasing with age up to 50% incidence in the very old. The patients in this series had the same incidence. In no case did patients with diverticulitis before commencement of therapy become worse later on. (d) Stricture associated with clinical symptoms has been observed in a few cases because of reduced distensibility (Table 1).

B. Complications giving rise to surgical intervention
Because of ileus or bleeding, seven patients (1.1%) have required operation. In four cases abdominal surgery likely to cause adhesions had previously been performed. The complications have occurred within three years of irradiation with a mean time of one and a half years (Table 2).

2. Complications in the Upper Urinary Tract

The series comprises a study of 111 patients, where both ureteric orifices received the same radiation dose in every instance.

The outflow through healthy orifices not infiltrated by tumour is not impaired by the radiation therapy.

TABLE 1

BLADDER CARCINOMA

COMPLICATIONS AFFECTING THE BOWEL

1957 - 1970

Reduced distensibility	10/130
Rectal irritation	3/130
Diverticulitis	3/130
Strictures not requiring surgery	3/130
Strictures requiring surgical intervention	7/598

TABLE 2

COMPLICATIONS REQUIRING SURGICAL INTERVENTION

Stage	Age Years	Previous Abdominal Surgery	Months After Irrad- iation	Compli- cation	Surgery
T2	42	-	18	adhesions	ileotransverse colostomy
T3	57	+	4	adhesions	entero- anastomosis
T3	64	-	10	stricture	colostomy
T3	56	+	14	stricture	transverse colostomy
T3	70	-	18	stricture	transverse colostomy
T3	57	+	30	stricture	ileotransverse colostomy
T3	59	+	36	stricture	ileal resection

An impairment in outflow after the treatment almost always reflects progression of the tumour (Edsmyr, Giertz and Nilsson 1967).

3. Vesico-Ureteric Reflux

Seventy-six patients have been examined with micturating cystography with roll film, taking one exposure every third second, using Urografin 17 per cent combined with Periodal Viscous 35 per cent as contrast medium. The time elapsing between therapy and the reflux study was up to seven years.

The frequency of reflux was low in patients whose orifices were without tumour growth (three of 44). In one of these an extensive resection had been performed around the contralateral orifice, with reimplantation of the corresponding ureter. It cannot be ruled out that changes in the anatomy of the bladder fundus, resulting from the operation, had been responsible for reflux on the opposite side.

Reflux was evident in a large proportion of the patients whose ureteric orifices were involved by the tumour growth.

Dilatation of the upper urinary tract was observed in three of 25 patients with reflux. No implantation metastases were discovered in the upper urinary tract (Edsmyr and Nilsson 1965).

4. Complications Involving the Femoral Neck

The bone mineral content of the femoral neck was determined by roentgen spectrophotometry in 12 patients before, during and after therapy. The mineral content was followed for an average of 6 months.

These patients received doses ranging from 2800 rads in 5 days (short time treatment) to 8400 rads in two months (superfractionation).

The mean reduction in the bone mineral content of 1.8 per cent is compared with the normal reduction with age. It seems that this type of treatment will not produce radiation injuries to the femoral neck, at least during the first year of treatment.

No fracture has been observed during over 10 years of follow-up in a series of 598 patients (Dalen and Edsmyr 1974).

5. Complications in the Inguinal Region

In 75 of 598 patients (13%) inguinal and sacral fibrosis have been observed. The patients had difficulty in moving and in bending down with swelling of the legs. The technique of therapy during the years has been:-

1957 - 1961	pendulum technique Co-60	2/50	or 4%
1961 - 1968	three-field technique Co-60	71/470	or 15%
1968 - 1970	three-field technique 6 MV X-ray	2/78	or 3%

The increased frequency of serious inguinal reactions in the group treated by the three-field technique using Co-60 as compared to the group treated by the 6 MV X-ray may possibly be explained by the difference in dose distribution. Due to a longer source-skin distance (SSD) and higher photon energy at the linear accelerator the relative depth dose is higher and therefore the dose given at each portal is lower, resulting in an increased skin sparing effect.

These conditions, illustrated in Fig. 1, show an example of the dose distribution in a tumour section. The left hand side illustrates the dose distribution for the linear accelerator at 100 cm SSD, the right hand the same for a Co-60 unit working at 80 cm SSD. The reference doses are approximately 25 per cent higher for the Co-60 plan and the subcutaneous maximum dose is for Co-60 approximately 95 per cent of the tumour dose while for the linear accelerator it is less than 85 per cent. This difference is probably responsible for the difference in results.

There is, however, another important factor which has to be considered. The irradiation technique is based on a "one field a day" scheme, which means an unfavourable fractionation at the areas where the beams enter, i.e. in the inguinal regions. This can be shown by applying the Ellis formula or a similar hypothesis for the fractionation.

Fig. 2 illustrates such a comparison for a Co-60 treatment. To the left the dose distribution in rads is given, to the right the biological effect curves in radiation equivalent units (reu), both expressed in per cent of the tumour dose.

The subcutaneous effect-maximum for the illustrated three-field technique might be reduced by 10 - 20 per cent by irradiating all three fields simultaneously instead of irradiating only one field daily. This change in fractionation should have a greater

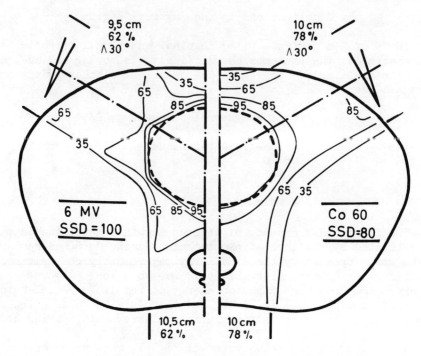

FIGURE 1

The dose distribution in a tumour section. The left hand side
illustrates the dose distribution for the linear accelerator at
100 cm SSD, the right hand the same for a Co-60 unit working at
80 cm SSD.

influence on the reaction in the inguinal region than the difference
in dose distribution between Co-60 and 6 MV X-rays. That is, of
course, if the fractionation hypothesis used is true.

SUMMARY

    An investigation has been performed to assess the complications
after radiotherapy in 598 patients with bladder carcinoma treated
at the Radiumhemmet in Stockholm from 1957 through 1970.

    The complications in the bowel are few and only in seven
patients has surgical intervention been necessary. The flow of
urine through healthy ureteral orifices not infiltrated by tumour
is not impaired by the radiation therapy and impairment always
reflects progression of the tumour.

    The frequency of reflux was low in the orifices without tumour

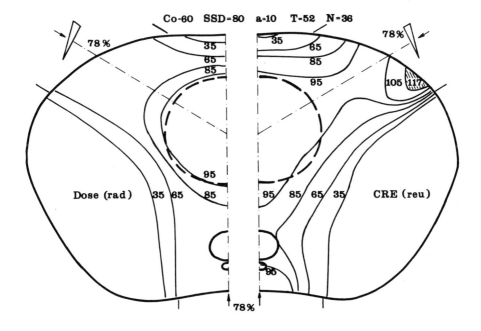

FIGURE 2

The irradiation technique based on a 'one-field a day' scheme. A
comparison for a Co-60 treatment: to the left the dose distribution
in rad, to the right the biological effect curves in reu, both
expressed in percent of the tumour dose.

growth but was evident in a large proportion of the orifices with
tumour.

The bone mineral content of the femoral neck shows no unexpected
reduction after therapy.

In our total series, inguinal fibrosis has been observed in
13 per cent. The majority of patients have been treated with a
three-field technique with Co-60, where one field has been
irradiated daily. The future recommendation will be irradiation
of all three fields every day to prevent these complications.

REFERENCES

1.   Dalen, N. and Edsmyr, F., Bone mineral content of the femoral
      neck after irradiation. Acta Radiol., 2, 97 - 101 (1974).

2.   Edsmyr, F. and Nilsson, A.E., Vesico-ureteric reflux in
     connection with supervoltage therapy for bladder carcinoma.
     Acta Radiol., 6, 449 - 456 (1965).

3.   Edsmyr, F., Giertz, G. and Nilsson, A.E., Effect of super-
     voltage therapy for carcinoma of the bladder on the outflow
     from upper urinary tract to bladder. Scand. J. Urol. Nephrol.,
     1, 247 - 252 (1967).

POST-DIVERSION, PRE-CYSTECTOMY IRRADIATION FOR TRANSITIONAL CELL CARCINOMA OF THE BLADDER

G RUTISHAUSER

Chief, Division of Urology, Department of Surgery

University of Basel, CH 4031 Basel, Switzerland

INTRODUCTION

The Division of Urology of the Surgical Department of the University of Basel treats about 70 patients a year with different stages of transitional cell carcinoma of the bladder on an in-patients basis (Table I).

In about half these patients the aim of the treatment is curative (patients with category T1-3 lesions). In four fifths of this group treatment consists of one or more sessions of trans-urethral resection (TUR) with or without postoperative irradiation.

TABLE I

PATIENTS WITH TRANSITIONAL CELL CARCINOMA OF

THE BLADDER TREATED IN 1974-76 (ALL STAGES)

	1974	1975	1976
TOTAL	60	84	87
Tis T1	19	32	38
T2 T3	34	42	38
T4	7	10	11

In about one fifth the decision for cystectomy is made. Since 1974 we have performed this operation in two stages. Cystectomy is preceded by some form of urinary diversion (usually by ileal-conduit) and high voltage irradiation of the bladder. Up to 1978, 20 patients have been treated by urinary diversion + 5500 rads pre-cystectomy irradiation delivered by a linear accelerator (8 MeV linac-photons) followed two to four weeks later by cystectomy. This paper gives a review of some problems with the first 12 patients of this group, treated in 1974 and 1975.

TREATMENT

This treatment is applied in the following way: first the usual staging-procedures (urography, cystoscopy, bimanual examination under general anaesthesia and lymphography) are performed followed by a diagnostic TUR during which the tumour is resected as radically as possible in one session. The urinary diversion is then carried out together with lymph node biopsy (iliac and external/internal iliac bifurcation).

Two to three weeks later, irradiation starts with daily doses of 180-200 rads up to a total dose of 5500 rads. Cystectomy is performed 3-4 weeks after the end of the irradiation.

In this first group of patients this treatment-concept has as yet brought no advantages in terms of survival since even though there was no post-operative mortality only 60% of the patients were alive after the first year. This is 10% less than with our conventional treatment of TUR and postoperative irradiation (Figure 1).

What are the main problems of cystectomy with preoperative irradiation?

One serious problem is the exact clinical assessment of the tumour-stage. We stand in admiration of all those who carry out this staging procedure with apparent ease and good results. In our hands it seems difficult and we understaged about two thirds of our patients. Overstaging was seen only in one case. In our opinion clinical staging remains one of the big problems in all statistical evaluation of bladder tumour treatment results.

Several authors have shown that prognosis in patients in whom preoperative irradiation reduces the tumour stage, is especially good. Van der Werf-Messing saw a five year survival rate of 70% and Prout of 60% in this special patient group.

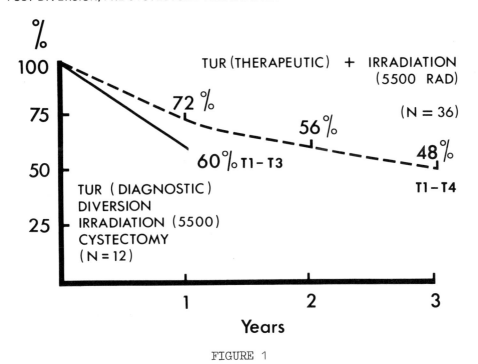

FIGURE 1

TCC OF THE BLADDER   SURVIVAL RATE 1-3 YEARS

In seven of our 12 cases we too got the impression of a stage reduction. But is this stage reduction really a consequence of irradiation or is it not rather, at least in part, the effect of the diagnostic TUR?

As yet we have not been convinced that the interpretation of Van der Werf-Messing, ie. of stage reduction by preoperative irradiation, is unchallengable.

If her views are correct and if stage reduction by preoperative irradiation does give a better prognosis we can only say that in our cases the impact of this stage reduction has not been as impressive as it is said to be (Figure 1). The problem, which concerns us much more than that of staging error, is the very high complication rate after cystectomy. This complication rate is definitely higher than is generally mentioned in the literature where figures between 20-30% are given. Exceptions are Miller (80%) and Genster. The latter told us personally that he also has a very high complication rate.

TABLE II

EARLY POSTOPERATIVE COMPLICATIONS IN 12 PATIENTS AFTER URINARY

DIVERSION, PRECYSTECTOMY IRRADIATION (5500 RAD) AND CYSTECTOMY

			PATIENTS
COMPLICATIONS			10 (83%)
TOTAL	SECONDARY WOUND HEALING	7	
	SEPSIS	1	
	INCISIONAL HERNIA + ILEUS	1	
	INTESTINAL PERFORATION	2	
	PYELONEPHRITIC ATTACKS	2	
NECESSITATING REOPERATION			7 (58%)
	MINOR OPERATIONS FOR DRAINAGE	8	
	FAECAL FISTULA		
	INCISIONAL HERNIA + ILEUS	1	

In our first group more than 80% had complications and 60% required at least one further operation (Table II).

This serious complication rate has to be lowered. Probably we will be obliged to reduce the irradiation dose. We hope that this meeting gives us ideas as to how better results can be obtained with precystectomy irradiation which theoretically should be superior to an adjuvant postoperative high voltage treatment.

SUMMARY

The urological division of the surgical department of the University of Basel hospitalises about 70 patients with bladder cancer each year. Only in half of them can curative treatment be attempted.

Over the past 20 years, different and newer methods of treatment (TUR, implantation of radio-gold seeds, cystectomy and betatron-irradiation) have not significantly improved the results and it seems that the tumour-stage at the moment of diagnosis is more important than the therapeutic method used.

Today, most of our patients (85%) are treated by TUR and external high-voltage irradiation with a linear accelerator. Only 15% have open interventions, some being treated by partial cystectomy in cases with special tumour localisation. The rest are treated by urinary diversion, followed by total cystectomy after preoperative high-voltage irradiation.

The three year results after TUR with irradiation, are fair and do not differ much from those presented in the literature. The results for cystectomy with rather heavy preoperative irradiation (5500-6000 rads) cannot yet be definitely analysed. As yet the trend in survival is no better than in the group with TUR and post-operative irradiation, whereas the complication rate is much higher and must be analysed very carefully. In addition, analysis of clinical "down-staging" after preoperative x-ray treatment must take into account the fact that these patients had quite a radical diagnostic TUR before their radiotherapy.

REFERENCES

1. Genster, H. G., Mommsen, S. and Hoisgaard, A., Zystectomie beim Blasencarcinom. Verhandlungsber. Dtsch. Ges. Urol. 1978, 29. Tagung Stuttgart 21, 24.9.77, 90-91. Springer Verlag, Heidelberg, Berlin, New York 1978.

2. Mahoney, E. M., Weber, E. T. and Harrison, H. J. J. Urol. 114, 46-49 (1975).

3. Miller, L. S. Cancer, 39, 973-980 (1977).

4. Prout, G. R., Slack, N. H. and Bross, J. D. J. Urol. 104, 116-121 (1970).

5. Prout, G. R., Slack, N. H. and Bross, J. D. J. Urol. 105, 223-230 (1971).

6. Van der Werf-Messing, B. Cancer, 32, 1084-1087 (1973).

7. Van der Werf-Messing, B. Cancer, 36, 718-722 (1975).

8. Whitmore, W. F., Front. Radiation Ther. Oncol. 5, 231-239 (1970).

TREATMENT OF MALIGNANT TUMOURS OF THE BLADDER BY IRIDIUM 192 WIRING

J AUVERT and H BOTTO

Hopital Henri Mondor

Creteil, Paris, France

INTRODUCTION

Frequent recurrences of malignant tumours of the bladder after transurethral resection or partial cystectomy have led to the use of complementary irradiation. In small cancers, showing early infiltration of the bladder wall, many attempts have been made to replace external by interstitial irradiation, which delivers a high radiation dosage to the pathological area but does not damage the whole bladder.

Radium needles were used in France by Darget before 1951 (5) but accurate dosage was difficult; the material was dangerous to the surgeon's hands and the procedure frequently led to bladder sclerosis. The technique is still used by Professor van der Werf-Messing in Rotterdam (15) and she strongly recommends pre-operative external irradiation (3 x 350 rads) to prevent implantation of tumour in the scar.

Further attempts using an intravesical balloon filled with a liquid radioisotope of Gold 198 or Cobalt 60 aimed against diffuse superficial malignant papillary tumours were abandoned due to radiation cystitis and subsequent contraction of the bladder. Recently Bloom and Wallace have used Tantalum 182 needles (3), which have a low energy and a short half life, for localised tumours.

Isotopic Iridium 192 wires have a similar activity to Tantalum and a half life of 7.4 days, a low energy gamma irradiation of 0.3 Mev and a Half Attenuation Constant of only 0.2 mm of lead (Table I). In addition the technique of inserting the wires is completely harmless to the surgeon's hands. For those physical

305

TABLE I

A COMPARISON BETWEEN Ra 226 - Au 198 - Ir 192 - Ta 182

	Half Life	Mev	H.tt.C. (mm Pb)
Radium	1620 years	1.4	1.2
Gold	2.7 days	0.4	0.3
Iridium	74 days	0.3	0.2
Tantalum	115 days	1.1	1

reasons and also because of the low price of this radio-isotope, Iridium 192 was chosen as the best interstitial irradiation agent for the treatment of small tumours of stage A or B1 (Jewett) - category T1-T2 (TNM), whose diameter does not exceed 4 cm, which are located in the mobile portion of the bladder and which show superficial infiltration of the bladder wall. When using the wires one should remember that the active zone is 1 cm broad (that is 5 mm each side of the wire).

TECHNIQUE

    This was first described in 1968 (10) and again in 1970 (14). After transurethral resection of the tumour for pathological examination and subsequent cystotomy plastic tubes are inserted into the bladder wall, with a big curved needle, on each side of the site of implantation of the tumour. Lead wires are secured at the place where the iridium wires will later be introduced. If a significant part of the tumour remains, a partial cystectomy is performed before the wiring. The ends of the plastic tubes lead out of the bladder through the cystotomy opening around a cystostomy tube. Following the Dutch recommendation, we irradiate the pelvis before operation by a two days' flash radiotherapy of twice 650 rads. Before opening the bladder we recommend a careful lymph node dissection of the pelvis for accurate staging. Lymph node dissection was carried out in 18 of the 26 cases in our series (Table II). Of these only one showed lymph node invasion (two lymph nodes were positive) and for this reason the patient also received post-operative irradiation (4,500 rads in four weeks) (Table III). In two cases the operation began by a prostatectomy after which the wiring was carried out. Three ureters required reimplantation into the bladder.

TABLE II

TREATMENT IN 26 PATIENTS

TUR Biopsy	26
Flash Radiotherapy (650 x 2 rads)	20
Cystotomy	26
Partial Cystectomy	16
Lymph Node Dissection	18

	N-	N+
	17	1
Post-op. Irradiation		1

Five or six days after operation the patient is transferred to the radiotherapy department. AP and lateral x-rays allow accurate computer calculation of the isodose (8,11). At this stage the inactive lead wires are replaced by active Iridium 192 wires and these are maintained in poistion for two to four days. During this time the target volume receives 7,000 rads. All the material is finally removed and the bladder closes spontaneously after indwelling urethral catheterisation for a few days. We have used the wiring technique only for the tumours of the mobile part of the bladder, ie. the dome or lateral walls. In our view, infiltrating tumours of the trigone are better treated by total cystectomy.

TABLE III

T-CATEGORY AND LYMPH NODE DISSECTION IN 26 PATIENTS WITH TUMOURS

OF THE MOBILE PORTION OF THE BLADDER TREATED BY IR 192 WIRING

Staging	No cases (26)	Lymph Node Dissection (18)	N-	N+
T1	15	8	8	0
T2	7	6	5	1
T3	2	2	2	
T2 - P3	2	2	2	

CLINICAL EXPERIENCE

Our clinical experience in six years includes 26 cases (23 males and three females). The most common age at presentation is between 50 and 60 years (12 cases). The treatment is suitable only for solitary tumours whose diameter must not exceed 4 cms and localised to the mobile portion of the bladder. Of the tumours treated, two were on the dome, 16 on the right lateral wall and eight on the left lateral wall. The left ureter was reimplanted on three occasions. In 15 patients the tumours were Jewett Stage A (Category T1), in seven Jewett B1 (Category T2) and in four cases Jewett B2 (Category T3). Most tumours were poorly differentiated (Category G2/3). After Iridium wiring the patients were followed up by cystoscopy every three months for the first year, then twice a year. When recurrence was suspected photography and biopsy were carried out.

RESULTS

Though considered as a simple surgical procedure, Iridium wiring of the bladder in our 26 cases was followed by two post-operative deaths during the first week (cardiac infarction - 1, pulmonary embolism - 1). Three other patients have since died of metastasis and one of cirrhosis (Table IV). Of these, the local tumour was controlled in the cirrhotic patient and in two of those with metastasis.

TABLE IV

FOLLOW-UP OF 26 BLADDER TUMOURS AFTER SURGERY + IRIDIUM 192 WIRING

	Years						
	0	1	2	3	4	5	6 7
No of cases (26)	26	24	17	16	11	7	3
Patient's first recurrence (5)		1	1	1	1	1	
Death (6)	2 Post-op	2 Metas-tases	1 cirrh-osis		1 Metas-tases		

Some complications were also observed including repeated encrustation on the irradiated area in one patient, persistent urinary infections in two (resolving within six months) and epididymo-orchitis following an indwelling urethral catheter for two weeks in one patient, for which castration was necessary. Also bladder contracture following wide partial cystectomy and post-operative external irradiation for pelvic lymphnode invasion occurred in one patient. In this unique patient a fistula occurred between the bladder and the sigmoid colon and cutaneous colostomy was necessary. After removal of the urethral catheter, septicaemia occurred in one patient due to E.coli. This rapidly resolved. A vesico-cutaneous fistula was observed once lasting for four months.

Iridium wiring has been in use in our Institution for more than six years and 24 of the 26 cases have now been followed up for more than one year. The recurrences are shown in Table V. On the five recurrences, three were at the site of wiring and two in another part of the bladder. Of the five patients showing recurrence, four were easy to cure with a good late result but in one with an infiltrating tumour of the dome death occurred due to brain metastasis (four years after iridium wiring) and one year after resection of the whole dome with ileocystoplasty. Metastases were observed in two other patients. Both patients died but without recurrence of tumour in the bladder.

CONCLUSION

Malignant tumours of the bladder, less than 4 cms in diameter and localised to the mobile portion of the bladder, showing a low stage of infiltration (T1 = A or T2 = B1) are well controlled by Iridium 192 wiring. The recurrence rate is low when compared to that of TUR alone in similar cases.

CARCINOMA OF THE URINARY BLADDER TREATED BY INTERSTITIAL RADIUM IMPLANT

B VAN DER WERF-MESSING

Rotterdam Radiotherapy Institute
Groene Hilledijk 297
Rotterdam, The Netherlands

SUMMARY

Six hundred and six patients with carcinoma of the bladder category T1, T2 and T3 not exceeding five centimetres in diameter were treated by radium implant at the Rotterdam Radiotherapy Institute. As a rule, preoperative irradiation to the category T2 and T3 lesions consisting of 3 x 350 rads is given. The preoperative irradiation does not significantly influence the prognosis in category T1 and T2 lesions but it completely prevents scar implants. In the T3 lesions it improves prognosis and also reduces the incidence of distant metastases in addition to completely preventing scar implants.

TABLE I

INCIDENCE OF LOCAL RECURRENCE, DISTANT METASTASES AND SECOND UROTHELIAL TUMOURS IN 606 PATIENTS WITH BLADDER CANCER

	T Category		
	T1	T2	T3
Patients	164	313	129
Local Recurrence	14	48	36
Distant Metastases	9	37	42
Second Urothelial Tumours	7	23*	5

* Two of these were ureteric.

In category T2 lesions the main diagnostic error is understaging: of 202 cases clinically T2, 30 turned out to be T3 when the
open bladder was palpated (all patients remained for statistical
analysis in the T2 category). These understaged T2 cases had a
prognosis comparable to the clinical T3 category.

The incidence of local recurrence, distant metastases and
second urothelial tumours is shown in Table I.

The operative mortality was 2% (12 of 606 patients).
Complications were seen in 42 patients (7%), 25 being of a temporary
and minor character.

The complete analysis has been published in International
Journal of Radiation Oncology, Biology Physics, 4, 373-378 (1978).

RADIOACTIVE SOURCE IMPLANTATION IN BLADDER TUMOURS

G S BARLAS

Department of Urology
Admiral Bristol Hospital
Istanbul, Turkey

ABSTRACT

Radiotherapy has been used for many years in the treatment of
bladder tumours and is now being used increasingly in combination
with surgery. It is important that the surgeon and the radio-
therapist decide together on the type of treatment to be offered.
One type of combined therapy includes the use of radioactive source
implantation after surgery. We used this procedure from 1963-66.

INTRODUCTION

There is a great variety of bladder tumours. Well
differentiated papillary tumours stay in the mucosa for a long time.
On the other hand anaplastic tumours infiltrate all the layers of
bladder and lymphatic and hematogenous dissemination occurs. Well
differentiated and pedunculated tumours have a good prognosis with
a five year survival of 70-75%. If tumour extension is present in
the submucosa and the muscularis the prognosis is worse. If all the
layers are infiltrated the death rate in five years is 90%. The
plan of treatment is decided according to the clinical classification
and the results of the biopsy. In our Department it is usual to
fulgurate the pedunculated mucosal lesions. If the tumour
infiltrates the muscle we perform a partial cystectomy if possible
and if not, carry out surgical removal of the tumour and radioactive
implantation. This technique is used for tumours of the base of the
bladder with infiltration of the submucosa and muscularis and without
involvement of the ureteral orifices.

The advantages of this treatment are that the tumour is
resected, surgery and radiotherapy are combined at the same time,
only the area of the lesion is radiated, the tumour free area is
less affected by radioactivity and since implantation is done under
vision, the area is well radiated.

Radioactive Gold (Au-198) grains and radioactive Tantalum
(Ta-182) wire are used for interstitial implantation. The advantages
of radioactive Tantalum over radioactive gold are that with the
Tantalum the radioactive source is implanted very accurately and if
implantation is not accurate it can be removed. Also the radiation
is homogenous and after the dose has been given the wires can be
removed. Also Ta-182 can be kept longer because its half life is
111 days. Despite this Au-198 is preferred in irregular tumours,
in patients with a narrow pelvis, and for tumours of the internal
urethral orifice.

CLINICAL MATERIAL

Twenty three patients with bladder tumours received radioactive implantation after surgery; of these 22 fitted our criteria.
In one case there were metastases to external and internal iliac
lymph nodes.

Au-198 was used in 20 cases but Ta-182 has been used only in
three cases because it was hard to import from England and we plan
to replace it with irridium 192 wire.

Of the 22 patients treated according to the criteria of
selection eight have died. Two died within the first three months,
four after total cystectomy for contracted bladder and a further two
of suicide and myocardial infarction. One patient had distant
metastasis treated with external radiation and is living after one
year. Thirteen patients were alive between five months and two
years without symptoms.

Radiation reactions were not severe. Most patients had dysuria
which disappeared after two months. In four patients this persisted
longer than three months associated with a reduced bladder capacity.

SUMMARY

Between 1963 and 1966 we treated twenty three selected patients
with bladder tumours using combined surgery and radioactive source
implantation. Our results are hopeful. At present we have been
using external radiation because of the difficulty of obtaining
sources.

REFERENCES

1. Bloom, H. J. G., Treatment of Carcinoma of the Bladder a
    Symposium. Treatment by Interstital Irradiation using Tantalum
    182 Wire. Brit. J. Radiol. 33, 471-79 (1960).

2. Nurlu, F., Uzel, R., Radioaktif Izotopla Tedave Edilmis Bir
    Mesane Tumor Vak'asi. Vakif Gureba Hastahanesi 1964 Yillik
    Bulteni s. 39-44.

3. Ozdilek, S., Urolojide Radioizotoplarin Kullanilisi. Ankara
    Numune Hastahanesi Bulteni 3: 753-769 (1973).

4. Riches, E., Malignant Disease of the Urinary Tract. Lancet
    2, 537-540 (1958).

5. Wallace, D. M., Tumours of the Bladder. Livingstone (1959).

INTRAVESICAL TREATMENT OF SUPERFICIAL URINARY BLADDER TUMOURS WITH ADRIAMYCIN

D MELLONI and M PAVONE-MACALUSO

Istituto di Clinica Urologia dell'Università di Palermo

Palermo, Sicily, Italy

ABSTRACT

Personal experience resulted in the observation that intravesical Adriamycin (ADM) is effective in some patients with multiple or diffuse papillary bladder tumours. A review of the literature shows that similar results have been obtained elsewhere, especially in Japan and Sweden. The response rate was higher if single doses of at least 50 mg were employed. Intravesical instillations of ADM appear to be valuable also in the treatment of carcinoma in situ and in prophylactic treatment after transurethral resection (TUR) of papillary bladder tumours.

CLINICAL EXPERIENCE

In 1971 when we started to study the action of intravesical ADM in the treatment of superficial transitional cell carcinoma (TCC) using very low doses (10 mg), we only obtained partial regressions in three out of five patients. Better results have been obtained by other workers who employed higher doses of ADM (Table I).

Of the 169 patients treated in the various centres the results differ according to the doses employed. This difference is shown in Table II. It is clear that the results are much better if doses of at least 50 mg are used since no patient failed to respond whilst greater than 90% or complete remission occurred in 30% of patients.

In a recent review Ozaki et al summarised the results obtained in 175 patients studied in different Japanese Universities. The response to intravesical ADM was influenced by the size, the histo-

317

TABLE I

INTRAVESICAL CHEMOTHERAPY WITH ADRIAMYCIN (DOXORUBICIN)

Author	Year	No. of Pts	Dose	Administration	RESULTS CR or PR >90%	PR >50%	PR <50%	No Change
PAVONE-MACALUSO	1971	5	10-20 mg/30 ml	weekly	0	0	3	2
CARAMIA et al.	1973	8	20 mg/30 ml	weekly	0	0	3	5
NIIJIMA	1975	5	20 mg/30 ml	daily for 3 days	2	2	1	0
		4	30 mg/30 ml	" " "	0	1	3	0
		2	60 mg/30 ml	" " "	2	0	0	0
MATSUMURA	1976	9	30 mg/30 ml	daily for 3 days	2	3	4	0
		17	60 mg/30 ml	" " "	4	11	2	0
FUJIWARA	1977	10	20 mg/20 ml	daily for 2 weeks	4	0	2	4
OZAKI et al.	1977	9	30 mg/30 ml	daily for 3 days (repeat after 1 week)	2	3	4	0
		25	50 mg/30 ml	" " "	7	11	7	0
		46	60 mg/30 ml	" " "	13	21	12	0
PAVONE-MACALUSO	1978	16	10 mg/30 ml	weekly x 4 then monthly	0	2	6	8
		10	20 mg/30 ml	" "	0	3	3	4
		3	40 mg/30 ml	" "	0	1	1	1

CR = Complete regression, PR = Partial regression.

TABLE II

CUMULATIVE RESULTS WITH TOPICAL ADRIAMYCIN: 169 PATIENTS

Dose	No. of Pts	CR or PR >90%	PR >50%	PR <50%	No Change
10-40 mg	79	10 (12%)	15 (19%)	30 (38.7%)	24 (30.3%)
50-60 mg	90	26 (28.9%)	43 (47.8%)	21 (23.3%)	0

logical grade and by the type of onset (primary or recurrent) of
the tumours. The response rate was slightly better in papilloma
than in TCC. The results were not significantly different whether
this dose was given by daily or by intermittent administration.
Preliminary results seem to show that local ADM administration is
effective in reducing the incidence of TCC recurrence after TUR.
The response rate was also better in multiple (67%) than in single
tumours (45%). The best results were obtained using a concentration
of ADM equal to 1.5-2.0 mg/ml and a total dose of at least 360 mg.

It is of interest that Edsmyr observed regression of carcinoma
in situ (CIS) after ADM instillations. Therefore, not only papillary
TCC but also CIS seem to respond to topical ADM.

TABLE III

SIDE-EFFECTS IN PATIENTS TREATED WITH INTRAVESICAL ADRIAMYCIN

Author	Year	No. of Pts	Dose (mg)	Pts with side-effects
CARAMIA et al	1973	13	10-20	0
NIJIMA	1975	11	20-60	9 (5 chemical cystitis, 4 alopecia)
IZBICRIN	1976	14	50	0
MATSUMURA	1976	26	30-60	2 (1 alopecia; 1 thrombo-cytopenia)
FUJIWARA	1977	10	20	10 (urethrocystalgia)
BANKS et al	1977	13	50	0
OZAKI	1977	80	30-60	25 (24 cystitis; 1 thrombo-cytopenia, alopecia and ECG impairment)
PAVONE-MACALUSO	1978	49	10-20	10 (1 moderate haematuria, 9 minor chemical cystitis)

The side-effects are shown in Table III. They were mainly
local and consisted of haematuria and chemical cystitis. They were
more frequent using the higher doses. Cystitis was always transient,
but occasionally required interruption of the treatment. No severe
systemic side-effects were observed. There was only one ECG abnormality, not clearly attributable to the treatment. Only two
cases of mild thrombocytopenia were reported. Six patients (4%)
developed temporary alopecia. This is a sign of absorption and of
systemic toxicity, but unfortunately no details are available on
these few patients in which alopecia developed. It is unknown
whether local conditions (such as recent TUR, inflammation etc)
were responsible for the enhanced absorption of ADM through the
bladder wall.

A more detailed analysis of local ADM treatment and a list
of references can be found in a previous report from our work (1).

REFERENCE

1.   Pavone-Macaluso, M., Intravesical treatment of superficial (T1)
      urinary bladder tumours. A review of a 15 year experience in
      Diagnostics and Treatment of Superficial Bladder Tumours.
      Montedison Lakemedel AB, Stockholm, Sweden, 21-36 (1979).

INTRAVESICAL THERAPY WITH ADRIAMYCIN IN PATIENTS WITH SUPERFICIAL BLADDER TUMOURS

F EDSMYR, T BERLIN, J BOMAN, M DUCHEK, P-L ESPOSTI,
H GUSTAVSON and H WIKSTRÖM
WHO Collaborating Centre for Research and Treatment of
Urinary Bladder Cancer, Stockholm and the
Department of Urology, Umea, Sweden

INTRODUCTION

Multiple, low grade papillomatous tumours of the bladder can be controlled by coagulation, transurethral resection or transvesical excision. In the event of frequent recurrences and/or extensive tumours, these methods are sometimes insufficient. Thus, there has been a search for other methods. The lesions suitable for such treatment include papillary tumours, carcinoma in situ (Tis) and secondary carcinoma in situ ("Tis"). Carcinoma in situ (Tis) means no visible tumour at cystoscopy/pre-invasive carcinoma/and untreated prior to instillation. Secondary carcinoma in situ ("Tis") means no visible tumour at cystoscopy but prior to instillation of Adriamycin treated by any of the mentioned methods.

Recently, Adriamycin has been tried as a topical agent in papillomatosis. Pavone-Macaluso (1972) reported four cases with partial regression of tumour growth in three. Banks (1976) published results after topical Adriamycin treatment in 13 patients with recurrent superficial bladder tumour with complete remissions in two cases.

TREATMENT

In this series 58 patients have been given intravesical instillation of Adriamycin for superficial bladder tumours in five institutions in Sweden.

Prior to Adriamycin instillation repeated transurethral resection/excision or radiotherapy with or without chemotherapy has

321

been performed in 44 patients. In 14 patients no treatment had
been given prior to instillation of Adriamycin. Before being given
Adriamycin therapy all patients had cytologically and/or biopsy
proven carcinoma of the bladder.

Adriamycin (80 mg) was dissolved in 100 ml physiological saline
and instilled into the bladder via a urethral catheter. The solution
was retained in the bladder for 60 minutes. The procedure was
repeated at monthly intervals. Complete disappearance of carcinoma
cells (cytological remission) in the Tis group occurred in nine of
11 patients. A partial effect, ie. the presence of atypical but not
malignant cells was seen in one of 11 patients in the same group.
In the corresponding group of secondary Tis ("Tis") patients the
figures were 11 of 19 with complete disappearance and three of 19
with atypia. Up to 26 courses of treatment have been given in the
Tis group and up to 20 courses in the group "Tis".

We conclude that at least four courses have to be administered
to each patient in group Tis and 11 in group "Tis" to achieve
complete disappearance of the carcinoma cells.

The bladder capacity at cystoscopy after treatment was unchanged
in most of the patients. Frequency, urgency and painful micturition
were seen in only three of the 58 patients; these disturbances were
transient.

No bone marrow depression or systemic toxic side effects were
observed.

CONCLUSIONS

In conclusion, we believe that topical intravesical
instillations of Adriamycin at monthly intervals for superficial
transitional cell carcinoma is therapeutically as effective as those
regimens that include conventional drugs such as Thiotepa and Epodyl
but without the side-effects and complications associated with these
agents. Adriamycin deserves further study as a drug for intravesical
use in the dose schedule outlined in the hope that these results
can be repeated.

The complete publication of this presentation has appeared in
Diagnostics and Treatment of Superficial Urinary Bladder Tumours.
Montedison Lakemedel AB, Stockholm, 45-53 (1979).

LOCAL TREATMENT OF UROEPITHELIAL BLADDER TUMOURS WITH ADRIAMYCIN

M DUCHEK

Department of Urology

University of Umeå, Umeå, Sweden

In this study 22 patients, 19 men and three women with uro-epithelial bladder tumours, were treated by local instillation of Adriamycin. Most of them had previously been treated by trans-urethral resection, other cytostatics and/or radiation therapy (Figure 1).

The lesions included carcinoma in situ, superficial forms of recurrent highly differentiated bladder cancer and superficial forms of poorly differentiated bladder cancer.

Treatment was started one month after the transurethral procedure. A dose of 80 mg Adriamycin in saline solution, the volume of which varied according to the bladder volume, was instilled once a month. The effect was evaluated after three such treatments. If it was judged to be favourable, three more instillations were performed before further evaluation was carried out.

Criteria of response in urinary bladder carcinoma in situ were:
1. for partial remission, alteration of cytology grade III to atypical cells,
2. for complete remission, to "normal" cells.

Criteria of response in superficial bladder carcinoma were:
1. for partial remission, 50% decrease of total tumour volume,
2. for complete remission, 100% decrease of all lesions, for a minimum time of three months.

The longest observation time is 30 months. In all cases treatment has been free of complications. No systemic side-effects have been noted. The patients had transient episodes of urinary urgency.

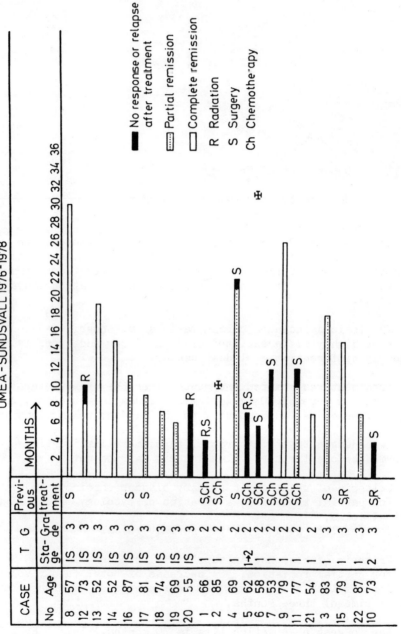

FIGURE 1

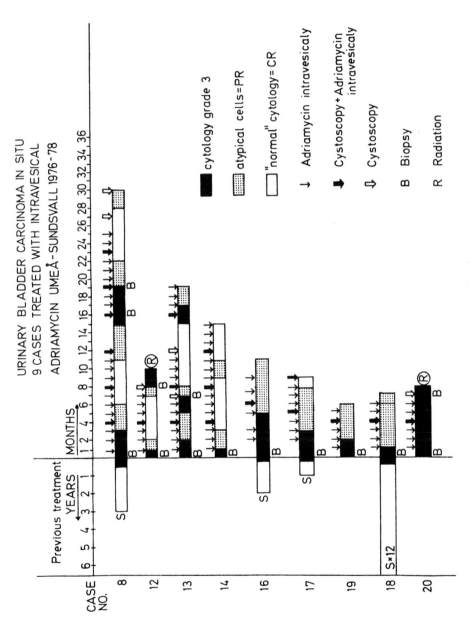

FIGURE 2

In the nine patients with carcinoma in situ complete remission
was attained in four; in one of these patients it was only
temporarily. Four other patients were judged to have attained
partial remission, and one has not responded to treatment.

Of the remaining 13 patients with an exophytic tumour, four
have attained complete remission and four partial remission. Two of
the latter, however, later relapsed; five failed to respond.

Figure 2 illustrates the course of the patients with carcinoma
in situ. Discontinuation of therapy often led to recurrence of
atypical cells in the bladder washings.

The optimal dosage, drug concentration and duration of therapy
remains to be determined.

ADRIAMYCIN THERAPY IN CARCINOMA IN SITU : A PRELIMINARY REPORT

G JAKSE and F HOFSTÄDTER

Department of Urology and Department of Pathology

University of Innsbruck, Innsbruck, Austria

INTRODUCTION

Cystectomy is recommended for cancer in situ of the bladder; as alternative treatment topical chemotherapy may be applied.

In this trial in six patients with in situ carcinoma 40 mg Adriamycin diluted in 20 ml saline was instilled every two weeks. Cytological preparations were obtained at each instillation and biopsies were taken every three months. The follow-up is now six to nine months.

RESULTS

In three of the six patients a tumour remission was obtained after six months. Tumour remission means that cytology was negative and that random biopsies revealed only mild dysplasia (Figure 1). None of the patients had local symptoms during or after treatment. No general toxic symptoms were noted.

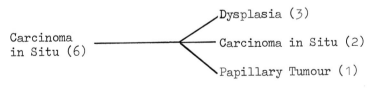

FIGURE 1

Results of Treatment for Six Months

Cytology correlated well with the histological specimens, ie. a negative cytology (Pap II) always corresponded with a positive response to the treatment and vice versa. Compared to the initially obtained cytology a decrease in the absolute number of desquamated cells by about one half and an increase in the ratio of superficial cells to basal cells was observed.

On **scanning** electron microscopy which was carried out on every specimen obtained prior to treatment and during treatment a re-organisation of the urothelium was noted. The number of basal cells was reduced and a normal layering with intermediate cells and superficial cells of the umbrella type were observed. However, there was no change in other tumour signs such as enlarged nuclei, thickened basement membrane or tumour vessels.

DISCUSSION

Our interpretation of these results if that Adriamycin slows down the cell cycle and gives more time for the basal cells to differentiate, resulting in a normal structure of the urothelium and less desquamation of the urothelial cells.

As yet we do not know what will happen to these "arrested" cells when treatment is stopped or the interval between Adriamycin instillation is changed.

BLADDER INSTILLATION OF ADRIAMYCIN IN MULTIPLE RECURRENT NON-INVASIVE PAPILLOMATOUS BLADDER TUMOURS

P A GAMMELGAARD, P MOGENSEN and F LUNDBECK

Herlev Hospital
University of Copenhagen
Denmark

INTRODUCTION

Attempts have been made to treat multiple non-invasive papillomatous bladder tumours with local instillation of Thiotepa and Epodyl. The results, however, have been disappointing.

Investigations using systemic Adriamycin treatment for bladder tumours show fairly good results, but side effects are not negligible. In order to minimise the toxic effect of the drug and to increase the local concentration we have started to instill Adriamycin into the bladder. This is a preliminary report concerning the results in the first 20 patients using instillations of 100 mg Adriamycin for one hour once a week in two series of eight weeks duration. Only patients with three or more non-invasive tumours with a diameter not exceeing two centimeters were treated. Histologically the tumours had to be grade I or II or carcinoma in situ grade III.

TREATMENT AND RESULTS

100 mg of Adriamycin dissolved in 100 ml of normal saline were instilled through a thin catheter which was then removed. One hour later the patient was asked to empty the bladder. The patients were treated as out patients and the instillations were carried out weekly in two series of eight week's duration. Cystoscopy was carried out after the first and second series in order to evaluate the effect of the treatment. If progression of the tumours occurred, treatment was discontinued.

Table I shows the results of the treatment. In four patients

TABLE I

RESULTS OF BLADDER INSTILLATION OF ADRIAMYCIN IN MULTIPLE,
RECURRENT NON-INVASIVE PAPILLOMATOUS BLADDER TUMOURS

Complete remission	4
Partial remission	11
No remission	3
Not evaluable	2

the tumours disappeared completely and in 11 patients, including
four who did not have the full treatment, more than 50% of the
tumours disappeared (partial remission). In three fully treated
patients the instillations had no effect. In the last two patients
treatment was discontinued early in the first series and the effect
therefore cannot be evaluated.

COMPLICATIONS

Table II shows the complications of treatment. Fourteen
patients had both series while treatment was discontinued in six
patients. In five of the 14 patients who had the full treatment no
side effects were shown. Four patients had temporary cystitis, ie.
moderate dysuria and voiding every second hour on the day of
treatment and the following couple of days. In eight of the patients
symptoms of severe cystitis occurred, ie. pain, frequency (voiding
once an hour) and often haematuria during most of the treatment. In

TABLE II

BLADDER INSTILLATION OF ADRIAMYCIN IN MULTIPLE, RECURRENT
NON-INVASIVE PAPILLOMATOUS BLADDER TUMOURS

		full treatment	treatment discontinued
Number of patients	20	14	6
Complications:			
none	5	5	–
temporary cystitis	4	4	–
severe cystitis	8	5	3
general symptoms	3	–	3

three of the eight patients treatment was discontinued for this
reason. The symptoms did not disable the patients until during the
second series of treatment. Two patients who had the full treatment
developed contracted bladder with a capacity below 100 ml. In three
old patients the treatment was discontinued due to general symptoms.
It is uncertain to what extent the symptoms were due to the
treatment.

SURVIVAL IN PATIENTS TREATED WITH EPODYL (1968-1978)

P RIDDLE

The Institute of Urology

University of London, London, England

This short communication follows the course of 63 patients treated with intravesical Epodyl between the years 1968-1978. The alternative with each of these patients was treatment of a radical nature, either surgery or radiotherapy.

The patients were finally placed in one of three groups:-

Group   I   Initial complete response; remained clear.

Group II   Initial complete response; recurred later.

Group III   Response not complete

The 63 patients were distributed in the three groups in roughly equal numbers. Approximately half the patients in Groups I and II were alive at the end of the review period 1978, whereas the majority in Group III were dead. It is significant that none of the patient deaths in Group I was associated with tumour, whereas nearly all were in Groups II and III.

TABLE I

SURVIVAL FOLLOWING TREATMENT WITH EPODYL

	Group I 19 Patients	Group II 20 Patients	Group III 24 Patients
Alive	7	10	4
Dead	8 None with tumour	9 All with tumour	16 13 with tumour
Lost to follow-up	4	1	4

333

The treatments these patients are currently undergoing or had received in the past are shown in Table II.

TABLE II

ALTERNATIVE TREATMENTS REQUIRED

	Group I	Group II	Group III
Still maintained on Epodyl	6	1	-
Cysto-diathermy	-	3	2
Radiotherapy	-	5	3
"Cystectomy"	-	10	13

It can be seen that the great majority of patients in Groups II and III underwent cystectomy, usually a radical cysto-urethrectomy; the remainder in this group, with the exception of six cases, had radiotherapy. The fate of both groups is shown in Table III.

TABLE III

OUTCOME IN PATIENTS TREATED BY CYSTECTOMY OR RADIOTHERAPY

	Alive	Dead	Lost to follow-up
Post-cystectomy	6	15	2
Post Radiotherapy	3	5	0

This paper demonstrates that although each case was initially one of widespread superficial disease, when this is no longer managable by local means the final outcome is very poor.

If the initial response to intravesical treatment is 100% and remains so on prophylactic treatment then the outlook is good. Should the patient fail to respond completely or fail to remain clear on continued treatment then radical surgery should be undertaken immediately and procrastination should cease.

A full review of this work is being published elsewhere by John Fitzpatrick and Peter Riddle of the Institute of Urology, University of London.

LONG-TERM INTRACAVITARY EPODYL® IN MULTIPLE OR EXTENSIVE PAPILLARY TUMOURS OF THE URINARY BLADDER

L Collste, T Berlin, I Granberg-Öhman, B von Garrelts and H Wijkström

Departments of Urology and Morphology
Huddinge Hospital, Stockholm, Sweden

Encouraging results using instillation of cytostatics in the urinary bladder have been reported. Ethoglucid (Epodyl^R ICI, England) is among the preparations used. It seems to lack toxicity and may be effective. We report here our experience with intra-cavitary Epodyl^R in seven patients. There was one woman and six men, 59-77 years of age, all with papillary tumours occupying the major part of the mucosa. Cytological and histological specimens showed that all were grade I or II (WHO) and of category T1 or T2 (TNM). One ml of Epodyl^R (1.13 g ethoglucid) was dissolved in 100 ml of sterile water. The solution was introduced via a urethral catheter and retained in the bladder for 1-3 hours. In no case was there any reason to discontinue the treatment on account of side-effects. Initially Epodyl^R was given once a week for three months. Thereafter the interval between treatments was increased to one month. Upon recurrence another series of weekly treatments was considered. One patient died of pneumonia one month after treatment was started. His clinical bladder status was unchanged. For the remaining six patients the periods of treatment were 4, 12, 18, 24, 24 and 24 months with a total number of treatments of 12, 16, 23, 26, 34 and 40 respectively. In one of the patients complete regression of visible lesions occurred. He has now been free of recurrence for 18 months (cystoscopy and cytology). Total regression occurred in another patient after the initial intensive treatment but there was recurrence within one year. One patient also having had an initial response, developed invasive grade III cancer after 24 months. The remaining three patients were at no time free of tumours. Patients with early complete regressions and a few recurrences may be considered for long-term Epodyl^R treatment.

SUMMARY

Intracavitary Epodyl^R (ethoglucid) was used for periods up to 24 months in seven patients with extensive papillomatosis of the urinary bladder. In one of the patients complete and long lasting regression of visible lesions occurred. Total regression occurred in another patient but there was recurrence within one year. One patient also having had an initial response, developed invasive cancer after 24 months. One patient died of pneumonia one month after treatment was started. His clinical bladder status was unchanged. The remaining three patients were at no time free of tumours.

TREATMENT OF MULTIPLE NON-INVASIVE BLADDER TUMOURS WITH INTRAVESICAL EPODYL®

A EK and S COLLEN

Department of Urology
University Hospital
Lund, Sweden

ABSTRACT

Twenty-three patients with multiple, recurrent bladder cancer grade I-II, category T1 were treated with regular intravesical instillation of Ethoglucid (Epodyl^R). In six of the patients the treatment had to be withdrawn because of severe and/or repeated cystitis. The therapeutic schedule has been completed or continued in 17 patients. In 16 patients the tumours were eradicated. Five of these patients continued the treatment on a prophylactic basis and were still without recurrence after 15-60 months. Myelosuppression was not observed but cystitis was a serious problem frequently jeopardizing the therapy.

INTRODUCTION

Local control of multiple, highly differentiated, superficial urothelial cancer by transurethral methods may occasionally be difficult, especially in patients with frequent recurrences. More radical procedures, such as cystourethrectomy seem to be too high a price to pay for a neoplastic disease that seldom infiltrates or establishes metastases. Topical treatment of these tumours with cytotoxic agents, eg. Thiotepa, has been utilised since the early 1960's (1,2,3,4,9,10). Although cure has been achieved in every second patient, serious side-effects, eg. myelosuppression, due to absorption of Thiotepa gives the method a certain disrepute and therefore it has never gained widespread popularity (1).

Ethoglucid (Epodyl^R) a radiomimetic with a higher molecular weight than Thiotepa and presumably less absorbable through the

337

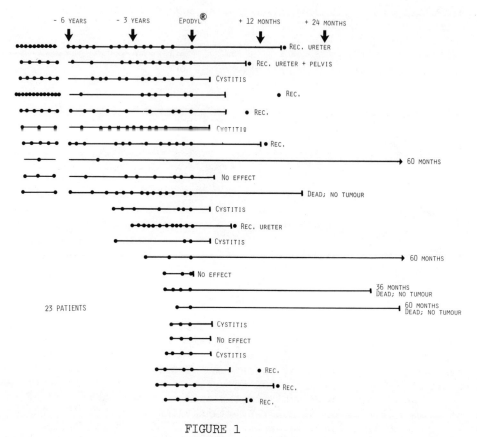

FIGURE 1

Survey of the 23 patients treated with Epodyl^R. Every line represents one patient and every point the date of new urothelial tumour.

bladder mucosa, was introduced by Riddle and Wallace in 1971 (6) for
the treatment of highly differentiated bladder tumours. We have used
intravesical Epodyl^R since 1973 and this report concerns the first 23
treated cases.

MATERIAL AND METHODS

The study comprises 16 males and seven females (mean age 70
years, range 54-82) with multiple, recurrent bladder cancer category
T1 (UICC) grade I-II (WHO) (5). Tumour classification was
established by urethrocystoscopy, bimanual palpation, cytological
evaluation of a mid-stream urine specimen and histological
examination of transurethrally obtained biopsy specimens. Six

patients had earlier undergone partial cystectomy with implantation of a Tantalum 182 needle in the resection area to achieve local tumouricidal radiation (8). Five of these patients and one other had vesicoureteric reflux. Most of the patients had suffered from frequent recurrences for several years, but in a few with widespread papillomatosis the history was shorter (Figure 1).

One hundred ml of 1% solution of Ethoglucid (Epodyl[R], obtainable from Imperial Chemical Industries Ltd., U.K.) was instilled into the empty bladder and retained for at least one hour before being voided. During the first three months the patients had one instillation weekly, during the following three months one every fortnight, for the next three months one monthly and after that one every third month.

During the first part of this study chemoprophylaxis against urinary tract infection was given continuously for the first three months and then for one week after each instillation; this schedule was later abandoned as it did not seem to reduce the incidence of cystitis. The instillations were given on an outpatient basis. Red cell, white cell and platelet counts were repeated every fortnight during the first three months. Urethrocystoscopy was performed every third month and at the same time specimens for urinary cytology were collected. An IVP was done once every second year during follow-up.

RESULTS

Treatment was terminated in six patients after two to five months because of severe and/or repeated cystitis (Figure 2). Despite the comparatively short period of treatment two of these patients became tumour free and remained so for 12 and 18 months respectively.

Seventeen patients tolerated the treatment and fourteen of these became tumour free. In three patients the tumours were not eradicated within six months and the treatment was therefore withdrawn. The follow-up of the 14 patients who tolerated the treatment and became tumour free was as follows:

  (i)   Five continued the treatment and were still without
        recurrence after 18-60 (mean 46) months.
 (ii)   Three patients discontinued treatment due to the
        appearance of new bladder tumours.
(iii)   In three, treatment was discontinued when tumour in
        the renal pelvis, the ureter or the urethra was
        discovered.
 (iv)   Three patients stopped treatment for non-medical reasons
        and tumour reappeared in the bladder within 6-9 months.

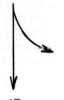

6 Discontinued; due to cystitis
(2 became tumour free)

17

3 Discontinued - Tumours not eradicated

14 Tumour free within 6 months:

5 Continued Treatment; still tumour free
after 18-60 (46) months

3 Discontinued Treatment; due to new tumour
in renal pelvis, ureter or urethra

3 Discontinued; due to new bladder tumours

3 Discontinued for non medical reasons and
developed new bladder tumours within 3-9
months.

FIGURE 2

23 Patients with Multiple Bladder Tumours T1 Grade I-II

Most patients experienced temporary dysuria after each
instillation; however, severe and persistent symptoms were recorded
only in six cases. This non-bacterial cystitis appeared during the
first three months of the schedule, ie. during the period of the
most intensive treatment.

The six patients with a severe reaction to Epodyl[R] had to
discontinue treatment, but nevertheless in some of them severe
symptoms persisted for more than a month after the instillations
were withdrawn. All symptoms eventually resolved and all patients
regained normal bladder capacity. Five of those with "Epodyl[R]
intolerance" were earlier treated with interstitial irradiation and
four had in addition vesicoureteric reflux.

No myelosuppression was recorded in any of the 23 patients.

DISCUSSION

In the present study of non invasive bladder tumours all lesions were eradicated in 75% of patients following Epodyl[R] instillations. This result equals that reported by Riddle (1973) (7) and is better than that achieved with Thiotepa instillations (1,10). Besides a higher therapeutic response a further advantage, as compared to Thiotepa, is the absence of systemic side-effects. In our study, however, local side-effects were a serious problem and resulted in every fourth patient discontinuing the treatment. This is a higher incidence than reported for Thiotepa (1,9,10) but also higher than reported for Epodyl[R] by others (6,7). In the present study most patients with severe cystitis had previously been treated with interstitial irradiation and/or had reflux which suggests that these factors are contraindications to Epodyl[R] treatment. Three of the 23 patients developed urothelial cancer outside the bladder not accessible to Epodyl[R] treatment and illustrate that the neoplastic disease of these patients does involve the whole urothelium.

Intravesical Epodyl[R] as a treatment for non-invasive, recurrent, widespread, highly differentiated urothelial cancer seems to be a good alternative to transurethral management, provided that the patient has not been previously irradiated, that the tumour responds to the treatment and that the neoplastic disease is confined to the bladder.

From our limited experience, it is not yet possible to draw any conclusions regarding the long term prophylactic effect of regular Epodyl[R] instillations.

REFERENCES

1.   Abbassian, A. and Wallace, D. M.   J. Urol. 96, 461-465 (1966).

2.   Esquivel, E. L., Mackenzie, A. R. and Whitmore, W. F. Investigative Urol. 2, 381-386 (1966).

3.   Jones, H. C. and Swinney, J. Lancet, 2, 615-618 (1961).

4.   Mitchell, R. J. Brit. J. Urol. 43, 185-188 (1971).

5.   Mostofi, F. K., Sobin, L. H. and Torloni, H. Histological typing of urinary bladder tumours. World Health Organisation, Geneva (1973).

6.   Riddle, P. R. and Wallace, D. M. Brit. J. Urol. 43, 181-184 (1971).

7.   Riddle, P. R. Brit. J. Urol. 45, 84-87 (1973).

8. Wallace, D. M., Stapleton, J. E. and Turner, R. C. Brit. J. Radiol. 25, 421-424 (1952).

9. Veenema, R. J., Dean, A. L., Roberts, M., Fingerhut, B., Chowhury, B. K. and Tarossoly, H. J. Urol. 88, 60-63 (1962).

10. Veenema, R. J., Dean, A. L., Uson, A. C., Roberts, M. and Longo, F. J. Urol. 101, 711-715 (1969).

THE TREATMENT OF SINGLE AND MULTIPLE PAPILLARY TUMOURS OF THE

BLADDER (Ta/T1 NX MO)

H R England, J P Blandy and A M I Paris

The London Hospital, Whitechapel

London E1, England

SUMMARY

Adverse change in stage or grade took place in only 34 out of a cohort of 275 superficial (T1) tumours followed over a minimum period of five years. In 37 cases Thiotepa was used in the immediate post-operative period after TUR or diathermy, and resulted in complete or near-complete clearance of the bladder in 30 (81%). Failure to respond to Thiotepa in seven cases was accompanied by multifocal malignant change in the upper tracts invasion of the prostate or distant metastases. It is suggested that response to Thiotepa can be used as an early means of distinguishing the small but important subgroup of T1 tumours which require more than endoscopic treatment.

INTRODUCTION

For the busy working urological surgeon the most important bladder tumours in terms of numbers of patients and the call upon endoscopic expertise are not the advanced T3 cancers but the more common single or multiple T1 tumours among which, as every surgeon knows, not all cases do well with conventional endoscopic resection and coagulation. In a given instance, what is the chance that these tumours will not respond and can the small group who do badly be predicted? These were the two questions to which we addressed ourselves when, some years ago, we began to collect on a prospective basis, a standard series of clinical and pathological data on all new cases of bladder cancer presenting to The London Hospital, among which about 80% initially fell into the T1 group.

MATERIAL

This study refers to a cohort of 275 patients all followed by regular endoscopic review for a minimum period of at least five years (Table I). In this group the overall survival was 86.5% at five years; among these deaths only 19 were known to have died with tumour, other causes of death being predictably common in this elderly group of patients.

TABLE 1

275 T1 BLADDER TUMOURS FOLLOWED 5 YEARS

Deaths from tumour   19   Non tumour causes   18

5 year survival 86.5% (excluding non-cancer deaths, 93.1%)

Deaths from cancer occurred in 9 G1, 7 G2, 3 G3 cases

When there was only a single tumour at first presentation (Figure 1) the bladder remained perfectly clear of tumour in a

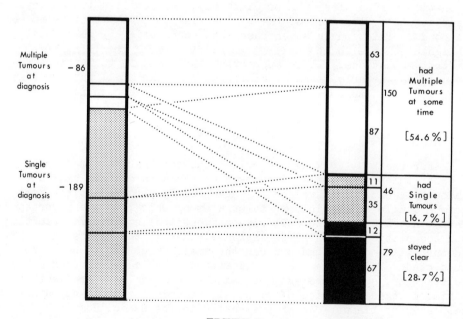

FIGURE 1

THE FATE OF 275 T1 BLADDER CARCINOMAS FOLLOWED UP FOR MORE THAN 5 YEARS.

substantial proportion (28.7%). A larger number grew single tumours from time to time in the follow-up period (16.7%) which posed no problem in treatment. Difficulty and hazards arose in the 54.6% of cases who developed, or persisted in developing, multiple tumours. Most multiple tumours were easy to deal with by means of trans-urethral resection or endoscopic coagulation, and in practice the difficult problem in management was posed only by those patients in whom the bladder appears to be more or less completely lined by unstable mucosa or multiple papillary tumours. In this group there was an undue preponderance of the higher grade tumours (G2 and G3).

An adverse change in tumour grade has been noted in six of these 275 patients in the five year period under study. A deterioration in tumours stage (T category) has been noted in 16 cases, 13 of whom ultimately died. Deterioration in both T and G categories has occurred in eight cases (2.9%). Tumours in the upper urinary tract have been noted in two patients (0.7%). Any or all of these adverse changes have been observed in 34 (12.4%) of the cohort of 275 cases. It should be noted that among these it has been unsuspected invasion of the prostate by transitional cell carcinoma (in six cases) which was responsible for the downstaging and the unhappy outcome.

For treatment of those T1 tumours which have deteriorated our policy has been to attempt a cure with radiotherapy in the first instance, and to offer cystectomy if the tumours persist, or if complications occur from post-radiotherapy bleeding or bladder con-tracture. The results of cystectomy in these 16 cases have been disappointing (Table II).

THIOTEPA AS ADJUVANT THERAPY TO TUR

We have used Thiotepa as an adjuvant to vigorous endoscopic resection of the multiple T1 tumours, relying on the persistent use of the resectoscope to clear the bladder as far as possible, even if three or four sessions of resection are required. Thiotepa has then been used in a dose of 30 mg in 50 ml saline alternate days for three doses, then three monthly after each check cystoscopy/biopsy.

Used in this way as an adjuvant to vigorous endoscopic treatment in 37 cases (Table III), Thiotepa seems to differentiate those who are going to do well from those who are going to do badly. In 30 cases the bladders were either entirely cleared of tumour, or were left, at check cystoscopy, with only one or two small tumours which were easily dealt with endoscopically. In seven cases (19%) the response has been poor. The failure to respond to Thiotepa has gone hand in hand with the development of upper tract tumours, tumour in the prostate, or distant metastases, suggesting that in these cases we are dealing with a different malignant disease potential. At the same time, these results seem to indicate that

TABLE II

CYSTECTOMY FOR FAILED RECURRENT T1 TUMOURS

G1 Pis	4	failed RT2, post RT bleeding 1	
		multiple tumours 1	
P1	4	post RT bleeding + single tumour 1	
		multiple, found to be G3 P4a (d) 1	
		multiple ⟶ Mets (d) 1	
		⟶ G2 P2, found to be P4a (d) 1	
G2 P1	7	contracted bladder after RT and	
		recurrence 1	
		after 4000 r 1	
		post RT bleeding, Mets (d) 2	
		G3 ⟶ P3 Mets, ⟶ P4a, (d) 2	
		post op (d) G3 P3 1	
G3 P1	1	recurrence after Radon 1	
Total	16		

RT = Radiotherapy,   (d) = death

TABLE III

RESULTS OF ADJUVANT THIOTEPA TREATMENT

GOOD

Bladder stayed completely clear
after 1 or 2 courses — or a
very active bladder only has 2   30 cases
or 3 tumours at check cystoscopy   (81%)
instead of usual 20+

BAD

Inadequate response, tumours in
kidney pelvis, worsening grade   7 cases
or distant metastases   (19%)

what is needed in such cases with a poor prognosis is an anticancer
agent which will act systemically, rather than upon the local disease
in the bladder.

ADJUVANT THERAPY OF T1 BLADDER CARCINOMA : PRELIMINARY RESULTS OF

AN EORTC RANDOMISED STUDY

C C SCHULMAN and EORTC Urological Group

Service d'Urologie
Hospital Universitaire Brugmann
Bruxelles, Belgium

ABSTRACT

This paper reports the preliminary results of an ongoing clinical trial in patients with Stage 1 bladder cancer who are randomised after transurethral resection to receive either Thiotepa, VM 26 or no treatment. While there are no significant differences between the three treatment groups with respect to the time until first recurrence, Thiotepa has significantly reduced the recurrence rate as compared to either VM 26 (P = .03) or no treatment (P = .04) among the 215 patients for whom follow-up information is currently available.

INTRODUCTION

Superficial bladder tumours (T1, P1 of the TNM classification (19) or Jewett Stage 0 and A) are often referred to as Stage 1 bladder carcinoma and are usually treated by transurethral resection (TUR). However, recurrence of the tumour after complete resection occurs in about 60% of the patients (9,10) with a significant percentage of these recurrences showing a higher degree of malignancy (10). In 10% of the cases the tumour progresses to invasive carcinoma (7) and the five year survival rate following TUR is about 62% (12).

Several adjuvant treatments to TUR have been advocated in an attempt to increase the survival rate, the duration of the disease free interval, and to reduce the recurrence rate. Thiotepa, Adriamycin, Epodyl, Bleomycin, BCG, Pyridoxine and VM 26 have all been suggested as intravesical agents of possible benefit (1,2,3,4,5,

347

6,8,11,13,14,21,22). Periodic instillation of Thiotepa, a cytotoxic alkylating agent, has been used for more than 15 years both for prophylaxis and for the treatment of recurrent stage 1 bladder tumours, but its true effectiveness remains to be demonstrated (8, 20,21). Staquet (18) has recently reviewed nine non-randomised studies with intravesical Thiotepa and found a success rate ranging from 24 to 100%.

OBJECTIVES OF THE STUDY

This randomised clinical trial was designed by the EORTC Genito-Urinary Tract Cancer Cooperative Group to compare:

1. the disease free interval,
2. the recurrence rate,
3. the number of patients with an increase in tumour grade in stage 1 carcinoma of the bladder after TUR alone or TUR followed by bladder installations of Thiotepa or VM 26 for one year (17).

SELECTION OF PATIENTS

Criteria for Admission

All patients with a biopsy proven primary or recurrent resect-able T1 papillary carcinoma of the bladder were considered eligible for the trial. T1 lesions are defined according to the 1974 TNM classification and represent tumours with no microscopic infiltration beyond the lamina propria (T1 Nx Mo P1). All visible lesions were completely resected. In addition, neither induration nor a mass could be palpated on bimanual examination under anaesthesia after TUR. In the case of urinary infection, the start of the trial was delayed until control of the infection. Criteria for exclusion are detailed in a previous report (17).

DESIGN OF THE TRIAL

Three weeks after TUR, the following treatments were randomly allocated to eligible patients after stratification for primary or recurrent cases : treatment group 1 : thiotepa instillation in bladder, treatment group 2 : VM 26 instillation in bladder, and treatment group 3 : no treatment.

Thiotepa and VM 26 were administered for one year starting one month after TUR. All patients entering the trial are followed for five years or until death, whichever comes first.

THERAPEUTIC REGIMEN

The drugs were instilled in 30 ml sterile water into the bladder and retained for one hour. The drug instillation was started one month after TUR, given every week for four weeks, and then once every four weeks for 11 months (total : 15 instillations) unless recurrence occurred (see next paragraph). Nitrofurantoin (Furadantine (R)) was given after each instillation at 3 x 100 mg/day for three days.

Thiotepa (Ledertepa (R)) 30 mg in 30 ml solution (diluted with distilled sterile water before use) was given to treatment group 1 according to the schedule given above.

VM 26 was provided by Sandoz in 50 mg vials at a concentration of 5 mg/ml and was diluted with 20 ml of normal saline. 50 mg in 30 ml solution was given to treatment group 2 according to the above schedule.

If a recurrence was observed during the instillation treatment a new complete schedule with the same regimen was repeated after TUR. Thus, one month after TUR, the drug instillation was started again every week for four installations and then once every four weeks. The total duration of treatment was limited to 12 months beginning after the first TUR.

EVALUATION OF THERAPY

1. Cystoscopy was repeated every 12 weeks during the first year every 16 weeks during the second year and then every 26 weeks during the following three years. All visible lesions seen on cystoscopy were biopsied.

2. Recurrence was confirmed by histologic examination of biopsy material. Cystoscopic examination was not taken into consideration for recurrence.

RESULTS

Three hundred and forty patients from 20 participating institutions in six different countries have been admitted to this protocol from November 1975 to April 1978. There are 215 patients for which follow-up is currently available. Kaplan-Meier curves are used to estimate the time until the first recurrence and differences between the curves are tested using the Logrank and Gehan Generalised Wilcoxon test procedures (15). Two-tailed significance levels are reported in the text. A comparison of the recurrence rates (number of recurrences per patient months of observation) is performed using a chi-square test statistic (16).

As indicated in the first line of Table I the number of patients entered on study as of April 1978 is 340. While the analysis which is presented here is based on the 215 patients for whom follow-up is available, a similar analysis yielding essentially the same results was made eliminating 16 ineligible or nonevaluable patients from the calculations.

The primary goal of the study was to increase the time until the first recurrence in patients treated with Thiotepa or VM 26. Hence, Kaplan-Meier curves giving the time until first recurrence have been calculated for each treatment group. Figure 1 gives a comparison of the time until first recurrence between primary and recurrent patients and the difference is significant at P = .01. The median time to recurrence is approximately 45 weeks for primary patients and 23 weeks for recurrent patients. If we compare the three treatment groups with respect to the time until first recurrence, we find that overall there is no significant difference between Thiotepa, VM 26 and no treatment. The same conclusion is valid among primary patients and among recurrent patients.

The number of patients in each treatment group with follow-up is indicated in the second line of Table I and the number of patients with recurrence per treatment group is given in line three. For the purposes of this paper the word "recurrence" will refer to a visit at which one or more tumours have reappeared in the bladder after having been removed previously by TUR. From this table we see that the percentage of patients with at least one recurrence is 49.3 for Thiotepa, 62.0 for VM 26, and 52.2 for placebo. Ignoring the time at which the first recurrence occurred, the difference between these percentages is not significant.

TABLE I

RECURRENCES BY TREATMENT (ALL PATIENTS)

	THIOTEPA	VM 26	NO TREATMENT	TOTAL
No. of Patients Randomised	115	116	109	340
No. of Patients with Follow-up	75	71	69	215
No. of Patients with Recurrences	37	44	36	117
Percent with Recurrences	49.3	62.0	52.2	54.4
Total No. of Recurrences	58	69	68	195
Total Months of Follow-up	837	682	682	2201
Recurrence rate/100 Patient Months	6.93	10.12	9.97	8.86

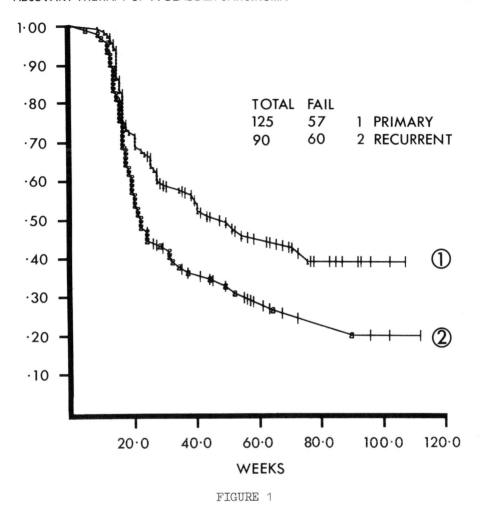

FIGURE 1

Kaplan-Meier curves for the time until first recurrence, a comparison of Thiotepa, VM 26 and no treatment in all patients.

In the lower part of Table I recurrence rates are determined for each treatment by dividing the total number of visits at which recurrence was present by the total patient months of follow-up for all patients in a treatment group. The average duration of follow-up for all patients is approximately 10 months; however, some patients have been followed for as long as two years. The recurrence rates per 100 patient-months of follow-up are 6.93 for Thiotepa, 10.12 for VM 26 and 9.97 for no treatment. Comparisons reveal that the recurrence rate for Thiotepa is significantly lower than that for either VM 26 (P = .03) or no treatment (P = .04) but there is no significant difference between VM 26 and no treatment. These

analyses for primary and recurrent patients are separate. In each
case the recurrence rate for Thiotepa is lower than that for no
treatment or for VM 26 but overall the differences are not
statistically significant (P = .11 for primary patients and P = .17
for recurrent patients).

The number of patients with recurrences showing a higher degree
of malignancy, that is an increase in G classification and the
number of patients with progression to a higher stage of the disease
(increase in T classification) was analysed. Also the number of
patients showing an increase in both the G and T classifications was
evaluated. Overall there are no significant differences between the
three treatment groups with respect to changes in the G and/or the
T classifications; however, among primary patients there has been a
higher incidence of increases in the T classification in patients
treated with VM 26 (P = .01).

DISCUSSION

The preliminary results from this study indicate that while
neither Thiotepa nor VM 26 significantly delay the time until first
recurrence as compared to no treatment, Thiotepa does appear to
decrease the overall recurrence rate. This result agrees with the
results of several previous studies (2) which advocate the prophylactic use of intravesical Thiotepa. However, since Thiotepa
failed to decrease significantly the number of patients who had
recurrences and does not delay the time until the first recurrence,
its activity can only be considered to be of minor importance. The
eventual effect of these drugs on the number of recurrence before and
after treatment was not considered in this preliminary report but
will be evaluated in the final analysis of the results when the study
will be completed. The full report of this analysis will appear in
Recent Progress in Cancer Research.

REFERENCES

1.   Abbassian, A., Wallace, D. M. J. Urol. 96, 461 (1966).

2.   Byar, D., Blackard, C. Urol. 10, 556 (1977).

3.   Drew, J. Marshall, C. J. Urol. 99, 740 (1968).

4.   Edsmyr, F., Boman, J. Acta Radiol. 9, 395 (1971).

5.   EORTC Cooperative Group for Leukemias and Haematosarcomas.
      Brit. Med. J. ii, 744 (1972).

6.   Esquival, E. C., Mackensie, H. R., Whitmore, W. F., Invest.
      Urol. 2, 381 (1965).

7. Greene, L. F., Hanash, K. A. and Farrow, G. M. J. Urol. 110, 205 (1973).

8. Jones, H. C., Swinney, J. Lancet, ii, 615 (1961).

9. Maltry, E. Med. Ex. Publ. Co. (1971).

10. Marshall, V. F. A Symposium. Philadelphia. J. B. Lippincott Company. p. 2 (1956).

11. Mitchell, R. Brit. J. Urol. 43, 181 (1971).

12. O'Flynn, J. D., Smith, J. M. and Hanson, J. S. Eur. Urol, 1, 38 (1975).

13. Pavone-Macaluso, M., Caramia, G., Rizzo, F. P. J. Radiol. Electrol. 55, 844 (1974).

14. Pavone-Macaluso, M., Caramia, G., Rizzo, F. P. and Messana, V. Eur. Urol. 1, 53 (1975).

15. Peto, R. et al. Brit. J. Cancer, 35, 1 (1977).

16. Potthoff, R. F. and Whittinghill, M. Biometrika, 53, 183 (196 (1966).

17. Schulman, C. C. et al. Eur. Urol. 2, 271 (1976).

18. Staquet, M. Eur. Urol. 2, 265 (1976).

19. UICC (International Union Against Cancer). TNM Classification of Malignant tumours, 2nd ed. Geneva. Imprimerie G. De Buren S. A. p. 79 (1974).

20. Veenema, R. J. et al. J. Urol. 88, 60 (1962).

21. Teenema, R. J., Dean, A. L., Uson, A. C., Roberts, M. and Longo, F. J. Urol. 101, 711 (1969).

22. Westcott, J. W. J. Urol. 96, 913 (1966).

PARTICIPANTS

J. Auvert (Hopital Henri-Mondor, Creteil, France)
C. Bollack (Hospices Civils, Strasbourg, France)
C. Bouffioux (Hopital de Baviere, Liege, Belgium)
G. De Clercq (A.Z. Middelheim, Antwerpen, Belgium)
L. J. Denis (A.Z. Middelheim, Antwerpen, Belgium)
S. Fantoni (University Hospital, Pavia, Italy)
R. Glashan (Royal Infirmary, Huddersfield, England)
A. Lachand (Hopital Henri-Mondor, Creteil, France)
B. Lardennois (CHU, Reims, France)
P. Lemaire (CHU, Reims, France)
D. Newling (Royal Infirmary (Sutton), Hull, England)
M. Pavone-Macaluso (University Hospital, Palermo, Italy)
W. Reinhardt (Hospices Civils, Strasbourg, France)
B. Richards (York District Hospital, York, England)
M. Robinson (Castleford, Normanton and District Hospital, Castleford,
   England)
C. C. Schulman (Hopital Universitaire Brugmann, Bruxelles, Belgium)
P. H. Smith (St James's University Hospital, Leeds, England)
M. Vandendris (Hopital Universitaire Brugmann, Bruxelles, Belgium)
G. Viggiano (Ospedale Civile, Mestre, Italy)

INTRAVESICAL CIS-PLATINUM IN BLADDER TUMOURS : TOXICITY STUDY

C C SCHULMAN, L J DENIS and E WAUTERS

University of Brussels

Brussels, Belgium

The Platinum compounds represent a new class of anti-tumour agents. Clinical trials have been restricted, to the investigation of Cis-Diamminedichloroplatinum (DDP), the most promising of these complexes and the only Platinum derivative sponsored for clinical trials by the Division of Cancer Treatment of the National Cancer Institute (1).

Systemic use of this drug in patients with invasive bladder tumour has given encouraging preliminary results (2,3). The main problem raised by the systemic use of this drug is nephrotoxicity and effect on auditory acuity (1). To avoid this problem, administration of Frusemide, Mannitol diuresis or high-fluid intakes have been recommended (4). Instillation of Cis-Platinum into the bladder for the treatment and prevention of recurrences of bladder cancer has to our knowledge not yet been used.

This preliminary study concerns a Phase I trial of intravesical Cis-Platinum to determine toxicity after repeated vesical instillations.

METHOD

Two different doses were used for intravesical instillation. One group received 50 mg DDP while the other received 100 mg. The drug was mixed with a volume of 50 cc of physiological solution and left in the bladder for 60 minutes. After this period the bladder was emptied and Frusemide (20 mg) was given intravenously. In patients with category T1 tumours the instillation was done between 1-12 hours after TUR. In patients with category T3-T4 bladder tumours, instillation was done at rest. It was repeated one and two months later.

TOXICITY TESTS

On days 0 - 1 - 4 - 15 - 45 after each instillation red blood cell count, platelets, urea and creatinine were checked. Audiometry was done prior to the first instillation and repeated 15 and 45 days after instillation. The total period for checking toxicity for each patient was 105   days after the first instillation.

CLINICAL MATERIAL

Twenty patients with histologically proven bladder tumours were selected for intravesical instillation. There were two groups, one receiving instillation of 50 mg DDP, the other 100 mg DDP. Ten patients were treated in each group. The 50 mg group includes eight patients with T1 tumours and two with T3-T4 lesions. In the 100 mg group, 10 patients were considered, six with T1 lesions and four with T3-T4 carcinoma.

RESULTS

No changes in any of the laboratory tests on the patients indicated toxicity.

A transient decrease in high tone hearing was noted on the audiogram in three patients in the 50 mg group but this returned rapidly to normal levels. No clinical signs of local or systemic toxicity became evident in any of the patients.

CONCLUSION

No local or systemic toxicity has been detected in this Phase I trial with intravesical instillation of 50 and 100 mg of DDP in patients with bladder tumours.

The therapeutic effect of the drug was not a prime consideration in this study. Recurrence was however observed only in one case with a T1 bladder tumour.

Further clinical studies should be encouraged to compare the effects of intravesical instillation of DDP with other drugs and with control groups in category T1 bladder tumours.

REFERENCES

1.   Rozencweig, M., Cis-diamminedichloroplatinum (II), a new
      anticancer drug. Ann. Int. Med. 86, 803 (1977).

2.   Yagoda, A., Future implications of phase II chemotherapy trials
      in ninety-five patients with measurable advanced bladder cancer.
      Cancer Res. 37, 2775 (1977).

3.   Merrin, C., Treatment of advanced bladder cancer with Cis-
      diamminedichloroplatinum (II N.S.C. 119875) : A Pilot Study.
      J. Urol. 119, 493 (1978).

4.   Hayes, D. M., Cvitkovic, E. and Golbey, R. B., High-dose Cis-
      Platinumdiamminedichloride : amelioration of renal toxicity by
      Mannitol diuresis. Cancer, 39, 1372 (1977).

Editorial Note (M P-M).   The indications for local chemotherapy
seem to widen. New drugs have been tested in recent years and nearly
all have been described as active in various open trials. The few
prospective randomised studies that have been completed or activated
do not, so are, confirm, the spectacular results of the early
studies, although Adriamycin and Thiotepa appear to be of some value.
Other drugs, allegedly very active, such as Epodyl and Mitomcyin C
have not yet been evaluated by randomised trials, to our knowledge.
A lot more needs to be done, with regard not only to clinical study,
but also in basic research in laboratory animals by in vitro cultures
and using other experimental models. Much is still uncertain and
controversial. Not only has the ideal drug not yet been discovered,
but much has to be learned about: a) absorption from the bladder -
and the related risk of systemic toxicity, b) fixation of the drugs
to the normal and neoplastic urothelial cells, c) the dosage,
concentration and contact time of the different drugs, d) the local
toxicity, e) the role of urinary pH bladder capacity, partial
urinary retention, vesico-ureteric reflux, previous treatments
including recent local chemotherapy; f) the duration of the treatment
and the frequency of the instillations which rank from one daily to
one three monthly in some reported series, g) the possible better
benefit from continuous irrigation as opposed to repeated instillation, h) the possible mutagenic or oncogenic effect of long term
treatment, i) the value of drug association in local chemotherapy.
It should be noted that the instillation regime for the local treatment of lesions,   such as carcinoma in situ or extensive T1
papillary tumours, may be quite different from those required if the
aim is chemoprophylaxis after TUR. Last but not least, the mechanism
of action of local chemotherapy is incompletely understood. Basic
research is therefore badly needed.

Editorial Note (C C Schulman).   The main questions raised in
the discussion concerned the choice of drugs and the duration of
treatment.

The importance of the recurrences of superficial bladder tumours
must be emphasised once again. Not only is the percentage of these
recurrences very high but also the evolution and the natural history
of these tumours must be underlined. Hence, 73% of the Mayo Clinic
patients experienced recurrences, half of them within a year; eight
patients however (more than 10%) had their first recurrence after
10 years only. In this respect, the question of different potential
diseases can be raised; some patients present with a high rate of
recurrence while others do not. In the Massachusetts General Hospital
series, 85% of the patients had recurrences in a five year follow-up.

The character of the adjacent urothelium likewise determines
the future course for in 35% of the patients with cellular atypia
next to overt tumour invasive carcinoma may develop.

The size of the initial lesion also exerts a definite influence
on the recurrence rate. Hence, 100% recurrences were noted in 15
Mayo Clinic patients who had lesions of 4 cm or larger. Thus when
considering the analysis of the results of chemotherapeutic adjuvant
therapy, the size of the initial lesion must be taken into
consideration. The number of recurrences prior to initiation of an
adjuvant chemotherapeutic treatment must also be noted since if one
patient for instance had multiple recurrences at a very high rate
(eg. 20 papillomata in one year) and if after one or two courses of
chemotherapeutic drugs the number of recurrences drops to one or two
a year, this result is significant and should be emphasised in the
analysis of the results.

In the analysis of the results, an exact comparison of
statistical data regarding survival rate and recurrence rate is
sometimes complicated by the grade of the lesion since 80% five year
survival is reported for Grade I lesions and only 39% for Grade II
lesions.

Considering the unpredictable potential of recurrences of the
disease, should chemotherapy be used for primary disease or limited
to recurrent lesions only? The general impression raised from the
discussion was that chemotherapeutic agents used as an adjuvant to
transurethral resection should be limited to the recurrent lesions.

The timing of intravesical adjuvant chemotherapy was also
discussed. Should intravesical agents be administered immediately
after TUR, or later? Some authors favour the immediate administration
of the agent into the bladder. Others, considering the potential
risk of higher intravascular absorption leading to a higher
concentration in the blood circulation, fear the immediate use of

the drugs and prefer to start the treatment after a few days. It was however generally considered that starting the treatment one month after TUR is too long a delay. General agreement was thus reached to advocate the use of intravesical agents one week after TUR but trials with immediate instillation after TUR must also be considered.

Length of Treatment. Several authors considered that either Thiotepa or Epodyl will separate "the sheep from the goats" and if the patients cannot be cured by these agents, the disease probably has a very high rate of recurrence and in these circumstances treatment should not be prolonged considering the potential risk of development of a more aggressive lesion necessitating aggressive and radical treatment such as cystectomy. In this regard the role of cytology was emphasised as probably the best method of monitoring the action of the treatment, perhaps stopping the treatment if no changes are seen after three to six months.

These patients represent those who will develop metastases at a later time or who will develop a higher degree of malignancy in subsequent recurrences. The impression was that in these patients, conservative treatment was commonly continued for too long and one should keep in mind that a fair number of these patients with T1 superficial tumours will develop a more aggressive lesion and die. Thus if treatment fails, a more aggressive approach should be recommended such as cystectomy or radiotherapy.

When the drugs work for how long should they continue to be used? No definite answer was given to this important question but some authors consider for instance that when Epodyl or Thiotepa bring significant results in a patient it should be maintained indefinitely.

The potential role of immunotherapy as an adjuvant to chemotherapy after TUR was also considered. For instance, the association of Levamisole or BCG with chemotherapeutic agents was advocated by some authors. Several studies have reported a decrease in tumour recurrence rate in patients receiving Levamisole after surgery for breast and lung carcinoma. Levamisole has an effect on immunopotentiation and might be of some help in a fair number of patients presenting a high rate of recurrence.

THE TREATMENT OF BLADDER CANCER WITH VITAMIN A

M C BISHOP

Department of Urology, Addenbrooke's Hospital

Cambridge, England

There is evidence that vitamin A in doses far beyond physiological requirements can inhibit carcinogenesis. This was first
demonstrated in organ culture (1) and later in whole animal experiments where it was found to exert a prophylactic and therapeutic
effect upon chemically induced skin tumours in mice (2) and
respiratory tract epithelial tumours in rats (3). In another series
of experiments vitamin A prevented the seeding of an highly immuno-
genic melanoma between strains of mice (4). The possibility that
the agent was acting as an immune adjuvant was reinforced by the
abolition of its anti-tumour action with anti-lymphocytic serum.
Furthermore, vitamin A can act synergistically with other forms of
treatment known to modify the immune response such as BCG (5).

In man systemic or local applications of vitamin A have been
very effective in the treatment of a number of dermatological
diseases including some which are pre-malignant or proliferative (6).
Papillary transitional cell tumours of the bladder were also partly
or completely destroyed in a trial conducted on a small number of
patients (7).

Unfortunately, the clinical use of vitamin A in large doses is
limited by its toxicity. Chronic overdosage affects most systems,
notably the skin, central nervous system and liver. The minimum
daily toxic dose is approximately 250,000 iu. given for two months
or a smaller dose given over a much longer period (8). Early on in
a course of treatment such side effects are reversible.

In the search for a less toxic preparation of vitamin A a range
of analogues of retinoic acid has been synthesised. Experimentally
they can favourably influence neoplastic changes in the same way as

the parent compound. For example a number of retinoids can reverse or prevent the dysplastic changes developing after treatment of explants of mouse prostate gland with methyl cholanthrene (9). Other workers have demonstrated this anti-neoplastic action on chemically induced bladder carcinoma in rats (10). A significant advantage in the use of retinoids may be a higher index of efficacy in relation to the minimum toxic dose than of the unmodified parent compound. Fortunately, the toxic and therapeutic effects of a wide range of retinoids seem to be dissociated (11).

There must now surely be a need for clinical trials of these compounds in bladder cancer. In Cambridge a trial of two retinoids - the ethyl ester and 13-cis derivatives of retinoic acid - has commenced on patients with multifocal non-invasive recurrent papillary tumours. Preliminary results of intracavitary application are encouraging, confirming their carcinostatic activity, even in very low concentrations.

REFERENCES

1.   Lasnitzki, I. Brit. J. Cancer, 9, 434-441 (1955).

2.   Bollag, W. Eur. J. Cancer, 8, 689-693 (1972).

3.   Cone, M. B. and Nettershein, P. J. Natl. Cancer Inst. 51, 1599-1606 (1973).

4.   Felix, E. L., Lloyd, B.,and Cohen, M. A. Science, 189, 886-888 (1975).

5.   Meltzer, M. S. and Cohen, B. E. J. Natl. Cancer Inst. 53, 585-588 (1974).

6.   Bollag, W. and Ott, F. Cancer Chemother. Rep. 55, 59-60 (1971).

7.   Evard, J. P. and Bollag, W. Schweiz. Med. Wschr. 102, 1880-1883 (1972).

8.   Muenter, M. D., Perry, J. O. and Ludwig, J. Amer. J. Med. 50, 129-136 (1971).

9.   Lasnitzki, I. Brit. J. Cancer, 34, 239-248 (1976).

10. Squire, R. A., Sporn, M. B., Brown, C. C. et al. Cancer Res. 37, 2930-2936 (1977).

11. Bollag, W. Eur. J. Cancer, 10, 731-737 (1974).

THE VETERANS ADMINISTRATION STUDY OF CHEMOPROPHYLAXIS FOR RECURRENT
STAGE I BLADDER TUMOURS: COMPARISONS OF PLACEBO, PYRIDOXINE AND
TOPICAL THIOTEPA

D P BYAR

Biometry Branch, National Cancer Institute

Bethesda, Maryland, USA

INTRODUCTION

At the first course on tumours of the genito-urinary apparatus
held in Erice in July of 1977, I presented preliminary results of
the Veteran's Administration randomised trial comparing placebo,
pyridoxine and topical thiotepa in preventing recurrence of Stage I
bladder tumours. Since that time, that trial has been completed and
reported in the literature (1). My purpose today is to review these
results with you particularly since they have stimulated a new trial
to be performed by members of the EORTC Urological Group, scheduled
to begin early in 1979.

The reasons for studying the two treatments compared to placebo
in this study were quite different. Thiotepa has been reported for
a number of years in uncontrolled series to be useful in treating
established bladder tumours when instilled directly into the bladder
(2,3). Since Stage I tumours can often be removed completely by
transurethral resection, but tend to recur in as many as 50% of the
patients within a period of two years, we were interested to see
whether instillations of thiotepa might retard the growth of these
tumours or cure them altogether. The rationale for studying
pyridoxine was based on epidemiological evidence that abnormalities
of tryptophan metabolism resulting in abnormally increased excretion
of certain metabolites of tryptophan occur in many patients with
Stage I bladder tumours (4). These same metabolites have been shown
in animal studies to be carcinogenic under certain conditions (5).
It is known that these abnormalities of tryptophan metabolism can be
corrected by the administration of 25 mg of pyridoxine daily by
mouth (6). It therefore seemed reasonable to determine whether the
regular ingestion of pyridoxine could reduce the frequency of

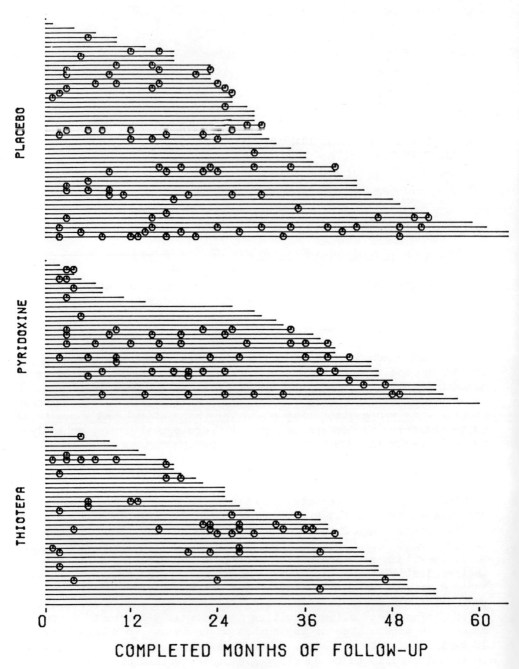

FIGURE 1

Basic data for the study. Lengths of lines represent duration of
follow-up and circles represent recurrences as defined in the text.

recurrence of superficial bladder tumours. It would have been
desirable to measure tryptophan metabolites following a tryptophan
load test in order to identify those patients who should have
benefited from this treatment. However, the logistic problems
involved in such an undertaking with a cooperative study of this
nature were deemed excessive and we elected instead to determine
first whether any empirical evidence could be obtained indicating
that pyridoxine might be useful. If so, in a later study more
detailed biochemical measurements could be made.

MATERIAL AND METHODS

Between November, 1971 and August 1976, 121 patients from 10
Veteran's Administration hospitals were admitted to the study. All
patients with either new or recurrent stage I bladder tumours were
eligible if the tumours could be completely removed by transurethral
resection (TUR). Patients having received previous radiotherapy or
chemotherapy, with carcinoma invading beyond the muscularis or
arising completely within the diverticulum, with bladder
papillomatosis, or who were in such poor physical condition that
the study would endanger their life were excluded.

All patients had stage I bladder tumours at the time they
entered the study, but these tumours were completely removed by TUR
and thus the diagnosis could be confirmed by histological examination.
Patients were assigned randomly to either oral placebo, oral
pyridoxine, or topical instillation of thiotepa. The 25 mg tablets
of pyridoxine were identical in appearance to the placebo tablets and
thus this portion of the study was double-blinded. Placebo and
pyridoxine tablets were taken daily by mouth. Thiotepa, 60 mg in
60 ml of water was instilled in the bladder for two hours once a
week for four weeks and once a month thereafter. All treatments were
to be compared for a period of two years. Patients were examined
cystoscopically every three months for recurrence of tumour and any
new tumours were removed.

In all three treatment groups, the average follow-up was about
31 months, but some cases may have been followed as long as five
years. Comparisons of rates of recurrence defined as the number of
recurrences per 100 patient-months of observation were performed
using an F-test (7). Actuarial curves were used to estimate the
time until first recurrence and differences between these curves
were tested using the Mantel-Haenszel chi-square (8). Responses
which could be treated as percentages were compared using the chi-
square for 2x2 tables. Since by hypothesis the two active treatments
were expected to decrease the recurrence rates, one-tailed
significance tests have been used throughout.

RESULTS

For the purpose of this study, a recurrence was defined as a
visit in which one or more tumours had reappeared in the bladder
after having been previously removed completely by TUR. It is
important to distinguish this terminology from the number of tumours
found at a single visit. The basic data are shown in Figure 1
where the lines represent the length of follow-up and the circles
represent recurrences as just defined. In Table I the number of
patients in the three treatment groups, the percent with recurrences
and the recurrence rates are shown. Although the numbers of patients
in the three groups are not the same, such numbers could easily
arise by chance since patients were randomised separately within
each of the ten hospitals. Patients in each of the three treatment
groups were comparable with respect to age, grade of tumours at
diagnosis, and number of tumours at diagnosis.

No significant difference was detected in the percentages
showing recurrence even though this number was a little higher for
the placebo group. Comparison of the recurrence rates shown in
Table I revealed that placebo and pyridoxine did not differ

TABLE I

RECURRENCES BY TREATMENT

| | Treatment | | | |
	Placebo	Pyridoxine	Thiotepa	Totals
No. of patients	50	33	38	121
No. without follow-up	3	2	0	5
Evaluable patients	47	31	38	116
No. (%) with recurrences	29 (61.7%)	15 (48.4%)	18 (47.4%)	62
Total No. of recurrences	87	57	45	189
Total patient months follow-up	1528	993	1183	3704
Recurrence rate*	5.694	5.740	3.804	5.103

*Expressed as recurrences/100 patient months follow-up

significantly but thiotepa differed significantly from placebo
($t=.012$) and from pyridoxine ($t=.019$). These results suggest that
while thiotepa does not cure these tumours, it does appear to
diminish their frequency somewhat.

Although some patients did not have recurrence of tumour during
the period of observation, other patients had as many as five or
more recurrences. The number of recurrences per patient in each of
the three treatment groups over the period of study is given in
Table II.

Since the ideal goal of treating a patient with recurrent
Stage I bladder tumours would be to prevent recurrence altogether,
the first recurrence is of greater importance than subsequent ones.
For this reason actuarial curves were constructed for time until
first recurrence. The results of this analysis are presented in
Figure 2. Pairwise comparison of these three curves reveal no
significant differences. However, the pattern of the curve for
pyridoxine suggests that almost all the pyridoxine treated patients
who were destined to recur during the period of study did so during
the first twelve months. The sharp fall in that curve between 42
and 45 months represents a single patient. Although it is sometimes
dangerous to over-interpret the shape of survival curves, this
impression would be consistent with the idea that some time is
required for pyridoxine to take effect and that it only affected a
subset of patients in this study, possibly those who had abnormalities of tryptophan metabolism. If we exclude all patients followed

TABLE II

NUMBER OF RECURRENCES PER PATIENT BY TREATMENT

Number of Recurrences per Patient	Placebo	Pyridoxine	Thiotepa	Totals
None	18	16	20	54
1	10	5	8	23
2	4	4	3	11
3	6	0	2	8
4	2	0	2	4
5	4	2	2	8
5	3	4	1	8
Totals	47	31	38	116

up less than 10 months and those who had recurrences during the
first 10 months, the comparison of pyridoxine with placebo is
significant (p=.03, one-tailed). In this analysis thiotepa did not
differ significantly from placebo nor did pyridoxine differ
significantly from thiotepa.

We also studied progression of disease as defined by increase
in the number of tumours seen on subsequent visits, development of
papillomatosis (defined as more than eight tumours present at any
one time), or an increase in tumour grade (Table III). Both
pyridoxine and thiotepa differed from placebo with respect to the
number of patients having an increased number of tumours compared
to the number initially present (p=.027 for pyridoxine, and p=.001
for thiotepa). These two treatments did not differ from each other
with regard to this endpoint. No differences were detected in the
proportion developing papillomatosis or increasing in tumour grade.

Hematological toxicity, defined as a white cell count falling
below 3,500 per cubic millimeter, or platelet count less than
100,000 per cubic millimeter, were each observed in five patients
treated with thiotepa. However, this toxicity was easily managed by
discontinuing the drug until recovery.

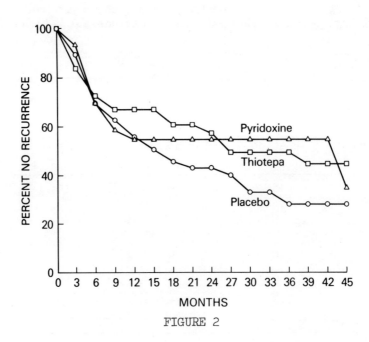

FIGURE 2

Actuarial survival curves for time until first recurrence.

TABLE III

PROGRESSION BY TREATMENT

Treatment	Number of patients	Increase in number of tumours	Development of papillomatosis	Increase of tumour grade
Placebo	47	22 (47%)	6 (13%)	13 (28%)
Pyridoxine	31	7 (23%)	5 (16%)	8 (26%)
Thiotepa	38	5 (13%)	2 (5%)	7 (18%)

* Figures in parenthesis are percent of total treatment group

DISCUSSION

The results for thiotepa suggest that this treatment may decrease the recurrence rate of Stage I bladder tumours, but it does not appear to cure the patient. The results for pyridoxine are interesting and suggest that further studies should be undertaken, particularly with respect to the hypothesis concerning tryptophan metabolism. The first goal of such a study should be to see whether or not these results can be repeated. If in such a study tryptophan load tests are given to all patients at entry, it may be possible to see if pyridoxine acts by altering abnormal tryptophan metabolism. It is conceivable that other mechanisms could explain the action of pyridoxine if in fact the results are confirmed. For example Romas et al (9) have shown that bladder cancer patients with abnormality of tryptophan metabolism showed a greater degree of unreactivity to cutaneous delayed hypersensitivity testing. There is some evidence suggesting that abnormalities of tryptophan metabolism may be unrelated to the development of bladder cancer. These abnormalities have been noted in a variety of other clinical states including Hodgkin's disease, rheumatoid arthritis, and breast cancer, and some workers feel that the abnormalities are produced by the cancer state rather than the reverse (10-12). Only further studies can resolve this issue.

REFERENCES

1.   Byar, D. P., Blackard, C., and the VACURG (Veterans Administration Cooperative Urological Research Group), Comparisons of placebo, pyridoxine, and topical thiotepa in preventing recurrence of Stage I bladder cancer. Urology, 10, 556 (1977).

2.   Jones, H. C. and Swinney, J., Thio-TEPA in the treatment of tumours of the bladder. Lancet, 2, 615 (1961).

3.   Veenema, R. J. et al, Bladder carcinoma treated by direct instillation of thio-TEPA. J. Urol. 88, 60 (1962).

4.   Price, J. M. and Brown, R. R., Studies on the etiology of carcinoma of the urinary bladder. Acta Un. Int. Cancer, 18, 684 (1962).

5.   Bryan, G. T., Brown, R. R. and Price, J. M., Mouse bladder carcinogenicity of certain tryptophan metabolites and other aromatic nitrogen compounds suspended in cholesterol. Cancer Res. 24, 596 (1964).

6.   Brown, R. R., Price, J. M., Satter, E. J. and Wear, J. B., The metabolism of tryptophan in patients with bladder cancer. Acta Un. Int. Cancer, 16, 299 (1960).

7.   Gehan, E. A., Statistical methods for survival time studies, in Staquet, M. J., Ed.: Cancer Therapy: Prognostic Factors and Criteria of Response, New York , Raven Press, 1975, p. 25.

8.   Mantel, N., Evaluation of survival data and two new rank order statistics arising in its consideration. Cancer Chemother. Rep. 50, 163 (1966).

9.   Romas, N. A. et al, Anergy and tryptophan metabolism in bladder cancer. J. Urol. 115, 387 (1976).

10. Gailani, S. et al, Studies on tryptophan metabolism in patients with bladder cancer. Cancer Res. 33, 1071 (1973).

11. Benassi, C. A. et al, The metabolism of tryptophan in patients with bladder cancer and other urological diseases. Clin. Chim. Acta 8, 822 (1963).

12. Teulings, F. A. et al, A new aspect of the urinary excretion of tryptophan metabolites in patients with cancer of the bladder. Int. J. Cancer 21, 140 (1978).

FLAT CARCINOMA IN-SITU OF THE BLADDER TREATED BY SYSTEMIC

CYCLOPHOSPHAMIDE - A PRELIMINARY REPORT

H R ENGLAND, E A MOLLAND, R T D OLIVER and J P BLANDY

Departments of Urology and Pathology, The London Hospital

and Department of Oncology, Institute of Urology, London

ABSTRACT

Nine patients with easily recognisable carcinoma-in-situ of the bladder have been treated with systemic cyclophosphamide. After therapy for six months no histological evidence of the disease could be found in eight patients and the extent of the involvement was markedly reduced in the remaining case. Five had severe "malignant cystitis" and four obtained rapid and complete relief. Longer term studies are needed to determine whether control will persist after discontinuing cyclophosphamide at one year.

INTRODUCTION

In the urinary tract the bladder is the most common site for flat carcinoma-in-situ (C.I.S.) but similar changes may be found in the urethra (Gowing et al, 1960), the prostatic ducts (Thelmo et al, 1974) and the ureters. Experience has shown that C.I.S. of the bladder is radioresistant and to date cystourethrectomy has been the only effective treatment. Examination of bladders removed because of high grade infiltrating tumours has revealed associated widespread C.I.S. in a high proportion of cases and the reported incidence of similar changes in the ureters has ranged between 8% and 50% (Skinner et al, 1974; Schade et al, 1971; Sharma et al, 1970 and Culp et al, 1967). Some patients with ureteric changes go on to develop transitional cell carcinoma of the upper tract following cystectomy (Skinner et al, 1974). Clearly then the ideal treatment for this disease is one which will favourably influence the urothelium as a whole. C.I.S. has a low tumour bulk and high tumour response to chemotherapy. In this study we have used systemic

371

cyclophosphamide to treat a small group of patients with C.I.S. of
the bladder and now report our early experience.

MATERIALS AND METHODS

TABLE I

Patients Treated - Details

Patients treated	9
Positive Cytology	8
"Malignant cystitis"	5
Duration of treatment	6-15 months

Nine patients have been treated so far (Table I). Multiple
biopsies from each were examined and the diagnosis of C.I.S. made
only when the abnormal epithelium was composed of cells showing
definite malignancy (Figure 1). Cases with atypical hyperplasia
and having less clear cut nuclear and cytoplasmic abnormalities were
not included. Two patients had not previously been treated for
bladder cancer. In three, C.I.S. persisted after radiotherapy had
successfully eliminated associated infiltrating tumours, and the
other four had developed C.I.S. two to five years after a T1 tumour
had been successfully treated.

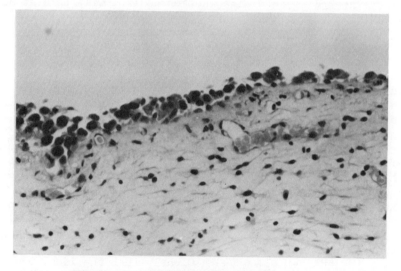

Figure 1   Definite Malignancy
Enlarged hyperchromatic nuclei disorderly pattern of
growth, no identifiable superficial cell layer.

Eight patients had positive urine cytology and five had significant symptoms of "malignant cystitis" consisting of frequency with urgency and often incontinence as well as bladder and genital pain.

The first patient was treated for 15 months but subsequently the plan has been to give cyclophosphamide i.v. every three weeks for six months, then every six weeks for a further six months in a dose of 1 g /m^2 of body surface area (Merrin et al, 1975). Multiple biopsies were taken every three months. Six patients have been followed six months and three others for 9, 12 and 15 months respectively. One patient refused further treatment at three months but has continued to be biopsied.

RESULTS

TABLE II

Summary of Results after Six Month's Therapy

in 9 patients

	Before	After
Cytology	8 Pos.	9 Neg.
Histology	9 Pos.	8 Neg.
Symptoms relieved	5 out of 5	

At six months urine cytology was negative in all nine patients (Table II). In eight, including the one who stopped treatment, no histological evidence of C.I.S. could be found (Figure 2). In the remaining patient the extent of the disease was reduced from florid C.I.S. in every biopsy to two tiny foci in six specimens (Figure 3). Patients followed longer than six months continued to display negative cytology and histology, but some sections at 12 and 15 months indicated that fibrosis of the lamina propria and muscle may be a significant side effect of continuing treatment (Johnson and Meadows, 1971).

Four patients had rapid and complete symptomatic relief. In the fifth, response was good but took place gradually over a period of 12 weeks, seemingly in keeping with persisting but diminishing C.I.S.

Histology showed two effects of treatment, the first being the effect of cyclophosphamide on C.I.S. and the second the changes of cyclophosphamide induced "haemorrhagic cystitis".

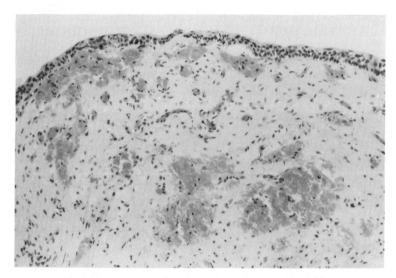

Figure 2   Intact Surface Layer of Cells
Thin but otherwise normal epithelium.

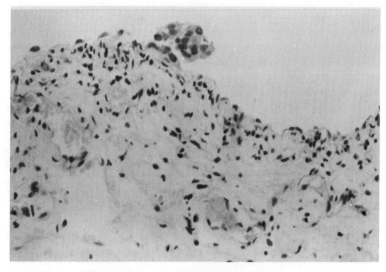

Figure 3   Denuded Surface -
Small Focus of C.I.S. Remaining at Three Months

1. Effect on Carcinoma in Situ

Early sections showed a surface either extensively denuded or lined by cells showing cyclophosphamide effects (Figure 3) but there was no evidence of C.I.S. In sections at 12 and 15 months there was re-epithelialization by thin but otherwise normal epithelium.

2. Cyclophosphamide "Haemorrhagic Cystitis"

At three months extensive areas were denuded and persisting cells showed marked enlargement with ballooning and vacuolation of cytoplasm. Nuclei were enlarged and irregular. The cell pleomorphism was stricking. In the lamina propria dilatation and congestion of capillaries was prominent and there were foci of recent haemorrhage.

Difficulties have been reported in distinguishing malignant epithelium from specific cyclophosphamide induced effects (Forni et al, 1964; Rubin and Rubin, 1966), but with the knowledge that the patient had received cyclophosphamide it was not difficult to distinguish the pleomorphic and rather bizarre changes due to that agent from the relatively uniform hyperchromatic cells of C.I.S.

CONCLUSIONS

In the short term and whilst treatment is continuing or has recently been stopped, cyclophosphamide has controlled C.I.S. of the bladder in eight of nine patients and has markedly reduced the extent of the disease in the remaining patient. Longer term studies are needed to determine how long control will persist after therapy has been stopped. It is very unlikely to persist and maintainence therapy will almost certainly be required. In that event it will be important to assess the extent of cyclophosphamide induced fibrosis and its relationship to dose and route of administration.

These early results are encouraging and demonstrate that C.I.S. of the bladder can be favourably influenced by chemotherapy. They justify further trials and a search for other effective agents.

REFERENCES

1.   Culp, O., Utz, D. and Harrison, E., Experiences with urethral carcinoma in situ detected during operations for vesical neoplasm. J. Urol. 97, 679-682 (1967).

2. Forni, A., Koss, L. and Geller, W., Cytological study of the effect of cyclophosphamide on the epithelium of the urinary bladder in man. Cancer, 17, 1348-1355 (1964).

3. Gowing, N., Urethral carcinoma associated with cancer of the bladder. Brit. J. Urol. 32, 422-438 (1960).

4. Johnson, W. and Meadows, D., Urinary bladder fibrosis and tolangicotasia associated with long term cyclophosphamide therapy. New Eng. J. Med. 281 (6), 290-294 (1971).

5. Merrin, C., Cartegena, R., Wajsman, Z., Baumgartner, G. and Murphy, G., Chemotherapy of bladder carcinoma with cyclophosphamide and adriamycin. J. Urol. 114, 884-887 (1975).

6. Rubin, J. and Rubin, R., Cyclophosphamide haemorrhagic cystitis. J. Urol. 96, 313-316 (1966).

7. Schade, R., Serck-Hanssen, A. and Swinney, J., Morphological changes in the ureter in cases of bladder carcinoma. Cancer 27, 1267-1272 (1971).

8. Sharma, T., Melamed, M.,and Whitmore, W., Carcinoma in situ of the ureter in patients with bladder carcinoma treated by cystectomy. Cancer, 26, 583-587 (1970).

9. Skinner, D., Richie, J., Cooper, P., Waisman, J. and Kaufman, J., The clinical significance of carcinoma in situ of the bladder and its association with overt carcinoma. J. Urol. 112, 66-71 (1974).

10. Thelmo, W., Seemayer, T., Madarnas, P., Mount, B. and MacKinnon, K., Carcinoma in situ of the bladder with associated prostatic involvement. J. Urol. 111, 491-494 (1974).

METHOTREXATE THERAPY FOR MULTIPLE T1 CATEGORY BLADDER CARCINOMA

R R HALL

Department of Urology
Newcastle General Hospital
Newcastle-upon-Tyne, England

INTRODUCTION

In our search for a more effective treatment of patients with extensive stage T1 bladder tumours, we are currently testing the action of Methotrexate against this disease.

According to the present understanding of the absorption, metabolism and excretion of Methotrexate, this drug is excreted largely unchanged in the urine. On this basis and given the normal range of daily urine production, it should be possible to obtain highly cytotoxic concentrations of Methotrexate in the urine by the oral administration of 50 mg Methotrexate. The possibility of treating superficial bladder carcinoma and possibly preventing recurrent superficial disease, by a non-toxic oral medication was an attractive one so we have embarked upon the following study.

METHOD

TABLE I

ORAL METHOTREXATE FOR MULTIPLE T1 CATEGORY TCC

INDICATORS:	Extensive or frequently recurring tumours
DOSE:	50 mg oral once every week
DURATION:	6 - 17 weeks

Patients presenting with very extensive multiple T1 category transitional cell carcinoma or who have had multiple recurrent tumours for more than one year, have been included in the study. After initial cystoscopic assessment and confirmation of normal renal function and peripheral blood count, patients have been treated with Methotrexate syrup 50 mg orally once every week for a minimum of six weeks after which time they have been re-cystoscoped to assess the extent of tumour necrosis.

RESULTS

Tumour Necrosis

In no patient has total tumour necrosis occurred. In three out of 11 patients more than 50% tumour necrosis has occurred, five have remained unchanged over a two to three month period and in three, tumour has become more extensive.

TABLE II

ORAL METHOTREXATE FOR MULTIPLE T1 CATEGORY, TCC

RESULTS: FIRST CYSTOSCOPY

Complete tumour regression	0/11
50% tumour regression	3/11
No change	5/11
Tumour progression	3/11

Follow-up, Six Months or more

Irrespective of the response to Methotrexate at the first follow-up cystoscopy, the bladder of each patient has been rendered tumour free by endoscopic resection, the latter being repeated after a few weeks if necessary to ensure complete tumour clearance. Thereafter patients have been maintained on Methotrexate therapy to assess its effectiveness in the prevention of a tumour recurrence. Of 10 patients who have been followed for six months or more, three have remained tumour free. In view of these patients' history this would appear to be a major achievement. In the remaining seven patients tumour has recurred. In three there have been only two or three small tumours but in two others their carcinoma has progressed and become deeply infiltrating.

TABLE II

ORAL METHOTREXATE FOR MULTIPLE T1 CATEGORY, TCC

RESULTS: FOLLOW   6/12 or more

Tumour Free   3/10

Tumour Recurred   7/10

Urine Methotrexate Levels

As the theoretical basis for our use of Methotrexate was not proven, we have measured the urinary excretion patterns of Methotrexate in our patients. It is generally accepted that a concentration of 10^{-7} M. is cytotoxic but levels of 10^{-6} M. are probably more desirable.

Fourteen of the 17 oral doses of 50 mg Methotrexate have achieved concentrations of 10^{-7} M. for an average of 10 hours after administration. Only five out of 17 doses achieved 10^{-6} M. for a much shorter period of less than two hours.

The total excretion of Methotrexate in the urine was surprisingly low, on average less than half of the 50 mg dose being retrieved in the urine.

TABLE IV

ORAL METHOTREXATE FOR MULTIPLE T1 CATEGORY, TCC

RESULTS: URINE METHOTREXATE LEVELS

5/17   Doses achieved 10^{-6} M. for 1 - 2.5 hours
        (Av. 1.7)

14/17   Doses achieved 10^{-7} M. for 3.5 - 30 hours
        (Av. 10.1)

Total excretion in urine was 21.7 - 96.5% (Av. 49.2%) of 50 mg oral dose.

CONCLUSIONS

1.   From our limited experience of the use of Methotrexate 50 mg orally every week, there is some evidence of anti-tumour effect.

2.   The regime has proved entirely non-toxic.

3.   The urinary excretion of Methotrexate has been surprisingly low.
This may contribute to our limited success and, more importantly,
implies a poorer absorption or higher metabolism of this drug than
has been recognised previously.

THE PLACE OF CHEMOTHERAPY IN THE TREATMENT OF PATIENTS WITH INVASIVE CARCINOMA OF THE BLADDER

R T D OLIVER

Senior Lecturer in Oncology, Institute of Urology

London, England

Most reports on the use of chemotherapy to treat patients with carcinoma of the bladder have used as evidence for activity the observation of greater than 50% reduction of measurable metastases in lungs, lymph nodes or soft tissues (1). Few of these reports have assessed the effect of these agents on primary tumours, principally because assessment of response of disease in the bladder, unless it is complete, is extremely difficult, particularly in patients who have already received radiotherapy to the pelvis. However, there have been anecdotal reports of complete disappearance of primary tumours in previously untreated patients (2,3). In an attempt to get more information on this problem, phase I studies using Methotrexate or Cis-Platinum, two single agents previously reported to be active against metastatic disease (4,5) and Adriamycin-Cyclophosphamide-Cis-Platinum, a highly active chemotherapeutic combination (6) were initiated to assess tolerance of these nephro-toxic drugs in patients with advanced pelvic disease. Allocations to these treatments was not random, but depended upon the avail-ability of Cis-Platinum and in the case of the combination treatment, whether the patient was clinically fit enough without evidence of ischaemic heart disease. All patients who were referred with recurrent of metastatic carcinoma of the bladder were entered on one of the treatment protocols. Table I gives details of the distribution of clinically demonstrable tumour in the patients and the treatment received. Seventeen of the 36 patients did not have any evidence of clinically or radiographically detectable metastases and of the patients with detectable metastases, only 10 of 19 had clearly measurable lesions ie. less than one-third of the total patient population. Only one of the 36 patients had previously had cystectomy.

TABLE I

DISTRIBUTION OF DETECTABLE DISEASE AT START
OF CHEMOTHERAPY

	Methotrexate 100 mg/m² weekly			Cisplatinum 50 mg/m² 3 weekly			Adriamycin 50 mg/m² Cyclophosphamide 150 mg/m² Cisplatinum 75 mg/m² 3 weekly		
	N	CR+PR	MR	N	CR+PR	MR	N	CR+PR	MR
Total Patient Group	22	3	9	10	2	3	4	1	1
Tumour in Bladder	17	3	6	8	0	2	4	1	1
Metastases:									
Bone	7	0	4	4	0	2	-	-	-
Node	-	-	-	2	2	0	-	-	-
Lung	4	0	0	3	0	2	-	-	-
Liver	1	0	0	-	-	-	-	-	-

N = Number of patients with tumour at site indicated.

Treatment was continued for a minimum of three months and
response was assessed by cystoscopy and examination under
anaesthetic. If there was evidence of response or no evidence of
disease progression treatment was continued for a further three
months. Table II gives the response of the patients to treatment
by site of disease and Table III gives the degree of response by

TABLE II

RESPONSE TO TREATMENT BY SITE OF DISEASE

	N	CR	PR	MR
Primary Tumour	30	3	1	9
Bone	11	-	-	6
Lymph Nodes	2	2	-	-
Lung	7	-	-	2
Liver	1	-	-	-
Overall	36	5	1	13

TABLE III

RESPONSE TO TREATMENT BY CLINICAL STAGE

		CR	PR	MR
T3 MO	8	3	1	-
T3 M+	10	1	1	4
T4 MO	9	-	-	5
T4 M+	9	-	-	4

clinical stage at the start of chemotherapy. Complete response means disappearance of all clinically measurable disease, partial response means greater than 50% reduction of measurable disease. Minimum response indicates either a subjective response such as loss of bone pain or reduction of outflow obstruction due to tumour at the base of the bladder. At this stage there was no indication of any difference in response to the three different treatment regimes. Relatively few of these patients (14%) showed clear objective evidence of response, though if the patients with relatively small amount of disease are considered (ie. the patients with the T3 tumours), six out of 18, ie. 33% did show objective evidence of tumour regression. The most impressive responses were the complete disappearance of primary tumours in three out of eight T3 patients who had persistent disease six to 18 months after treatment with radiotherapy and the two instances where supraclavicular lymph node metastases completely disappeared.

From the point of view of drug toxicity there were no serious haematological or renal complications after treatment, though all patients receiving cis-platinum vomited four to six hours after each treatment. Treatment had to be stopped in only one patient due to development of an allergic skin reaction to methotrexate, which rapidly resolved after stopping the drug.

DISCUSSION

Evidence for response to chemotherapeutic agents in patients with solid tumours usually depends on measurement of metastatic lesions. It is clear from the data presented here that less than one third of patients with carcinoma of the bladder have measurable metastatic lesions. To restrict study of the use of chemotherapy in bladder cancer to these patients means that two-thirds of the patients will not be studied. At present phase II studies of chemotherapeutic agents are restricted to these patients with measurable metastatic lesions. It is possible that this could produce mis-

leading information when attempts are made to use these drugs in
phase III trials treating all patients with bladder cancer, as
experiments with animal tumours have demonstrated that clones of
cells with metastatic potential have biological properties which
distinguish them from those without metastasising potential (7).
It is also clear from these studies that the major clinical problem
with invasive carcinoma of the bladder is management of the primary
disease as more than 80% of these patients had clinically symptomatic
recurrence of primary tumour in their bladder (8). There is
obviously an urgent need for additional methods such as urine
cytology, computerised axial tomography or carcinoembryonic antigen
measurements in the urine to evaluate response of the primary tumour
in patients receiving chemotherapy.

Nevertheless, despite all these problems and the advanced state
of disease in the patients treated in this study it is clear that
these drugs are active in advanced carcinoma of the bladder as has
been reported by others and it is necessary to consider how the drugs
may be integrated into their primary management of this disease. As
the survival of patients who show complete disappearance of a tumour
after treatment with radiotherapy is so good (approaching 70% at
five years)(8), it would probably be wise in the first instance to
restrict use of these drugs in a systematic way to those patients
who fail to respond to primary radiotherapy treatment or develop
recurrence after treatment with radiotherapy, 50% of whom will be
dead in less than 12 months (8). The high cost of these drugs, the
risks involved in using drugs which may in themselves increase the
incidence of second malignancy or cause death due to renal or
haematological toxicity, are all factors which make this approach
the most reasonable one to be considered at the present time. Only
those agents or combinations which prolong survival of these patients
should be considered for adjuvant therapy in previously untreated
patients.

SUMMARY

    A phase I examination of the use of either methotrexate, cis-
platinum or the combination of adriamycin, cis-platinum and cyclophosphamide in patients with carcinoma of the bladder who fail
primary treatment with radiotherapy has confirmed that these agents
do demonstrate some activity. However, it has also emphasised the
difficulties of evaluating response in patients who have persistent
primary tumour and shown that to restrict studies of these drugs to
patients with measurable metastasis means that more than two-thirds
of patients will not be studied. Better methods of evaluating
response of primary tumour are clearly urgent priorities for the
future as are prospective randomised trials treating all patients
who have failed primary treatment.

ACKNOWLEDGEMENTS

I am grateful to J. P. Blandy, P. R. Riddle, H. E. England,
P. Worth, H. J. G. Bloom, R. Morgan, W. F. Hendry, M. Singh and
J. P. Williams for referring patients.

REFERENCES

1.   Carter, S. K. and Wasserman, T. H.   Cancer 36, 729-747 (1975).

2.   Hall, R. R., Bloom, H. J. G., Freeman, J. E., Nawrocki, A.
      and Wallace, D. M.   Brit. J. Urol. 46, 431-438 (1974).

3.   Cross, R. J., Glashan, R. W., Humphrey, C. S.,
      Robinson, M. R. G., Smith, P. H. and Williams, R. E.   Brit.
      J. Urol. 48, 609-615 (1976).

4.   Turner, A. G., Hendry, W. F., Williams, G. B. and
      Bloom, H. J. G.   Brit. J. Urol. 49, 673-678 (1977).

5.   Yagoda, A., Watson, R. C., Gonzalez-Vitale, J. C., Grabstald, H.
      and Whitmore, W. F.   Cancer Treat. Rep. 60, 917-923 (1976).

6.   Sternberg, J. J., Bracken, R. B., Handel, P. B. and
      Johnson, D. E.   J.A.M.A. 238, 2282 (1977).

7.   Fidler, I. J. and Kripke, M. L.   Science, 197, 1076-1082 (1977).

8.   Oliver, R. T. D., Hope Stone, H. F., Blandy, J. P.,
      England, H. E.   In preparation.

CHEMOTHERAPY IN THE TREATMENT OF INVASIVE BLADDER CANCER

P H SMITH

Department of Urology
St. James's University Hospital
Leeds, England

Survival for the patient with invasive bladder cancer, whether treated by surgery, radiotherapy or a combination of both is by no means satisfactory. For the patient with a category T3 lesion five year survival following cystectomy alone rarely exceeds 20% (Bowles and Cordonnier 1963; Poole-Wilson and Barnard 1971; Pearse, Reed and Hodges 1978). Up to 30% of patients survive following radiotherapy (Frank 1970) and using the combination of pre-operative radiotherapy and cystectomy the figure rises to 40-50% (Wallace and Bloom 1976; Van der Werf-Messing 1973; Whitmore et al 1977).

Until recently the fact that approximately 40% of such patients die within the first year of diagnosis, whatever the treatment, has been largely ignored. Some idea of the cause of this high death rate has been given by Prout (1977) who found that, of 59 cystectomies for Stage B, C, D, (T2-T4) bladder cancer distant metastasis was the first sign of failure in 24 patients (40%) and that 85% of their metastases was seen in the first year after surgery. Such figures must imply that local treatment is ineffective and demand systemic treatment possibly by cytotoxic chemotherapy. Such adjuvant therapy is usually restricted to patients with a poor prognosis but as De Kernion (1977) observes - "Invasive bladder cancer fulfils this criterion".

It seems that further refinements of surgical or radio-therapeutic technique are unlikely to influence the survival in the critical first year after treatment. The use of additional therapy at this time is likely to prove the most rewarding method of attack.

Such logic encourages consideration of the possible role of adjuvant chemotherapy which has already proved so successful in certain solid tumours in children and in tumours of the testis.

In 1975 Carter and Wasserman showed that only three agents -
Adriamycin, 5-Fluorouracil and Mitomycin C has been investigated and
that remissions were seen in 25-35% of patients. Since that time
information has become available on a further six agents - Bleomycin,
Cisplatinum, Cyclophosphamide, Methotrexate, Neocarzinostatin and
VM 26. The results of a recent computer search of the use of
cytotoxic agents in bladder cancer is shown in Table I. The list
of drugs which have not been evaluated is shown in Table II and from
this it is clear that much work remains to be done to identify
agents which may be effective and subsequently to combine them for
clinical usage (Smith and YUCRG, 1979).

TABLE I

CYTOTOXIC DRUGS ACTIVE IN BLADDER CANCER

DRUGS EVALUATED	REMISSION RATE	
	Alone	In Combination
Adriamycin	40/168	40/111
Bleomycin	5/36	5/5
Cis-Platinum	8/23	11/18
Cyclophosphamide	18/47	14/39
5-Fluorouracil	39/90	23/49
Methotrexate	29/77	-
Mitomycin C	13/51	-
Neocarzinostatin	14/17	-
Vincristine	3/10	-
VM 26	5/30	5/27

The EORTC Urological Group and the Yorkshire Urological Cancer
Research Group have already undertaken studies in this field (Cross
et al 1976; EORTC Group B 1977; Glashan et al 1977; Richards, Akdas
and YUCRG 1978). These will be referred to later in this session.

Some early results of the use of adjuvant chemotherapy in
patients with bladder cancer treated either by cystectomy or radical
radiotherapy (Merrin and Beckley 1978; Richards, Akdas and YUCRG
1978) strongly suggest that chemotherapy has much to offer in moving
the survival curve to the right and in transforming the outlook for
the patient.

Urologists have a decision to make. Do we accept the evidence
now available that chemotherapy is an existing part of urological
practice or alternatively continue to use existing treatments which
are known to be unsatisfactory?

TABLE II

CYTOTOXIC DRUGS NOT YET EVALUATED IN BLADDER CANCER

ALKYLATING AGENTS

N_2 Mustard
Chlorambucil
Melphalan
Busulfan

MITOTIC INHIBITORS

Vinblastine

ANTIMETABOLITES

6 Mercaptopurine
6 Thioguanine
Cytosine Arabinoside

RANDOM SYNTHETICS

B.C.N.U.
C.C.N.U.
Methyl C.C.N.U.
Streptozotozin
D.T.I.C.
Hexamethylmelamine
Dibromodulcitol
Procarbazine
L-Asparaginase

ANTITUMOUR ANTIBIOTICS

Actinomycin D
Mithramycin

(BLAISE - February 1978)

REFERENCES

1. Bowles, T. W. and Cordonnier, J. J. J. Urol. 90, 731-735
    (1963).

2. Carter, S. K. and Wasserman, T. H. Cancer, 36 (Supp), 729-747,
    (1975).

3. Cross, R. J., Glashan, R. W., Humphrey, C. S.,
    Robinson, M. R. G., Smith, P. H. and Williams, R. E. Brit. J.
    Urol. 48, 609-615 (1976).

4. De Kernion, J. B. Cancer Res. 37, 2771-2774 (1977).

5. EORTC Urological Group B. Eur. Urol. 3, 276-278 (1977).

6. Frank, H. G. Clin. Radiol. 21, 425-430 (1970).

7. Merrin, C. and Beckley, S. J. Urol. 119, 62-63 (1978).

8. Pearse, H. D., Reed, R. R. and Hodges, C. V. J. Urol. 119,
    216-218 (1978).

9. Poole-Wilson, D. S. and Barnard, R. J. Brit. J. Urol. 43
    16-24 (1971).

10. Smith, P. H. and YUCRG. J. Roy. Soc. Med. (In Press) (1979).

11. Prout, G. R. Jr. Cancer Res. 37, 2764-2770 (1977).

12. Richards, B., Akdas, A. and YUCRG. Recent Results in Cancer
    Research, Springer-Verlag, Berlin, Heidelberg. G. Mathe.
    (In Press).

13. Van der Werf-Messing, B. Cancer, 32, 1084-1088 (1973).

14. Wallace, D. M. and Bloom, H. J. G. Brit. J. Urol. 48, 587-594,
    (1976).

15. Whitmore, W. F. Jr., Batata, M. A., Ghoneim, M. A., Grabstald,
    H. and Unal, A. J. Urol. 118, 184-187 (1977).

5-FLUOROURACIL AND ADRIAMYCIN IN LOCALLY RECURRENT AND/OR

METASTATIC BLADDER CANCER

C-E LINDHOLM, W MATTSSON, P LANGELAND AND I GYNNING

Department of Oncology

Malmö General Hospital, Malmö, Sweden

SUMMARY

Ten patients with locally recurrent and/or metastatic bladder cancer were treated with 5-Fluorouracil on day 1-3 and Adriamycin on day 4, every three to four weeks up to a maximum dose of Adriamycin of 500 mg/m^2.

Four objective regressions were obtained. In addition there was good relief of severe pain in three patients and disappearance of haematuria and frequency in three and two patients respectively. Side effects during treatment, though sometimes pronounced, were transient.

CLINICAL MATERIAL

The age of the ten patients ranged from 59-84 years (median 70 years). Previous treatment included full dose radiotherapy (66 Gy in six and a half weeks) in seven patients, full dose radiotherapy followed by cystectomy in two patients and trans-urethral resection in one patient.

At the start of chemotherapy there was locally recurrent tumour in 10 patients and disseminated metastases in three (in bone in two and in skin and lymph nodes in one). Locally palpable tumour was found in 9/10 cases and tumour seen at cystoscopy in 5/7 cases. Morphological proof of malignancy was obtained in all ten patients by histology from biopsy specimens in 7/7, by cytological examination of fine needle aspiration biopsies in 2/2 and by exfoliative urinary cytology in 7/7 patients. According to WHO-malignancy grading three

TABLE I

TREATMENT SCHEDULE

Day 1   5-FU   15 mg/kg Body Weight in 500 cc 5.5% Glucose in
                    6 hours iv. infusion

Day 2   5-FU   30 mg/kg Body Weight in 1,000 cc 5.5% Glucose,
                    divided in 2 x 6 hours iv. infusion

Day 3   5-FU   30 mg/kg Body Weight in 1,000 cc 5.5% Glucose,
                    divided in 2 x 6 hours iv. infusion

Day 4   Adriamycin 40 mg/m^2 body surface by iv. bolus injection.

Treatment repeated every three to four weeks to a maximum dose of
Adriamycin 500 mg/m^2.

patients had greade II lesions, six patients grade III tumours. In
one the G category was uncertain. The treatment schedule is shown
in Table I.

RESULTS

The results are shown in Table II.

Palpable tumour regression was noted in two patients and in one
of them a regression of lymph nodes and cutaneous metastases also
occurred, lasting for five months. In two further patients malignant
urinary cytology returned to normal. The survival of these four
responders was 6-17 months compared to 4-11 months in non responders.
Subjective improvement was observed in four patients for three to
nine months (pain relief in three, disappearance of frequency in
two).

At autopsy persistent local tumour was found in 7/9 patients
together with disseminated metastases in six of these. In two
patients who died from other causes and who underwent autopsy no
remaining tumour was found, only marked local fibrosis. In these two
patients superficial bladder cancer recurrences were proven before
chemotherapy by urinary cytology in both and by transurethral
resection biopsy in one but in neither was infiltrating tumour
proven.

In the two patients whose urinary cytology became normal during
chemotherapy their palpable tumour was unchanged. In these two
cases there may have been post radiotherapy fibrosis before chemotherapy plus superficial urinary bladder cancer recurrences, cured by

TABLE II

TREATMENT RESULTS

NUMBER OF COURSES	DISAPPEARENCE OF SYMPTOMS	DURATION MONTHS	PALP TUMOUR REGRESSION	NORMALISATION OF CYTOLOGY	SURVIVAL MONTHS	AUTOPSY FINDINGS
1	NO	–	NO	NO	4	NO AUTOPSY
2	NO	–	NO	YES	6	FIBROSIS
4	NO	–	NO	–	4	CANCER
4	YES	3	NO	–	11	CANCER
5	NO	–	NO	–	4	CANCER
5	NO	–	NO	NO	7	CANCER
7	NO	–	NO	YES	17	FIBROSIS
7	YES	5	YES	YES	8	CANCER
11	YES	6	NO	–	10	CANCER
14	YES	9	YES	NO	11	CANCER

the chemotherapy.

SIDE EFFECTS

All patients had alopecia, transient nausea and diarrhoea (sometimes rather disabling) during treatment. Stomatitis was observed in one patient but there was no serious myelosuppression. In one responding patient with a previous history of peptic ulcer haematemesis occurred during treatment. Another patient developed a paralytic ileus during treatment.

ADJUVANT CHEMOTHERAPY FOLLOWING PRIMARY IRRADIATION IN T3 BLADDER

CANCER

B RICHARDS and the Yorkshire Urological
    Cancer Research Group

York District Hospital
York, England

SUMMARY

This paper presents the early survival figures of a study
designed to evaluate the toxicity of Adriamycin and 5-Fluorouracil
combined with irradiation in the primary treatment of T3 bladder
cancer. Fifteen of 18 patients survived one year. These results
are better than would be expected. Adjuvant chemotherapy in T3
bladder cancer deserves further evaluation.

INTRODUCTION

The main thrust of urological endeavour against carcinoma of
the bladder has been directed towards improving the treatment of
the primary disease; these efforts have been reasonably rewarded
as long as the disease is superficial. However, when the cancer has
infiltrated deeply the situation is much less agreeable. While there
are significant differences in the survival rates in series of
patients treated with primary radiotherapy (5,6), primary surgery (7)
or a combination (6,7), these differences are insignificant compared
to the number of patients who die whatever treatment is employed
Irrespective of the primary treatment, 40% of the patients diagnosed
as having T3 bladder carcinomas are dead in a year, 50% in two years,
and 70% in five years.

Adjuvant chemotherapy has been advocated by Prout (4) and
De Kernion (2), the disadvantage being that at present the drugs which
which are available for use in advanced bladder cancer are not very
effective, are toxic and expensive. It has been argued that it is
unethical to treat patients with toxic and possibly ineffective drugs

when some of them will survive without treatment. But there is surgical prejudice here, as relatively few urologists hesitate to submit their patients to a total or radical cystectomy which causes a significant mortality and morbidity despite the fact that it fails to cure at least two thirds of cases and is unnecessary in one fifth who would have had a prolonged survival without it. In round figures, 100% have the operation, 70% die anyway, and 20% would have survived without it and are thus overtreated. Only 10% benefit.

YORKSHIRE UROLOGICAL CANCER RESEARCH STUDIES

Impressed by the combination of Adriamycin and 5-Fluorouracil in advanced bladder cancer (1), the Yorkshire Urological Cancer Research Group decided to undertake a randomised prospective study evaluating these drugs as adjunctive therapy to primary irradiation. As the combination of radio- and chemotherapy might have been toxic, a preliminary study was carried out on 18 patients with T3 bladder cancers to see whether it was safe and tolerable (3). The toxicity was acceptable. The initial survival in this group of patients is better than predicted. Fifteen of 18 (83%) were living at one year as opposed to 60% in larger studies of conventional therapy. It must be emphasised that the numbers are small, entry was uncontrolled, that this was a toxicity study only, and that the difference does not persist at two years. The results, however, suggest that adjuvant chemotherapy in these patients is unlikely to reduce survival, and that it is appropriate to initiate a randomised controlled trial to assess whether it is beneficial. Such a study is now in progress in the Yorkshire Urological Cancer Research Group.

REFERENCES

1. Cross, J. R., Glashan, R. W., Humphrey, C. S., Robinson, M. R. G., Smith, P. H. and Williams, R. E., Treatment of advanced bladder cancer with Adriamycin and 5-Fluorouracil. Brit. J. Urol. 48, 609-615 (1976).

2. De Kernion, J. B., The chemotherapy of advanced bladder carcinoma. Cancer Res. 37, 2771-2774 (1977).

3. Glashan, R. W., Houghton, A. L., Robinson, M. R. G., A toxicity study of the treatment of T3 bladder tumours with a combination of radiotherapy and chemotherapy. Brit. J. Urol. 49, 669-672 (1977).

4. Prout, G. R., The role of surgery in the potentially curative treatment of bladder cancer. Cancer Res. 37, 2764-2770 (1977).

5. Rider, W. D. and Evans, D. H., Radiotherapy in the treatment of recurrent bladder cancer. Brit. J. Urol. 48, 595-601 (1976).

6. Wallace, D. M. and Bloom, H. J. G., Management of deeply infiltrating (T3) bladder carcinoma: controlled trial of radical radiotherapy versus pre-operative radiotherapy and radical cystectomy. Brit. J. Urol. 48, 587-594 (1976).

7. Wajsman, C., Merrin, C., Moore, R. and Murphy, G. P., Current results from treatment of bladder tumours with total cystectomy at Roswell Park Memorial Institute. J. Urol. 113, 806-810 (1975).

8. Whitmore, W. F., Batata, M. A., Ghoneim, M. A., Grabstald, H., and Unal, A. Radical cystectomy with or without prior irradiation in the treatment of bladder cancer. J. Urol. 118, 184-187 (1977).

9. Whitmore, W. F., Batata, M. A., Hilaris, B. S., Reddy, G. N., Unal, A., Ghoneim, M. A., Grabstald, H., and Chu, F. A comparative study of two preoperative radiation regimens with cystectomy for bladder cancer. Cancer 40, 1077-1086 (1977).

5-FLUOROURACIL IN THE TREATMENT OF RECURRENT CANCER OF THE URINARY BLADDER

M DUCHEK[*], F EDSMYR and I NÄSLUND

Department of Urology and Radiumhemmet

Karolinska Hospital, Stockholm, Sweden

In a current series of trials of various chemotherapeutic agents to treat advanced recurrent cancer of the urinary bladder following full-dose radiation therapy - conducted at Radiumhemmet in Stockholm in collaboration with the urology clinics in that city during 1974 and 1975 - 5-Fluorouracil was chosen as the first preparation to be tested. When 5-Fluorouracil had no objective effect on the tumour tissue, a combination of 5-Fluorouracil, Adriamycin and Vincristine was used.

METHOD

Two different routes of administering 5-Fluorouracil were chosen: orally on an out patient basis and by intravenous drip to hospitalised patients.

The dose was 500 mg 5-Fluorouracil per day for 10 days. Five cycles were fiven at intervals of one month.

Cystoscopy and cytological examination of bladder washings were carried out initially before the start of chemotherapy; cytology was repeated before the third and fifth cycles and cystoscopy before the fifth cycle. Intravenous urography was performed initially and prior to the fifth cycle. Fifteen patients were treated in each group.

RESULTS

In each group there was partial regression of the local tumour in one patient. In the other patients no objective regression could

be seen, either of the local tumour or of metastases. The side
effects were slight nausea and mild diarrhoea in a couple of
patients. Two patients who received 5-Fluorouracil by intravenous
drip had episodes of gastric bleeding, which perhaps may be
attributable to the treatment given.

CONCLUSIONS

5-Fluorouracil in a dose of 500 mg per day, given in five cycles
of 10 days duration at intervals of one month to patients with
advanced recurrent cancer of the urinary bladder following full-dose
radiation therapy had virtually no effect.

* Present address: Department of Urology, University of Umeå, Umeå,
                     Sweden

RADIOTHERAPY, CHEMOTHERAPY AND IMMUNOTHERAPY FOR CARCINOMA OF THE BLADDER

P A GAMMELGAARD, F LUNDBECK, I S CHRISTOPHERSEN

Herlev Hospital
University of Copenhagen
Denmark

INTRODUCTION

In the period from July 1976 19 patients with invasive cancer of the bladder have been included in a Phase II trial to assess the value of radiotherapy and simultaneous chemotherapy with subsequent Levamisole therapy. Fourteen patients were newly diagnosed and five had received surgical treatment prior to the start of the trial. The patients were T-staged according to UICC (September 1975) and the grading follows Bergkvist's classification. Table I shows the T-category and histological grade of the patients.

Histology showed transitional cell carcinoma in 18 patients and a mixed lesion in one. Tumour size ranged from 2 x 2 - 7 x 12 cm and the age from 29-70 years (mean 54 years). Patients over the age of 70 were excluded from the trial.

TABLE I

T-CATEGORY AND HISTOLOGICAL GRADE IN 19 PATIENTS

CATEGORY	GRADE
T1 - 1	II - 2
T2 - 5	III - 14
T3 - 10	IV - 2
T4 - 3	Not Known - 1

TREATMENT

Radiotherapy and chemotherapy were initiated simultaneously. A total dose of 60 Gy (6,000 rad/24 fractions/6 weeks) (CRE: 1855 reu. 106, 5 TDF. 8 MeV lin. acc.) was delivered via one anterior and two lateral portals, the whole field including the small pelvis and the obturator and iliac nodes.

The chemotherapy consisted of seven cycles of three weeks duration without intervals, followed by eight weeks of Levamisole therapy. In each cycle Adriamycin 60 mg/m^2 iv. was given on day one, 5-Flurouracil 12 mg/kg orally was given on day one and eight and finally Levamisole 2.5 mg/kg was given each week on two consecutive days, starting on day one.

RESULTS

The results are shown in Table II.

TABLE II

THE THERAPEUTIC EFFECTS IN 19 PATIENTS

Time of Evaluation	RESPONSE					NO. OF PATIENTS		
	CR	PR	NR	PRO	REL	Cystoscopy performed	Cystoscopy not performed	Deceased
After 4 weeks radiotherapy 4 Gy (4,000 rads)	2	5	2	1		10	9	
3 months after completion of radiotherapy	14	3	1			18		1
6 months after completion of radiotherapy	11	1			1	13	2	2

CR = Complete Remission   PR = Partial Remission   NR = No Response
PRO = Progression   REL = Relapse

Only 10 patients were evaluated at 40 Gy. Two patients showed complete remission at this stage and received no further radiotherapy. Five patients showed partial remission and in two patients no response was found. One patient was severely affected by the tumour before the start of the treatment. In this patient the tumour progressed, and he died four weeks after the start of the combined treatment.

Eighteen patients were examined three months after the completion of the radiotherapy. Fourteen patients showed complete remission and three patients partial remission. One patient showed no response and cystectomy was then performed on this patient.

At the next cystoscopy, ie. six months after the completion of radiotherapy, 13 patients were evaluated. Two patients had died since the last examination, one from a pulmonary embolism, the other as a result of dissemination of the cancer. This patient had bone metastases at the start of the treatment.

Eleven patients showed complete remission and one patient partial remission. One patient had relapsed. Two patients were not examined as they had not been observed for six months after completion of radiotherapy.

Twelve patients received 75% of the scheduled Adriamycin dose and only two received 100%. The 5-Fluorouracil dose was not reduced to the same extent, and 9 patients received 100%. The Levamisole dose has not been reduced, and only four patients felt slight nausea in connection with the treatment with Levamisole. One patient, however, developed agranulocytosis five weeks after completion of the Adriamycin and 5-Fluorouracil treatment and died of septicaemia. This was attributed to Levamisole since the bone marrow had regenerated sufficiently three weeks after the last Adriamycin dose was given.

TABLE III

DOSE REDUCTION DURING CHEMOTHERAPY

Chemotherapy Doses	Adriamycin	5-Fluorouracil
100%	2	9
75%	12	7
50%	3	3
25%	2	0
Number of Patients	19	19

CONCLUSIONS

In all, 17 patients have responded to the treatment, evaluated
three months after completion of radiotherapy, and 15 patients have -
at some time - shown a complete remission. Six patients were
addmitted to hospital for two weeks for treatment of side effects.
Neither ileus nor intestinal perforation have been seen. The
scheduled chemotherapy appears to be at the upper limit of patient
tolerance and probably should be reduced to 75% of the suggested
level in future studies.

INTEGRATED THERAPY FOR INVASIVE BLADDER CARCINOMA

J A MARTINEZ-PIÑEIRO

Service of Urology, La Paz Clinic

Faculty of Medicine, Autonomous University, Madrid, Spain

INTRODUCTION

The results of the treatment of infiltrating bladder carcinoma continue to be less than satisfactory. The failure to obtain acceptable survival rates by surgery alone in patients with T3 - T4, No - N1 Mo category tumours has emphasised the necessity of exploring new treatment strategies, including combinations of radiotherapy, chemotherapy and immunotherapy; that is, of integrated therapy.

Two controlled clinical trials (1,2) designed to compare the results of radical radiotherapy and of preoperative radiotherapy plus radical cystectomy in T3 tumours, have shown that the combined treatment affords a significant improvement in survival rates in comparison with radical irradiation alone, and also in comparison with those yielded by cystectomy alone in other series (3-7). A similar conclusion was also obtained by many others in non-controlled studies (6-25). The most impressive finding of all these studies was that the five year survival rates, for the patients whose tumours had experienced a radiobiologically induced T - reduction (or down-staging) were more than twice as great as those for the patients which did not show a significant response, reaching 70-80% five year survival rates in patients whose tumours were ablated (Po). Unfortunately, only 40-50% of T3 bladder cancers show a substantial response to preoperative irradiation with a dose of 4,000-4,500 rads, which has been considered as a safe dose from the view-points of post-operative morbidity and mortality, and which is nevertheless adequate to eliminate moderate disease in the bladder, perivesical space and pelvic nodes (20). A second relevant finding, either in cases treated with combined radiotherapy and cystectomy or with

radical cystectomy alone (1,2,6,7,21), was that the most frequent
cause of failure was disseminating disease, a fact which supports
the current feeling that invasive bladder cancer should be regarded
as a systemic disease, and that local treatment alone is not
sufficient to eradicate the disease (2,6,7,21).

Protocols contemplating systemic treatments as part of
integrated therapy programs are under study by different groups, who
are trying to ascertain whether the use of adjuvant cytotoxic
chemotherapy will increase the success rate. The rationale of these
programmes is supported by two possible actions of adjuvant therapy:
(i) Improvement of the rate and degree of local regression, and
(ii) destruction of distant micrometastases present at the time of
treatment. A preliminary toxicity trial carried out by Glashan et al
(26) in order to assess whether the combination of radical radiotherapy and chemotherapy with Adriamycin plus 5-Fluorouracil was safe
and could be tolerated by the patient, suggested the acceptability of
this combination. The drugs were administered one to three months
following the completion of radical radiotherapy to the bladder, at
three weekly intervals and, providing the therapy was limited to four
cycles, there was no serious toxicity.

An important drawback of any multimodal therapy may, however, be
the induction of immunological depression in the host with enhancement of residual tumour growth, as a result of the immunosuppressive
effects of radiation (27-30) and cytotoxic chemotherapy (31,32). To
minimise the possible risk of enhancement of distant micrometastases
during the period of immunodepression induced by these agents it
seems appropriate to include immunostimulation as part of any future
programme of integrated therapy; whether this stimulation should be
specific-active or passive or non specific still remains to be
determined. Some authors (33,34) report that BCG is relatively safe,
easy to use and appears to be effective in terms of obtaining
remissions and prolonging survival. This suggests that this non-
specific stimulant should be one of the treatments to be tried in
future studies. In summary the ideal modality of integrated therapy
for invasive bladder carcinoma has yet to be defined, but in theory
it should combine surgery, radiotherapy, chemotherapy and immunotherapy. However, before implementing trials with this complex
combination, its possible toxicity has to be determined. Herein
we report the results of a study carried out by our service, in an
attempt to ascertain the toxicity and immunologic side-effects of a
combination of simultaneous radiotherapy - chemotherapy -
immunotherapy - and diverse surgical procedures.

PATIENTS AND METHODS

Two studies were undertaken successively. The first combined
cytotoxic chemotherapy with Adriamycin (ADM) and 5-Fluorouracil

(5-FU), plus telecobalt therapy 4,000-6,000 rads plus BCG immunostimulation, and non-radical surgery - either TUR or urinary
diversion - or no surgery at all, as specified in Table I; the
patients who entered this study were not considered candidates for
radical surgery either due to local extension (T4 one case) low
stage (T2 two cases), disseminated disease or advanced age (two cases
each) or intercurrent illness.(three cases).   Table II, shows the
age, sex, stage and modality of treatment.

The second study combined the same inegrated therapy and a
radical cystectomy, as specified in Table III.   Fourteen patients
entered the study, but four did not undergo cystectomy for different
reasons, leaving ten patients available for assessment:
three of these patients did not receive BCG for the purpose of
comparison as specified in Table IV.

TABLE I

DESIGN OF STUDY No. 1

A.   1.   TUR, complete or palliative, followed four weeks later
          by simultaneous integrated therapy with:

     2.   a.   Telecobalt-irradiation, 4,000-6,000 rads.

          b.   Adriamycin 50 mg/m^2 plus 5-Fluorouracil 500 mg/m^2.
               One cycle every three weeks, starting on first day
               of irradiation, until progression of the disease or
               until a total dose of 550 mg/m^2 of ADM.

          c.   Immuno BCG Pasteur vaccine, 150 mg scarifications, at
               a weekly interval during one month, and on day 14 of
               each cycle thereafter.

B.   1.   Urinary diversion, either four weeks before or four weeks
          after telecobalt irradiation.

     2.   a.   Telecobalt irradiation 2,500-6,000 rads.

          b.   As in A) except that ADM and 5-FU are discontinued
               four weeks before surgery and started again four
               weeks after surgery.

          c.   As in A)

C.   1.   No surgery, except diagnostic TUR.

     2.   a, b, and c as in A).

TABLE II

CASES ENTERED INTO STUDY No. 1

10 Patients, 8 Males - 2 Females

Ages 42-82 (mean 70.2)

TUR Group (6 cases)	2 - T2 Mo
	3 - T3 Mo
	1 - T3 M1b N4
Urinary Diversion	1 - T3 Mo
Group (3 cases)	1 - T4 Mo
	1 - T4 M1c
No Surgery (1 case)	1 - T4 M1b

Pre-treatment studies of the patients entering both trials included a complete physical and urological examination, blood and urinalysis, liver and renal function tests, bone and liver scans, chest x-ray, ECG, bimanual palpation under anaesthesia and deep TUR biopsy or total resection when feasible, and delayed sensitivity skin tests (DNCB, PPD, candidine, epidermophyton, Tricophyton, streptodornase-streptokinase).

TABLE III

DESIGN OF STUDY No. 2

A. 1. Telecobalt-irradiation, 4,000 rads in four weeks.

　　2. a. Radical cystectomy with lymphadenectomy four weeks after telecobalt-irradiations.

　　　　b. ADM 50 mg/m^2 plus 5-FU 500 mg/m^2 at four weekly intervals. The first cycle is administered on the first day of irradiation and the second on the last day. The third cycle is withheld until the patient has recovered from radical cystectomy (4-7 weeks). Therapy is continued until progression of the disease or until a total dose of ADM of 550 mg/m^2.

　　　　c. Immuno BCG Pasteur vaccine, 150 mg scarifications at a weekly interval during irradiation and at four weekly intervals thereafter (on day 14 of each chemotherapy cycle).

B. 1, 2a and 2b as in A.　　　　2c. No BCG is administered.

TABLE IV

CASES ENTERED INTO STUDY No. 2

10 Patients, 9 Males - 1 Female

Age 46-73 (mean 62.4)

BCG Group (7 cases)   5 - T3 Mo
                         2 - T4a Mo

No BCG (3 cases)   3 - T3 Mo

During the treatment, cardiac, liver, renal and haematological toxicity was monitored by means of ECG and blood analysis performed on day 14 and the day before each chemotherapy cycle; if cardiac toxicity was detected, ADM was discontinued until the ECG returned to normal. In some cases when the ECG remained abnormal it was stopped indefinitely. For haematological toxicity persisting the day before a new cycle, the drug dosage was reduced to 50% or administration delayed until the platelets were above 75,000 mm^3 and/or the leukocyte count above 3,000 mm^3.

Skin tests were repeated immediately after completion of irradiation.

The patients were fully assessed three months later and every six months afterwards, carrying out the pretreatment studies, excluding cystoscopy in cystectomised patients.

RESULTS

Survival

Eleven patients (55%), four of study No. 1 and seven of study No. 2 are presently alive; the follow-up period ranging between three months and 18 months; three of the four survivors of study No. 1 are free of disease more than one year later (2 - T2, 1 - T3) and the seven survivors of study No. 2 (6 - T3, 1 - T4a) are free of disease between three months and one year. The current survival rate is 50% for the TUR group, 33% for the diverted group, 0% for the non-operated patient of study No. 1 and 70% for the cystectomy group.

Mortality

Study No. 1   One patient (11.1%) died postoperatively (15th

day) after an ileal loop diversion for a T4a tumour due to leakage
of the uretero-ileal anastomosis, wound infection and paralytic
ileus. He had received 2,500 rads postoperatively and two cycles
of ADM and 5-FU.

Three patients died at two and a half, five and 13 months
respectively due to progression of metastases and local disease.
Two patients died at four and 13 months, of intercurrent illness,
but were free of malignant disease (T3 Mo, 4,000 and 6,000 rads, TUR,
four cycles of chemotherapy each, eight and 18 scarifications
respectively).

Study No. 2   Three patients (30%) died postoperatively; one
of septic shock, renal and hepatic failure and disseminated intravascular coagulation (16th day), one of peritonitis due to ureterocolic leakage (9th day), and one of massive gastro intestinal
bleeding (36th day).

The overall mortality in both groups attributable to the
integrated therapy was therefore 20% (four of 20 cases).

TOXICITY AND COMPLICATIONS

Eighteen patients (90%) presented side effects and/or
complications caused by the treatment, eight of study No. 1 and ten
of study No. 2. The complications resulted in the death of the
patient in four cases, were major in five other patients and minor
in the remaining nine. Table V shows the morbidity related to the
treatment regime.

Surgical morbidity (Table VI) amounted to 76.9%; none of the
TUR patients had complications but they will not be taken into
consideration to evaluate the rate of surgical complications, because
all of them were operated before the start of combined therapy. Ten
of the 13 patients undergoing open surgery presented postoperative
complications, which proved fatal in four of them. The most frequent
cause of morbidity was infection, which affected the wound in six
cases, resulting in septicaemia in three of them and leading to death
in two; ureterocolic anastomotic dehiscence was the primary cause of
infection in two of these cases.

Twelve patients (60%) developed subjective or objective signs
of drug toxicity (Table VII) which were severe in four cases (20%)
and moderate in eight (40%). These toxic effects appeared more
frequently (80% versus 40%) in No. 1 trial patients, probably
because of the shorter interval between the cycles (three versus
four weeks) but were of lesser importance.

TABLE V

Surgical Complications

TUR	0/6	0%	
Urinary Diversion	2/3	66.6%	Fatal in 1 patient
Radical Cystectomy	8/10	80%	Fatal in 3 patients
Total	10/19	52.1%	

Cytotoxic Drug Toxicity

Study No. 1	8/10	80%	Severe in 1 patient
Study No. 2	4/10	40%	Severe in 3 patients
Total	12/20	60%	

Telecobalt Side-effects

Study No. 1	2/10	20%	Severe in 1 patient
Study No. 2	5/10	50%	
Total	7/20	35%	

BCG Side-effects

Study No. 1	0/10	0%	
Study No. 2	1/7	14.2%	Severe in 1 patient
Total	1/17	5.8%	

Eight patients suffered from gastro-intestinal side-effects, severe enough in two to necessitate a 50% dose reduction.

Although all the patients showed a fall in the leukocyte and platelet count, with a nadir at two meeks, only two (10%) developed significant myelo-depression (2,000 and 520 leukocytes/mm^3, respectively) making it necessary to postpone and adjust the following cycles.

One patient suffered a reactive hepatitis caused by Adriamycin after only two cycles and radical cystectomy had to be delayed for two months until SGOT and SGPT returned to normal. In spite of this, his postoperative course was stormy and he died on the 16th day of septic shock, renal failure, hepatic failure (bilirubin 7 mg%) and disseminated intravascular coagulation. Another patient also had transient liver dysfunction with a rise of bilirubin to 3 mg% after the first cycle; the dose was reduced to 50% on the second cycle and was again raised to 100% on the third and fourth cycles without further signs of liver toxicity.

In one patient cardiotoxicity (ventricular extrasystoles with acute heart failure) was found after seven cycles, necessitating definitive interruption of cytotoxic therapy. He is living, disease free 18 months later.

TABLE VI

SURGICAL COMPLICATIONS

	Study No. 1 2/3 pts (1)	Study No. 2 8/10 pts	Overall rate in 13 patients	Degree
Wound Infection	1	5	46.1%	3 major 3 minor
Sepsis	1	2	23%	2 fatal 1 severe
Renal Failure	–	1	7.6%	1 fatal
Uretero-Intestinal Anastomotic Leak	1	1	20%	1 fatal 1 severe
Peritonitis	1	1	15.3%	1 fatal 1 severe
Incomplete Intestinal obstruction	–	1	7.6%	1 fatal
Thrombophlebitis	1	–	7.6%	1 minor
Pneumonia	–	1	7.6%	1 minor
Upper gastro intestinal haemorrhage	–	1	7.6%	1 fatal
Hepatic failure	–	1	7.6%	1 fatal
Disseminated Intravescular coagulation	–	1	7.6%	1 fatal

(1) Only the three patients who underwent a urinary diversion are
evaluated here. Transurethral resections were performed before the
start of integrated therapy, and had no influence upon the assessment
of complications due to the same.

Apart from minor local discomfort and in some cases fever, BCG
scarifications were tolerated remarkably well. One case, however, a
woman of 62 years, developed fever, asthenia and coughing four months
after radical cystectomy, when she had received five chemotherapy
cycles and 10 BCG vaccinations. A chest x-ray showed a basal right
lung consolidation and acid-alcohol fast bacilli were detected in the
sputum. Whether it was a reactivation of an old pulmonary TB or a
new lesion caused by the Calmette-Guerin bacillus is difficult to

TABLE VII

CYTOSTATIC-DRUG TOXICITY

	Study No. 1 8/10 pts	Study No. 2 4/10 pts	Overall rate in 20 pts	Degree
Gastro-Intestinal	6	2	40%	6 Minor 2 Major
Oral Ulceration	2	1	15%	3 Minor
Haematologic (1) (WBC $<$ 3,000 ml Platelets $<$75,000 ml)	1	2	15%	2 Minor 1 Major
Hepatic	1	1	10%	2 Minor
Cardiac (2)	1	-	5%	1 Minor

(1)   50% dosage reduction and/or postponement
(2)   Chemotherapy suspended permanently

tell, but either or both situations can probably be attributed to
BCG therapy. Her skin reactivity to PPD was + before commencing
the treatment, ++ after completing telecobalt-therapy and two cycles
of ADM + 5-FU and four BCG scarifications, and + at the assessment
performed three months after cystectomy; her DNCB test was ++. She
has been admitted to another hospital for specific treatment;
chemotherapy and immunostimulation have been interrupted.

Radiotherapy induced cystitis was suffered by five patients,
four having received not more than 4,000 rads and one 6,000 rads.
In two cases it was severe and resisted treatment. One other patient
developed signs of radiotherapy induced proctitis which became worse
following radical cystectomy and uretero-sigmoidostomy; one year
later he still has rectal frequency.

There did not seem to be any correlation between the performance
status of the patients and the frequency or seriousness of the
therapeutic ill-effects.

IMMUNOLOGIC RESPONSE

A patient's delayed cutaneous hypersensitivity, and thus his
cell mediated immune response, was considered normal when the result
of the DNCB test was ++++ or +++, impaired when it was ++ or +; when
the test was negative the patient was considered anergic. The

results of the skin tests with recall antigens often did not
correlate with those of the DNCB test and were not taken into
consideration when assessing the immune response. Nonetheless the
PPD test was considered with respect to BCG therapy; in seven PPD-
negative patients, the injection of 1 mg BCG intradermally with
weekly intervals reversed the test to + in two or three weeks,
allowing the scarifications programme to start in all of them.

    Table VIII shows the results of the DNCB test before treatment
and during the follow-up. Only 25% of the patients had a normal
response before treatment which improved to 50% immediately after
irradiation and up to 55% in subsequent assessments. Conversely,
the rate of negative responses decreased from 55% before treatment
to 30% after irradiation and to 20% in the following months.

    The total lymphocyte count is peripheral blood was considered
normal ($>$1,500 ml) in 75% of the patients before commencing the
treatment. After telecobalt irradiation plus cytotoxic chemotherapy
and BCG therapy, the rate of normal counts decreased to 35%, later
improving to 42.8% (Table IX). In general the lymphocyte level
remained lower than before treatment for periods of up to one year.

TABLE VIII

DNCB Test - 20 patients

	Normal ++++ or +++	Abnormal ++ or +	Negative
Before Treatment	5	4	11
After Irradiation	10	4	6
On last follow-up	11	5	4

TABLE IX

Peripheral blood lymphocyte count below 1,500 mm^3

Before Treatment	5/20	25%
After Irradiation	5/20	65%
On last follow-up (x) (3-18 months)	8/14	57.1%

(x) Unknown in six cases

The improvement rate of the skin reactivity to DNCB was a little higher (47% versus 33%) in patients treated with BCG and the impairment of the lymphocyte count was also less frequent in patients receiving BCG, as shown in Table X.

TABLE X

INFLUENCE OF BCG UPON IMMUNE RESPONSE

| | Improvement | | | | Impairment | | | |
	BCG		No BCG		BCG		No BCG	
DNCB Test	8/17	47%	1/3	33.3%	1/17	5.8%	0/3	0%
Lymphocyte count	1/17	5.8%	0/3	0%	6/17	35.2%	2/3	66%

It seems, therefore, that the patients who were stimulated with BCG, had a slight immunological advantage over those not stimulated; however, because of the small number of patients not receiving BCG, the difference cannot be considered significant.

There was a clear direct correlation between the status of immune response following treatment and the outcome in the patients. 75% of the disease free living patients have a normal DNCB test and,

TABLE XI

CORRELATION BETWEEN SURVIVAL AND RESULT OF DNCB TEST
FOLLOWING TREATMENT

| | ALIVE | | DEAD | | |
	Disease Free	With Disease	Disease Free	Progression	Postoperative
Normal 11 patients	6	0	1	1	3
Abnormal 5 patients	3	1	1	0	0
Negative 4 patients	1	0	0	2	1
Total	10	1	2	3	4

TABLE XII

CORRELATION BETWEEN SURVIVAL AND PERIPHERAL BLOOD LYMPHOCYTE
COUNT, FOLLOWING TREATMENT

Lymphocyte Count	ALIVE		DEAD		
	Disease Free	With Disease	Disease Free	Progression	Postoperative
> 1,500 ml 7 patients	3	0	1	1	2
< 1,500 ml 13 patients	7	1	1	2	2
Total	10	1	2	3	4

conversely, 66.6% of the survivors who died later of their malignant
disease did not react to DNCB (Table XI).

A similar correlation was not found between the lymphocyte
count and the course of the disease (Table XII).

TUMOUR RESPONSE TO INTEGRATED THERAPY

The local tumour response to the combination of simultaneous
radiotherapy cytotoxic drug-BCG was evaluable in the 10 patients of
Study No. 2 who underwent a radical cystectomy (Table XIII).

In five patients (50%) tumour could not be found in their
bladder specimen, but two of them (40%) had one regional node
invaded, supporting the case in favour of radical cystectomy with
lymphadenectomy even in those cases where radiotherapy has eradicated
the tumour from the bladder.

In another case the tumour showed a stage reduction from T3 to
P2 No; this raises to six (60%) the figure of responders to therapy.
Four of these responders had received BCG.

Among the four non-responders, three (75%) also had invaded
regional nodes and these had received BCG, while the one patient
free of node invasion had not received it. Three of these non-
responders are alive one died postoperatively. As far as BCG
adjuvant therapy is concerned, four of seven patients receiving BCG
therapy were responders, two were completely free of tumour, one
still had tumour in the bladder, and one had tumour in one regional
node. Two of three patients not receiving BCG were also responders,

TABLE XIII

LOCAL TUMOUR RESPONSE TO IRRADIATION, CYTOTOXIC THERAPY, BCG

T Category Before Treatment	P, N categories in Radical Cystectomy Specimen		Downstaged	
T3 8 Patients	Po No - 2 patients Po N1 - 1 P2 No - 1 P3 No - 1 P3 N1 - 1 P3 N2 - 2		4	50%
T4a 2 Patients	Po No - 1 patient Po N1 - 1		2	100%
Total 10 Patients	Po - 5 P2 - 1 P3 - 4 Tumour ablation in 5 bladders - 50%	No - 5 N1 - 3 N2 - 2	6	60%

one was completely free of tumour and one had one regional node
invaded.

None of the three patients of study No. 1 with disseminated
disease showed objective regressions of their metastases and all
died between two and a half and five months. Two were anergic before
and following treatment and one showed a transient improvement but
reverted to anergy before death.

DISCUSSION

The findings of the particular group of patients of study No. 1
who underwent only a TUR or no surgery at all, suggest that the
combination of simultaneous irradiation plus ADM and 5-FU, plus BCG
is safe. Toxicity or side-effects were of minor importance in all
the cases. Moreover, when considering the whole series of the 20
patients in the two studies, drug toxicity was really significant in
four patients (20%) and minor in eight (40%), a frequency that is
comparable to that of other studies (26,35).

Of the 20 patients treated, BCG side-effects were remarkable
only in one patient and severe bladder and rectal side-effects of
telecobalt radiation appeared in two cases; however, the wound

infection rate (46%) and the incidence of uretero-intestinal anastomotic leak (20%) were significantly higher than in other irradiated series (6,8,11,14,16,23,24,36,37,38) suggesting that cytotoxic chemotherapy plus irradiation add their effects, accounting for impaired healing, less resistance to infection and postoperative deaths. In fact, the radical cystectomy mortality (30%) and morbidity (60%) rates were inordinately high and unacceptable in comparison to our 16.4% mortality in other series (45), or to the 9-19% ratos in tho world litoraturo (2,4,5,6,13,15,16,18,25). Apart from the usual complications of radical cystectomy, wound infection and sepsis were a major problem among our patients, despite broad spectrum antibiotic coverage. The postoperative stay of the survivors was also very long (22-60 days, mean 37.2 days), indicating that the recovery after cystectomy was affected by prior irradiation-chemotherapy.

Besides these negative findings, some positive aspects emerged from our study. On one hand, integrated therapy did not seem to have suppressor effects upon the cell-mediated immune response, as assessed by the DNCB test. Five (25%) of the anergic patients reverted to normal and five normal patients remained normal during and following the treatment. Whether this is to be attributed to BCG immunostimulation or to a decrease of the tumour burden is a matter of speculation; the slightly better improvement rate of DNCB test in patients receiving BCG dose not afford any proof to resolve the doubts, but the reported immuno-depression found following other regimes (27-32) suggest either that the DNCB test is not trustworthy as a measure of the immune status, or that BCG has played a significant role in sustaining the immunologic competence in our patients. The last hypothesis seems more plausible to us, in view of the world wide acceptance of the DNCB test for the assessment of the host's immune response (39,44).

The behaviour of the peripheral blood lymphocyte count did not correlate with the skin tests, as it should theoretically have done. In 58% of the whole series, the count remained below 1,500 ml for a year or more after the start of therapy, the decrease being more likely to be attributed to irradiation than to the cytotoxic drugs (27,28,32). The importance of a low count is as yet not fully understood; contrary to the findings of Amin and Lich (45) we did not observe any correlation between lymphocyte count and outcome of our patients.

BCG seemed to be effective in preventing this lymphocyte depletion (as demonstrated by the 35.2% rate of impairment, against 66.6% in patients not receiving BCG), though its main action is supposed to be exerted upon the monocytes or macrophages.

A second positive aspect of this study is the very high rate (50%) of tumour ablation in the bladder specimen achieved by simultaneous irradiation-chemotherapy, in comparison to the 24-25% range in the literature (2,6,7,9,10,12,14,15,16,17,24,25). This improvement is likely due to the action of the cytotoxic drugs, which may be two-fold, on the one hand destroying tumour cells and on the other increasing their sensitivity to radiation.

In spite of the positive aspects of our findings, we feel nevertheless that the combination of radical surgery plus radiation and systemic therapy as used in this study is not acceptable, and that the combination is safe only for patients who will not undergo an open surgical procedure.

Therefore, another less aggressive programme of integrated therapy has been designed recently to compare postoperative therapy with ADM plus 5-FU versus nil in patients treated primarily by 1,500 rads flash high energy-radiation and radical cystectomy.

CONCLUSIONS

Simultaneous telecobalt-irradiation plus chemotherapy with ADM and 5-FU, plus BCG immunotherapy, is safe and acceptable as an integrated therapeutic regime for patients in whom conservative. surgical approaches have been carried out previously for the treatment of high grade T2 tumours, and/or T3 - T4 tumours in patients not fit for radical surgery. However, it is not safe in association with a radical cystectomy undertaken four to six weeks after completion of irradiation. The heavy burden which cystectomy imposes upon elderly patients is aggravated by prior radiotherapy plus simultaneous systemic cytotoxic therapy, converting radical surgery into an extremely high risk procedure.

REFERENCES

1.   Miller, L. S. and Johnson, D. E.   Natl. Cancer Conf. Proc. 7, 771 (1973).

2.   Wallace, D. M. and Bloom, H. J. G.   Brit. J. Urol. 48, 587 (1976).

3.   Cox, C. E., Cass, A. S. and Boyce, W. H.   J. Urol. 101, 550 (1969).

4.   Lange, J., Lange, D., Phelippot, J. L. and Valentine, F.   J. d'Urol. Nephrol. 79, 99 (1973).

5.   Pearse, H. D., Reed, R. R. and Hodges, G. V.   J. Urol. 119, 216 (1978).

6. Whitmore, W. F. Jr., Batata, M. A., Ghoneim, M. A., Grabstald, H. and Unal, A. J. Urol. 118, 184 (1977).

7. Prout, G. R. Cancer Research, 37, 2764 (1977).

8. Whitmore, W. F. Jr. J.A.M.A. 207, 349 (1969).

9. Van der Werf Messing, B. Eur. J. Cancer, 7, 467 (1971).

10. Van der Werf Messing, B. Cancer, 32, 1084 (1973).

11. Poole-Wilson, D. S. and Barnard, R. J. Brit. J. Urol. 43, 16 (1971).

12. Bloom, H. J. B. International Bladder Cancer Conference, Leeds (1971).

13. Edsmyr, F., Moberger, G. and Wadstrom, L. Scand. J. Urol. Nephrol. 5, 215 (1971).

14. Prout, G. R., Slack, N. H. and Bross, I. D. S. J. Urol. 105 223 (1971).

15. Blackard, C. E., Byar, D. P. and the VACURG. J. Urol. 108, 875 (1972).

16. Veenema, R. J., Guttmann, R., Uson, A. C., Senyszyn, J. and Romas, N. A. J. Urol. 109, 397 (1973).

17. Prout, G. R. Jr., Slack, N. H. and Bross, I.D.J. Natl. Cancer Conf. Proc. 7, 783 (1973).

18. Richie, J. P., Skinner, D. G. and Kaufman, J. J. J. Urol. 113, 186 (1975).

19. Reid, E. C., Oliver, J. A. and Fishman, I. J. Urol. 8, 247 (1976).

20. Caldwell, W. L. Urol. Clin. N. Amer. 3, 129 (1976).

21. Caldwell, W. L. Cancer Research, 37, 2759 (1977).

22. De Weerd, J. H. and Colby, M. Y. Jr. J. Urol. 107,51 (1972).

23. Galleher, E. P., Young, J. D. Jr., Campbell, E. W. Jr., Wizenberg, M. J., Jacobs, J. A. and Millstein, D. I. J. Urol. 118, 179 (1977).

24. De Weerd, J. H., Colby, M. Y. Jr., Myers, R. P. and Cupps, R. E J. Urol. 118, 260 (1977).

25. Daughtry, J. D., Susan, L. P., Stewart, B. H. and Straffon, R. A. J. Urol. 118, 556 (1977).

26. Glashan, R. W., Houghton, A. L. and Robinson, M. R. G. Brit. J. Urol. 49, 669 (1977).

27. O'Toole, C., Perlmann, P., Unsgaard, B., Moberger, G. and Edsmyr, F. Int. J. Cancer. 10, 77 (1972).

28. O'Toole, C., Perlmann, P., Unsgaard, B., Almrgaard, L. E., Johansson, B., Moberger, G., and Edsmyr, F. Int. J. Cancer, 10, 92 (1972).

29   Catalona, W. J., Potwin, C. and Chretien, P. B. J. Urol. 112, 261 (1974).

30. McLaughlin, A. P. III, Kessler, W. O., Triman, K. and Gittes, R. F. J. Urol. 111, 233 (1974).

31. Hitchings, G. H. and Elion, G. B. Pharmacol. Rev. 15, 265 (1963).

32. Catalona, W. J. J. Urol. 112, 802 (1974).

33. Morales, A. and Eidinger, B. J. Urol. 115, 377 (1976).

34. Martinez-Piñeiro, J. A. and Muntañola, P. Eur. Urol. 3, 11 (1977).

35. EORTC Urological Group B. Eur. Urol. 3, 276 (1977).

36. Kursh, E. D. Rabin, R. and Persky, L. J. Urol. 118, 40 (1977).

37. Johnson, D. E. and Lamy, S. M. J. Urol. 117, 171 (1977).

38. Bredin, H. C. and Prout, G. R. Jr. J. Urol. 117, 447 (1977).

39. Catalona, W. J., Taylor, P. T., Rabson, A. S. and Chretien, P. B. New. Engl. J. Med. 286, 399 (1972).

40. Catalona, W. J., Smolev, J. K. and Harty, J. K. J. Urol. 114, 922 (1975).

41. Brosman, S., Hausman, M. and Shacks, S. J. J. Urol. 114, 375 (1975).

42. Martinez-Pineiro, J. A., Muntanola, P. and Hidalgo, L. Eur. Urol. 3, 159 (1977).

43. Adolphs, H. D. and Steffens, L. Eur. Urol. 3, 23, (1977).

44.   Klippel, K. F., and Jakse, G.   Aktuelle Urologie, 9, 205
       (1978).

45.   Amin, M. and Lich, R. J.   J. Urol. 111, 165 (1974).

46.   Martiñez-Pineiro, J. A.   Lecture at the meeting of the
       Asociacion Española de Urologia, 7 Feb, 1976, Madrid.

CANCER CHEMOTHERAPY, WITH SPECIAL EMPHASIS ON THE ROLE AND INFLUENCE OF CLINICAL TRIALS[*]

J H MULDER

Department of Internal Medicine
Radio-Therapeutic Institute
Rotterdam, The Netherlands

ABSTRACT

New methods of treatment are regularly compared with existing methods. The aim of doing clinical trials is to improve the standard treatment regimens. Important aspects of this process are the trial protocol, trial organisation and the impact of clinical research on the medical treatment in general.

INTRODUCTION

Two decades ago, the medical treatment of cancer patients was quite simple. The physician had a limited number of drugs and the criterion for success was tumour regression without too much toxicity. As more new agents were discovered and extensive basic knowledge was obtained on the mechanism of action of the various drugs, highly sophisticated drug shedules were designed. As a consequence, a more or less standard treatment can be described for each tumour type. Everyone who is familiar with medical treatment of cancer patients, however, knows that the so called standards treatment of today does not imply that this treatment is always very successful. For instance, one could state that Adriamycin in combination with 5-Fluorouracil is a generally accepted treatment for advanced bladder carcinoma. However, the number of patients who will have a long lasting benefit from the treatment is negligible. The cytostatic drug treatment of bladder carcinoma as well as of other urological tumours needs substantial improvement (Table I).

* Supported by the "Koningin Wilhelmina Funds" of the National Cancer League.

TABLE I

CYTOSTATIC DRUG TREATMENT OF UROLOGICAL TUMOURS: A TREATMENT POLICY
FOR PATIENTS TREATED IN A GENERAL HOSPITAL

Tumour Type	Suggested Treatment
Renal cell carcinoma	No chemotherapy
Bladder carcinoma	Adriamycin + 5 FU, but only if there are objective tumour parameters. No adjuvant chemotherapy
Prostatic carcinoma	No cytotoxic chemotherapy
Testicular carcinoma	Refer to a cancer centre for curative treatment

Medical treatment in some malignant diseases has dramatically improved the prognosis. The development of chemotherapy for testicular tumour patients demonstrates this very clearly. Because clinical trials have played such an important role in the improvement of the results, it seems appropriate to opt for a similar strategy in bladder, prostate and renal cell carcinoma. How do we initiate clinical trials in these diseases?

TABLE II

RELATIONSHIP BETWEEN KIND OF PHASE STUDY AND TUMOUR TYPE

Standard treatment has not been established; therefore, there is a need for Phase II drug screening studies in:

- Renal cell carcinoma, inoperable or metastatic
- Bladder carcinoma
- Prostatic carcinoma, chemotherapy

Standard treatment more or less accepted; Phase III, controlled clinical trials needed in:

- Prostatic carcinoma, hormonal therapy
- Testicular carcinoma and seminoma

Adjuvant chemotherapy attractive; an urgent need for Phase IV, combined modality trials in:

- Testicular carcinoma

THE TRIAL PROTOCOL

The clinical investigations are organised into Phase study formats:

Phase   I : dose and toxicity investigations,

Phase II : antitumour response measurements,

Phase III : controlled clinical trial,

Phase IV : combined modality treatment with and without
             adjuvant chemotherapy.

The first essential to improve medical cancer treatment is the design of a trial protocol. Without a well written protocol, it is impossible to start clinical research. The contents of the various chapters of the protocol should be formulated as exactly as possible. These chapters are:

Aims of the study : Define the questions that are being asked,

Selection   : which patients are eligible,

Treatment   : is it a drug screening study or will two
                     treatments be compared?

Evaluation   : What are the tumour response criteria and
                     are additional investigations required?

Organisation   : What is the minimum number of patients to
                     be included according to the statistician?
                     Who is in charge of the data processing?
                     Are there study forms to be filled in?
                     How are the patients informed?

THE AIMS OF THE TRIAL

In the first chapter the aims of the study are stated as shortly and clearly as possible. If no effective drug is known for a particular disease, the aim of the study will be to find one. A typical example of a Phase II study could be: what is the effect of chlorozotocin in advanced renal cell carcinoma? If, however, a more or less standard treatment is available and it is decided to improve the standard therapy, a Phase III controlled clinical trial should be organised; then the critical question is: which treatment is more effective, the existing or the new one? The question raised in an adjuvant trial is far more complex than in the Phase II and III studies. Chemotherapy can be considered in "high risk" patients immediately after the primary treatment, whether surgical or radiotherapeutic. If the risk of occult micrometastases is high, early cytostatic treatment may sterilise these small tumour foci. Since it is not certain that the cytoxtatic drug treatment will be of real advantage to the patient, the results obtained in the treated

patients will be compared with those of not treated or control
patients. The first question to be answered in a Phase IV adjuvant
trial is whether the disease free time interval between primary
treatment and tumour recurrence is increased. Another question is
where the tumour will eventually relapse, loco-regionally or at a
distance from the primary tumour area. These types of data can have
a great impact on the design of the subsequent combined modality
trial. Apart from tumour response, the patient survival time can
be used as a study parameter. The survival time, however, is a
rather crude method of treatment evaluation. The next question is
what the treatment policy should be when the patient's tumour
relapses during or after the end of adjuvant chemotherapy. Finally,
the clinical investigator should take into account the morbidity of
the treatment. Social, economic, psychological and physical "side
effects" will be taken increasingly into account when adjuvant trial
results are discussed.

THE SELECTION OF PATIENTS

The second paragraph of a trial protocol concerns the selection
of patients. In a Phase II screening study, this should be simple.
Are there any objective tumour parameters and is the physical
condition of the patient reasonably good. The selection in a Phase
III study is much more complicated. The diagnosis must be certain,
the presence of an objective tumour parameter is a condition sine
qua non and the Karnofsky index indicating the clinical condition of
the patient must be relatively high. But these selection criteria
are not sufficient. Clinical experience as well as retrospective
analyses have shown some clinical factors to be highly correlated
with patient prognosis. The consequences of these prognostic factors
are that patients should be stratified according to the most
important factors. The purpose of stratification of patients is to
balance treatment groups as accurately as possible. All of the
differences among the results observed in the groups can then be
attributed to the treatment and not to a biased patient selection.

The selection of patients in a Phase IV adjuvant trial is even
more complicated. No one should receive unjustified cytostatic
treatment and each patient in an adjuvant trial should have a high
risk of tumour recurrence. Until we have tumour markers to detect
subclinical disease the tumour recurrence risk has to be calculated;
tumour size, histological grade, extent of tumour infiltration and,
most important, the presentation of histologically proven lymph node
metastases are the most commonly used prognostic factors. Not all
these factors are well established and not all are of equal
importance. A valuable spin-off of any well designed trial is the
search for the most important prognostic factors.

TREATMENT

The third element in a trial protocol is the treatment. In a
Phase I study, the choice of drug will be influenced by what the
experimentalist will suggest from his animal data. In such a study,
the highest tolerable dosages are established and the most important
side effects evaluated. The dose and schedule of the drug determined in the Phase I study is used in the Phase II screening trial.
Here after two or three courses of treatment the antitumour response
is measured using the objective tumour parameters. The procedure
in a Phase II study is therefore really very straightforward.

The situation is totally different in a Phase III controlled
clinical trial. Before the study starts the investigators should
establish the optimal existing treatment. This may take some time.
Then, someone has to suggest something new which is at least as
effective as the generally accepted standard treatment. In Phase IV
adjuvant trials, a comparison will be made between chemotherapy and
regular postoperative follow-up. The adjuvant treatment should be
simple to administer and the total length of treatment time should
not be too long. For instance, to give a patient cytostatic agents
each month for a year is not a simple task either for the patient or
for the clinician.

EVALUATION OF THE RESULTS

The last important medical aspect of a protocol concerns the
tumour response evaluation. Complete remission is self explanatory
and the definition of partial response is simple:- a tumour volume
reduction equal to or more than 50% of the volume before treatment.
The interpretation of response in certain areas eg. bone metastasis
in patients with prostatic cancer, is more difficult and it is
probable that extramural review of all of the clinical data,
organised by the study coordinator is more important than endless
discussions on how to define tumour response.

ORGANISATION OF A TRIAL

After designing a good trial protocol the next requirement for
improving the medical treatment of cancer is a well organised plan of
action. Here professional statistical advice is essential as to how
many patients are needed in a study if the conclusions are to be
statistically significant. For instance to enter 200 patients in a
Phase III study, several centres should cooperate. This implies
that, before the trial is activated, the possibility of recruiting
it should be ascertained.

Another aspect of organisation is the problem of clinical
follow-up accompanying a trial. The most extreme example will be
encountered in an adjuvant trial: "Usually we had a simple check
during the surgical follow-up period but since this adjuvant business
started....", is a common complaint of surgeons. In the adjuvant
format, we have to know exactly how the surgical treatment was
performed and how many lymph nodes were histologically investigated.
Copies of pathological reports will be requested by the investigator.
Then comes the patient selection and stratification. Next the
randomisation procedure, that is to say, in the controlled trials the
choice of treatment is by chance. At the trial data centre, a sealed
envelope is deposited containing information on the type of treatment
the patient will receive. In contrast to follow-up without medical
treatment, the clinical investigator has to inform the patient of
what he plans to do. All of this takes considerable time. Then, the
treatment starts with all the accompanying minor and sometimes major
toxic side effects. At the end, all the study forms should be filled
in as accurately as possible. Who wants to do the job? Who has time
to do this type of clinical research? Who will finance the project?
All of these are matters of organisation and should be discussed
before starting. The final requisite to improve the medical
treatment of cancer is obviously the publication of results.

INFLUENCE OF MEDICAL CANCER RESEARCH ON DAILY PRACTICE

If the general public cannot immediately benefit from the
results obtained from medical cancer research, then the whole project
is a waste of money. Not every physician can or wants to participate
in, for instance, an EORTC clinical trial. But anyone who treats
patients with antitumour agents wants to be sure that he is applying
the cytostatic drug arsenal in the optimal way. A beneficial effect
of initiating a clinical trial is the fact that the investigators
have to analyse what is occurring in routine practice.

Is the treatment of symptoms or hormonal treatment perhaps as
good as or even better than chemotherapy in renal cell carcinoma?
Is combination chemotherapy really more effective than single drug
therapy in bladder carcinoma? Is an aggressive treatment of late
testicular carcinoma recurrences not as good as early adjuvant
chemotherapy.

If we wish to improve the quality of medical oncology, we must
discuss these questions in general, especially with those clinicians
who are not in a position to do clinical research. In this way, all
patients who will not be treated according to a particular trial
protocol will at least get the best standard treatment. As soon as
the clinical investigator has shown without a doubt that something
is significantly better, the new regimen will be advocated. A result
of this policy the difference in the quality of treatment between
trial and non-trial patients will be as minimal as possible.

Part 3
Prostatic Cancer

OESTROGEN - ANDROGEN BALANCE IN HUMAN BREAST AND PROSTATE CANCER

L CASTAGNETTA

University of Palermo
"M Ascoli" Oncological Hospital
Palermo, Sicily, Italy

Although we conventionally categorise the hormonal steroids as oestrogens, progestins, corticoids or androgens it is more realistic to consider that the steroids exhibit a continuous spectrum of biological effects.

Certain classes of steroids may either synergise or neutralise the expected effects of other steroids (24). Numerous interactions occur among the oestrogens and the androgens (Table I): ie. testosterones will in some species exert the type of uterotrophic action usually attributed to the oestrogens (42).

Administration of oestrogens suppresses the release of LH by negative feedback on the pituitary-hypothalamic axis thereby curtailing the secretion of testosterone and reducing the circulating concentrations of plasma-androgens (19,35).

Mammary tumours contain receptors for androgen in addition to those for oestrogen, progestin and glucocorticoid, so one assumes that the androgen effect is receptor-mediated (30,33). It has been proved on human prostatic carcinoma cells that both the action of E_2 (28) and that of cyproterone acetate (CA), an effective antiandrogen in the treatment of prostatic cancer (20) are achieved through inhibition of the androgen receptor, while diethylstilboestrol (DES), according to very recent studies, has a different mechanism of action.

The possible metabolic transformation of androgen to yield oestrogenic hormones, by the oestrone-pathway is well known.

Only in the last years have studies been carried out on the

TABLE I

SOME ASPECTS OF STEROID INTERACTION

1. STEROID LEVELS INTERACTIONS

    Both of oestrogens and/or androgens (24,42)
    Increase of corticosteroids secretion (4,5)
    Reduction of circulating androgens (22,34)

2. INTERFERENCE BY MECHANISM OF ACTION ON CYTOPLASMIC
    AND NUCLEAR RECEPTORS

    Differentiate actions of E_2, CA and DES (21,28,30,33)

3. DIRECT INTERACTIONS

    Metabolic aromatisation of androgens in peripheral
    tissues (19,35)
    Regulation of FSH and LH by catechol oestrogens (21,36)

4. NON SPECIFICALLY MEDIATED INTERACTIONS

    Other biochemical mechanisms
    Cyclic AMP and oestrogens (13,32,38)

5. THE OPPOSITE ROLE OF OESTROGEN AND ANDROGEN

    a) On SBbetaG of human plasma (25,37,43)
    b) In the digestive and urinary tract carcinogenesis
        induced in rats by BBN (31,46)

    The role of oestriol : protection - The role of
    testosterone : enhancement

direct formation of oestrogens from circulating androgens (2,17).

There is now good experimental evidence of the conversion of
androgens to oestrogens in peripherical tissues. We refer, above
all, to catechol oestrogens which can be produced by conversion of
androgen to oestrogens (19,35).

Testosterone but not DHT can be metabolised to oestradiol
17beta in certain regions of the brain (44).

Peripheral oestrogen production by aromatase enzymes (36) is an
important source of oestrogens in both men and post-menopausal women.
Moreover recent evidence suggests that this reaction may be important
in gonadotropin regulation (16,21).

The non-specific interactions of the various classes of steroid hormones refer to actions mediated by biochemical effectors, eg. to cyclic adenosine monophosphate (C-AMP). We know that C-AMP is essential for the normal function and growth of steroid-sensitive cells (32,38) and we also know the opposite actions on growth-control mechanism of E_2 and C-AMP (13). This is another example of hormone interference: oestrogens may condition the growth of prostatic cancer cells not only through the receptors.

Lastly (15) we draw attention to the opposite actions of E_2 (37) and androgens (43) on the steroid binding beta globulin (SB-beta-G) of human plasma (increase after oestrogen and decrease after androgen administration). Likewise the action of testosterone (favouring) and that of E_3 (counteracting) the carcinogenetic action induced by bis-butyl-nitrosamine (BBN) in experimental tumours in rats show an opposite behaviour (46). This is a further demonstration that it is necessary to distinguish clearly between biological and biochemical action, and reject outdated classifications on active and inactive oestrogen metabolites.

ADVANCED BREAST CANCER EXCRETION PATTERNS

The parameters selected through studies on advanced and metastatic breast cancer in postmenopausal women shown in Table II (7,9,10) are four in addition to: 1) the three classical oestrogens (oestrone, oestradiol, oestriol, ie. E1 + E2 + E3); 2) the oestriol ratio (E3/E1 + E2); 3) those which we have defined as unusual oestrogen metabolites, relative both to the ketol fraction and the non-ketol fraction; and lastly; 4) the ratio of classical oestrogens to unusual metabolites (ie. pattern index = PI).

TABLE II

SELECTED PARAMETERS OF OESTROGENS

1 Classical Oestrogens	3 Unusual Metabolites	EXCRETION PATTERNS OF OESTROGENS ▼
2 Oestriol Ratio	4 Pattern Index	PROGNOSIS IN HORMONE TREATMENT

These four parameters shown in Table II defined as oestrogen metabolic pointer, (OE. M.P.) can indicate the degree of abnormality of the oestrogen patterns (10).

A larger number of abnormal characteristics are positively correlated with a more advanced stage of cancer both in terms of size and spreading of metastasis (10).

Studies on postmenopausal patients with advanced breast cancer undergoing hormone adjuvant therapy have shown a negative correlation between positive response to therapy and the reduced pattern index. A negative correlation between response and negative oestrogen metabolic pointers was also shown (10).

These results enable us to envisage the possibility of using oestrogen excretion patterns and their selected parameters as a guide for prognosis of hormone treatment of advanced human breast cancer (11).

In our studies in advanced postmenopausal breast cancer a decrease in androgen metabolites excretion appears positively correlated with an abnormal oestrogen excretion (Table III).

TABLE III

URINARY OESTROGENIC OUTPUT IN POSTMENOPAUSAL

ADVANCED BREAST CANCER (n=72)

	CLASS OEST.	E3 RATIOS	CLASS OEST. / UNUS. MET. RATIOS	UNUS MET.	WHOLE OEST.	17 KST / WHOLE OEST. RATIOS
Group I	− (+)	− (‡)	−− (‡)	+++ (‡)	+++ (‡)	− (+)
Group II	++ (‡)	+ (‡)	− (+)	++ (+)	+++ (‡)	−− (‡)

+ p < 0.05   Postmenopausal Age: Group I : n = 26

‡ p < 0.01   from 3 to 15 years   Group II : n = 46

‡ p < 0.001

The relationship between excretion levels of all the selected androgens (=17 oxosteroids = 17 KS) and of all the selected oestrogens (whole oest.) is defined as oestrogen-androgen balance (= OE - A balance). It is dependent upon androgen excretion level (normally about 100 times as much as that of oestrogen).

Increased OE-A balance was positively correlated with both the reduced pattern index and the negative oestrogen metabolic pointers.

Moreover, in patients with postmenopausal breast cancer responding to hormone therapy, the OE-A balance, which had increased

significantly, mainly because of a reduction in androgen excretion
tends to return to normal values; while in the group of patients not
responding to endocrine therapy, the OE-A balance remains
significantly close to normal control values of healthy postmenopausal women.

TABLE IV

STEROID HORMONE PATTERNS

Plasma Concentrations

	T	DHT	E2	E1	E3	E2/T
Breast Cancer Group (n = 72)	+(=)		=	=	=	=
Prostatic Cancer Group (n = 17)	=(+)	=	=	=(+)	=	=

Excretion Levels

	Andr. (9)	Oest. (7,8)	P1 (10)	OE-A BAL (10)	17 OHCS (40)
Breast Cancer Group (n = 72)	−	+	−	+	+
Prostatic Cancer Group (n = 17)	−	+	−	+	+

PLASMA CONCENTRATIONS AND EXCRETION LEVELS OF STEROIDS

Our studies refer to steroid excretion patterns determined in a
24 hour urinary specimen. This is a more consistent indicator of
abnormal steroid production than the measurement of "spot" plasma
values as emphasised by James (17) with reference to "spot" plasma
values of cortisol in relation to the 17 - OHCS 24 hour urinary
excretion values. Alternatively, the evaluation of the 24 hour
mean values according to Zumoff'(24) can be made.

We have also studied both the androgens and the oestrogens by
gas-chromatography and, if necessary, by mass spectrometry. The
urinary excretion profiles of the steroids (7,8), the excretion
levels of certain selected metabolites and their ratios (9) and
comparisons of the androgen and oestrogen excretion of these metabolites were also investigated (10).

For almost all the parameters studied by us, the plasma values were not significantly different from the normal control group both for all three groups and for most of the parameters studied, ie. DHT (3), Androsterone (A), E2 (23), E3 and for the E2/T ratio (see Table IV).

In particular T and E1 were sometimes significantly increased (T in group 3; E1 in groups 1 and 3) in prostatic cancer patients (Tablo V).

TABLE V

ANDROGEN EXCRETION PATTERNS (7,9) IN PROSTATIC CANCER (n = 17)

	A	E	D	11KA	11KE	11OHA	11OHE	17KS	17OHCS
Group 1 <65 yrs	+	-	-	+	=	+	+	-	+
Group 2 >65 yrs	-	=	-	=	=	=	+	-	=
Group 3*	=	+	-	+	+	=	-	-	+

A: Androsterone; E: Aetiocholanone; D: Dehydro Epiandrosterone; 11 KA: 11 Keto Androsterone; 11 KE: 11 Aetio-cholanone; 11 OHA: 11 Hydroxy Androsterone; 11 OHE: 11 Hydroxy etiocholanone; 17 KS: 17 Oxosteroids; 17 OHCS: 17 Hydroxy-corticosteroids.
* Group 3 : patients with advanced disease regardless of age.

These data too appear to be perfectly consistent with those of many authors (39, 47, 48). Different results have been obtained, however, by some other authors (3).

PROSTATIC CANCER EXCRETION PATTERNS: PRELIMINARY REPORT

Our evaluation of steroid excretion enables us to point out some abnormal characteristics common to two hormone dependent types of human cancer: breast and prostate.

1)   Unbalanced or inverted pattern index, ie. the ratio between classical oestrogens and unusual metabolites in many of the patients studied, above all in those of groups 1 and 3 in whom the excretion levels of unusual oestrogen metabolites were higher.
2)   Oestrogen metabolic pointers: abnormalities of the oestrogen metabolites obtained with these parameters were significant, especially in the patients of group 3. This is consistent with a worse prognosis in older patients (48).
3)   Oestrogen-androgen balance: the oestrogen-androgen ratio was significantly higher in prostatic cancer patients both because

of a considerable reduction of androgen excretion and of a major
increase in the excretion of total oestrogens. The values were
significantly different, from the statistical point of view, from
the normal control group.

These abnormal characteristics of oestrogen metabolism are
present in most patients with prostatic cancer. The composition
of group is given in Table V. It should be noted that the number
of patients in each group is relatively low.

CONCLUSIONS

The data obtained with RIA tests on the plasma concentrations
of the oestrogens E1, E2 and E3 are not homogeneous in the three
groups, so that there is only partial agreement with previous reports
by other authors (3,4,23,39,47,48).

In any case, it may be utopian to expect homogeneous results in
patients differing so widely with regard to clinical state, type and
spreading of metastasis, age and performance status.

This may explain the discrepancies between the results obtained
by various authors (4,48). The same can be said of the excretion
levels of E1, E2 and E3 considered individually (1).

On the other hand, the excretion patterns of both androgens and
oestrogens give a homogenous indication, for most prostatic cancer
patients, of abnormal and atypical oestrogen metabolism.

Probably:

A)   high oestrogen levels explain the high S B-beta-G levels
found in prostatic cancer patients;

B)   the fact that the peripheral production of oestrogens from
androgens - via testosterone - is an alternative to that of DHT,
explains the abnormal metabolism of oestrogens evidenced by us and by
others (9,18) together with reduced T concentration (group 1) and
reduced 17-KS excretion levels, and draws attention to the oestrogen-
androgen-balance;

C)   the therapeutic action of DES in prostatic cancer patients
may be explained by the hypothesis that its action mechanism inter-
acts with oestrogen metabolism (12).

Several attempts have been carried out so far: a) to correlate
urinary excretion with clinical status (6); b) to estimate endocrine
modification for the hormonal control of cancer (45) and c) also
after surgical treatment (26), in breast and prostatic cancer

patients. We have long had experimental evidence of abnormal steroid
excretion patterns both in breast and in prostatic cancer (4,41).

Attempts at comparative studies between different cancers in
the same area of hormone-sensitivity have been very few (29); nevertheless this can be a very important source of information provided
that we select the correct parameters: the oestrogen-androgen
balance (14) proves to be one of these.

SUMMARY

These studies on breast and prostatic cancer patients concern
the excretion patterns and plasma concentrations of both androgen
and oestrogen. Although the plasma concentrations were scarcely
contributory, evaluation by excretion patterns makes it possible,
with the parameters used by us, to observe abnormal steroid
excretion, as well as some anomalous characteristics common to
postmenopausal breast and prostatic cancer patients. The evidenced
characteristics are: a) abnormal oestrogen excretion patterns and
b) reduced total 17-KS excretion levels, clearly indicated by
oestrogen-androgen balance. This reduced excretion seems to
correlate positively with the abnormal oestrogen excretion, as well
as with the less favourable prognosis for prostatic cancer patients
with advanced disease.

REFERENCES

1.   Adlercreutz, H., Luukkainen, T. and Svanborg, A., Ann. Med.
     Exp. Fenn. 45, 277-286 (1967).

2.   Ball, P. R., Knuppen, R., Haupt, M. and Breuer, H. J. Clin.
     Endocrin. Metab. 4, 736-746 (1972).

3.   Bartsch, W., Steins, P. and Becker, H. Eur. Urol. 3, 47 (1977).

4.   Blackard, C. E., Byar, D. P., Seal, U. S. and VACURG. J. Urol.
     113, 517-525 (1975).

5.   Briggs, M. Biochemical effects of oral contraceptives. In :
     Advances in Steroid Biochemistry and Pharmacology. Vol. 5
     (Academic Press London, 1976).

6.   Bulbrook, R. D., Franks, L. M. and Greenwood, F. E. Brit. J.
     Cancer, 13, 45-58 (1959).

7.   Castagnetta, L., Traina, A., Agostara, B., D'Alessandro, A. M.,
     Tesat, G., Brucoli, G and Paparopoli, G. In Proceedings of
     International Symposium on metastasised Human Breast Cancer,

(Cancer Centre "M. Ascoli" Palermo, 1976).

9. Castagnetta, L., Paparopoli, G., Traina, A., Agostara, B.
    and Brucoli, G. In Prevention and Detection of Cancer Part I,
    Vol. 1 Marcel Dekker Inc. New York and Basel, (1977).

10. Castagnetta, L., Agostara, B. and Traina, A. In Proceedings of
    Advances in Cancer Chemotherapy. (E. Majorana Centre Erice,
    1977).

11. Castagnetta, L., Traina, A., Agostara, B. and Grant, J. K.
    In Abstracts of Symposium on Pharmacological Modulation of
    Steroid Action (Turin, 1978).

12. Castagnetta, L., Traina, A., Agostara, B., Russello, T. and
    Paparopoli, G. In Abstracts of Symposium on Pharmacological
    Modulation of Steroid Action (Turin, 1978).

13. Cho-Chung, Y. S. and Gullino, P. M. Science, 183, 87-88
    (1974).

14. Chopra, I. J. and Tuchinsky, D. J. Clin. Endocrin. Metab. 38,
    269-276 (1974).

15. Corvol, P. L., Chrambach, A., Rodbard, D. and Bardin, C. W.
    J. Biol. Chem. 246, 3435-3443 (1971).

16. Davies, I. J., Naftolin, F., Rian, K. J., Fishman, J. and
    Siu, J. Endocrinology, 97, 554-557 (1975).

17. Fishman, J. and Norton, B. Endocrinology, 96, 1054-1058
    (1975).

18. Farnsworth, W. E. and Brown, J. R. In Prevention and Detection
    of Cancer Part I Vol. 1 Marcel Dekker Inc. New York and Basel
    (1977).

19. Gelbke, H. P., Ball, P. and Knuppen, R. In Advances in
    Steroid Biochemistry and Pharmacology, Vol 6 (Academic Press
    London, New York, San Francisco, 1977).

20. Geller, J., Vazakas, G., Fruchtman, B., Newman, H., Nakao, K.
    and Loh, A. Surg. Gynaec. Obstet. 4, 748-756 (1968).

21. Gethmann, U., Ball, P. and Knuppen, R. In Abstracts of
    Symposium on Pharmacological Modulation of Steroids Action
    (Turin, 1978).

22. Goodwin, D. A., Rasmussen-Taxadai, O. S., Ferreira, A. A. and
    Scott, W. W. J. Urol. 86, 134-142 (1961).

23.   Harper, N. E., Peeling, W. B., Cowley, T., Brownsey, B. G.,
      Phillips, M. E. A., Groom, G., Fahmy, D. R. and Griffiths, K.
      Acta Endocrinol. 81, 409-418 (1976).

24.   Hertz, R. In Steroid Hormone Action and Cancer (Plenum Press
      New York and London, 1976).

25.   Heyns, W. In Advances in Steroid Biochemistry and Pharmacology
      Vol. 6 (Academic Press, London, New York, San Francisco, 1977).

26.   Huggins, C. and Hodges, C. U. Cancer Res. 1, 293-297 (1941).

27.   James, V. H. T. and London, J. In Recent Advances in
      Endocrinology (Churchill, J. and A. London, 1968).

28.   Jungblut, P. W., Hughes, S. F., Gorlich, L., Gowers, U. and
      Wagner, R. K. Hoppe Seyler's Z Physiol. Chem. 352, 1603-1608
      (1971).

29.   Kaul, P., Prasao, G. C., Gupta, R. C. and Udupa, K. N.   Indian
      J. Cancer, 11, 162-167 (1974).

30.   King, R. J. B. Essays in Biochemistry, 12, 41-76 (1976).

31.   Lemon, H. M. Cancer Res. 35, 1341-1353 (1975).

32.   Liao, S. and Liang, T. In Hormones and Cancer (Academic Press
      New York and London, 1974).

33.   Lippman, M. In Breast Cancer. Trends in research and
      treatment. (Raven Press, New York 1976).

34.   Mainwaring, W. I. P. In Steroid Hormone Action and Cancer.
      (Plenum Press, New York, 1976).

35.   Naftolin, F., Ryan, K. Y., Davies, I. J., Reddy, V. V.,
      Flores, F., Petro, Z., Kuhn, M., White, R. Y., Takaoka, Y.
      and Molin, L. Res. Prog. Horm. Res. 31, 295-319 (1975).

36.   Paul, S. M. and Axelrod, J. In Abstracts of Symposium on
      Pharmacological Modulation of Steroid Action (Turin, 1978).

37.   Pearlman, W. H. and Crepy, O. J. Biol. Chem. 242, 182-189
      (1967).

38.   Radhey, L., Singhal, M. R., Parulekar, M. R., Vijayvargiya, R.
      and Robison, G. A. Bioch. J. 125, 329-342 (1971).

39.   Robinson, M. R. G. and Thomas, B. S. Br. Med. J. 4, 391-402
      (1971).

40.   Silber, R. H. and Porter, C. C.   In Methods of Biochemical
      Analysis, Vol 4 (Interscience, New York, 1957).

41.   Stern, E., Hopkins, C. E., Weiner, J. M. and Harmorston, J.
      Science, 145, 716-719 (1964).

42.   Velardo, J. I.   In Hormonal Steroids, Vol 1 (Academic Press,
      New York, 1964).

43.   Vermeulen, A., Verdonck, L., Van Der Straeten, M. and Orie, N.
      J. Clin. Endocr. Metab. 29, 1470-1480 (1969).

44.   Vertes, M., Barnea, A., Linder, H. R. and King, R. J. B.
      In Receptors for Reproductive Hormones (Plenum Press, New York,
      1973).

45.   Wotiz, H. H., Shane, R., Vigersky, and Brecher, P. I.   In
      Prognostic Factors in Breast Cancer (E. and S. Livingstone
      Ltd., Edinburgh and London, 1968).

46.   Yamamoto, R. S. and Weisburger, E. K.   Rec. Prog. Horm. Res.
      33, 617-653 (1977).

47.   Young, H. H., II, and Kent, J. R.   J. Urol. 99, 788-795 (1968).

48.   Zumoff, B.   In Endocrine Control in Neoplasia (Raven Press,
      New York, 1978).

STEROID RECEPTORS IN HUMAN PROSTATIC TISSUE

H J DE VOOGT

Reader in Urology, University Hospital Leiden

Rijnsbergerweg 10, Leiden, The Netherlands

INTRODUCTION

Though the methodological problems of receptor determination
have been largely resolved by Wagner's agar-gel-electrophoresis,
some difficulties in relation to collection of adequate tissue,
problems with the variable amounts of cells and stroma in cancer
tissue, and in the interpretation of results, still remain. First
we did experiments, largely on tissue showing benign prostatic
hypertrophy (BPH), to decide whether the small amount obtained by
needle biopsy could be used for receptor determination. Secondly
we compared pieces obtained by surgical dissection and by transurethral resection (TUR) from the same prostatic adenoma and found
roughly the same quantities of receptor (not statistically
different).

From these results we concluded that both needle-biopsies and
TUR-material can be used for determining the presence or absence
steroid-receptors. Receptors were regarded as present if the concentration was equal to or higher than 20 fmol/mg tissue protein

RESULTS

Our results in 68 patients with BPH and 35 patients with
prostatic cancer are shown in Table I.

There is a striking difference in DHT-R-content between BPH and
carcinoma. After oestrogen treatment much more DHT-R can be found,
probably because more free receptor-sites are present when endogenous
androgens are suppressed. However we did not find much difference in

TABLE I

PRESENCE OR ABSENCE OF DHT-R AND E2-R IN HUMAN PROSTATIC CYTOSOL

	DHT-R		E2-R	
	N	% positive	N	% positive
BPH	66	27	68	97
Carcinoma 1	20	60	20	95
2	15	73	15	80
3*	12	50	12	58

1 = Untreated, 2 = Treated with Oestrogens for a long period,
3 = Treated with Oestrogens for six months.

* These patients also appear in Group 1.

TABLE II

SPEARMAN CORRELATIONS BETWEEN DHT-R AND E2-R AND SOME CRITERIA
FOR RESPONSE TO ENDOCRINE THERAPY

DHT-R

tumour regression	0.34	18	0.16	-0.50	15	0.060	-0.15	12	0.63
patient complaints	-0.09	18	0.70	-0.12	15	0.64	0.05	12	0.86
laboratory examinations	0.01	18	0.98	-0.28	15	0.30	0.59	12	0.051
final evaluation	-0.10	18	0.67	0.17	15	0.52	0.53	12	0.079

E2-R

tumour regression	-0.08	18	0.75	-0.14	15	0.59	0.04	12	0.88
patient complaints	0.10	18	0.69	-0.25	15	0.35	0.16	12	0.60
laboratory examinations	-0.18	18	0.45	-0.12	15	0.65	-0.17	12	0.58
final evaluation	-0.10	18	0.67	0.04	15	0.88	0.53	12	0.080

E2-R presence between the groups. We looked at several criteria for
response to endocrine treatment but could not find any statistically
significant correlation (Table II).

However, all these assessments were done without making
allowance for the very heterogenous composition of most prostatic
carcinomatous tissues. For instance when we looked at the grade of
malignancy (differentiation) of the carcinoma, we found a positive
correlation between E2-R and grade of malignancy, E2-R being found
almost exclusively in well-differentiated carcinoma.

Finally when we considered the epithelial and stromal components
of the various tissues examined, which can vary greatly from one
piece to the other, a positive correlation between E2-R values and
large amounts of stroma was evident (Table III). This indicates the
possibility that E2-R at least is found more in the stroma
(connective tissue) than in the epithelial cells, which gives support
to some recent developments in the research in this field.

TABLE III

SPEARMAN CORRELATIONS BETWEEN EPITHELIUM/STROMA

AND STEROID-RECEPTOR VALUES

	DHT-R			"E2-R"		
	r	N	P	r	N	P
group 1	-0.045	19	0.85	-0.107	19	0.65
group 2	-0.180	14	0.52	0.525	14	0.058

HORMONAL RECEPTORS IN HUMAN PROSTATE : A COMPUTERISED STUDY OF NORMAL AND PATHOLOGICAL TISSUE SAMPLES*

E Bercovich, M Soli

Clinica Urologica dell'Università di Bologna

Bologna, Italy

ABSTRACT

The authors report the results of a computerised study on hormonal receptor assessment in normal and pathological human prostate. Analysis and interpretation of receptor profiles for DHT, 17βE, Progesterone and Cortisol are discussed.

INTRODUCTION

Prostatic carcinoma is a hormone-sensitive neoplasm, but Huggins' theory of prostatic malignancy seems to us an over simplification of the facts.

In our five years experience we have not shown any noteworthy alteration of plasma levels of androgens in patients with cancer of the prostate (Ca P).

Also in our opinion animal research is useless when considering hormone dependence since, in some hormone dependent tumours in animals, the withdrawal of a hormone stops the growth of the neoplasm and even allows its total regression and vice versa whilst such a direct hormone dependence has not yet been demonstrated in human beings. Therefore, our attention has focused on the very centre of the problem, the prostatic cell. If we think in terms of the

* This work was carried out in collaboration with Drs S Grilli, M C Galli, C DeGiovanni (Istituto di Cancerologia dell'Università di Bologna)

cell and hormone dependence it becomes natural to investigate hormonal receptors and we believe that receptor assessment can provide a biological base for a less empirical interpretation of this phenomenon.

The data which we have tried to elicit with our technique are as follows:-

1. Information on hormone dependence
2. Correlations between:
    a)   hormone dependence and histology
    b)   hormone dependence and hormonal levels
3. Information on hormonal changes during evolution of Ca P.
4. Early predictability of response to therapy.

METHODS

The important points to keep in mind when a receptor assessment is performed are:-

1. 400 mg of tissue (100 mg/receptor) is required,
2. patients must not have received endocrinological therapy and then they should have a thorough endocrinological screening. It is important to obtain and preserve the tissue samples with great care to allow reproducibility of the measurements.

Our trial includes the following sequential steps:

1. Measurement of palsma androgens.

2. Excision of prostatic tissue for receptor measurement, histological examination and, for patients with carcinoma:

3. staging

4. bilateral subcapsular orchidectomy

5. therapy with cyproterone acetate

6. periodical follow-up.

Prostatic tissue samples have been obtained by adenomectomy for benign hypertrophy (BPH), perineal biopsy and transurethral resection (TUR) for tumour tissue and after cystoprostatectomy in patients with bladder carcinoma, to obtain normal prostatic tissue.

Each sample was divided into two parts, one for histological examination and the other, after being freed from impurities, was used for the determination of receptors for dihydrotestosterone (DHT), oestradiol, progesterone and cortisol. We used a modified dextran coated charcoal method. Parallel determinations of plasma androgens testosterone, dihydrotestosterone and Δ4 - androstenedione were undertaken.

The data obtained was processed by a data machine. The level of confidence was 95% and we report only statistically significant data. We have investigated 58 patients from whom we obtained specimens of prostatic tissue which was normal in eight, showed BPH in 20 and cancer in 30 (grade I - 12, grade II - 12 and grade III - 6).

RESULTS

The values of DHT and cortisol receptors are shown in Table I.

As can be seen, DHT receptors are found in large amounts in benign hypertrophy, and decrease significantly in carcinoma, with a minimum in grade III lesions.

This information confirms the known clinical behaviour of prostatic carcinoma, in which the more differentiated the lesion the more probable is its androgen dependence.

Carcinoma of grade II in particular shows a variable behaviour. It can have large or small amounts of DHT receptors and, therefore, potentially great or small androgen responsiveness. Furthermore, if we compare the response to therapy, we find a positive trend between the presence of receptors for DHT dihydrotestosterone and the response to therapy ie. the greater the amount of DHT receptors, the better the response to therapy.

TABLE I

VALUE OF RECEPTORS FOR DHT AND CORTISOL IN 58 PATIENTS

RECEPTORS

	DHT fmol/ g DNA	Cortisol fmol/ g DNA
Normal Prostate	2.17 ± 0.55	9.93 ± 4.26
BPH	3.82 ± 0.94	8.81 ± 2.00
Ca P Grade I	1.36 ± 0.37	2.80 ± 1.24
Ca P Grade II	1.50 ± 1.43	3.60 ± 1.81
Ca P Grade III	0.06	0.54

Receptors for 17β-oestradiol and progesterone have been found in benign hypertrophy, but they are practically absent in carcinoma. Cortisol receptor profiles reach their highest levels in normal and in hypertrophic prostate (Table I).

Among the carcinomas they show a regression pattern, as we have seen for dihydrotestosterone receptors.

CONCLUSIONS

We can summarise our findings as follows:-

1. the correlation between prostatic neoplastic pathology and hormone dependence is confirmed;

2. the hormone dependence is correlated with the quantity of receptors for dihydrotestosterone;

3. the dihydrotestosterone receptors decrease in frequency and quantity with dedifferentiation;

4. the effectiveness of antiandrogenic therapy seems to increase proportional to the quantity and frequency of dihydrotestosterone receptors.

5. The cortisol receptor level could be assumed as a molecular index, which we can call "cellular normality".

6. The cell in benign prostatic hypertrophy contains all four receptors analysed with peaks for dihydrotestosterone and cortisol receptors; therefore, a multiple pharmacological approach may be appropriate.

Receptor measurement is an advanced research technique in studies of prostatic cancer and demands a research team and a complex clinical and laboratory structure. The data must be compared in order to elaborate final theories.

REFERENCES

1. Lippman, M., Bolan, G. and Huff. K., The effects of androgens and antiandrogens on hormone-responsive human breast cancer in long-term tissue culture. Cancer Res. 36, 4610-4618 (1976).

2. Galli, M. C., Gola, G., Orlandi, C., Rocchetta, R., Nanni, P., Grilli, S. and De Giovanni, I. R. C. S., Steroid hormone receptors in normal and neoplastic human ovary. Med. Sci. (1978) In Press.

3.   Pichon, M. F. and Milgrom, E., Characterisation and assay of progesterone receptor in human mammary carcinoma. Cancer Res. 37, 464-471 (1977).

4.   Liskowski, L., Rose, D. P., Dondlinger, T. and Olenick, J. S., The determination of progesterone receptors in breast cancer and their relationship to oestrogen receptor. Clin. Chim. Acta, 71, 309-318 (1976).

5.   Baxter, J. D., Schambelan, M., Matulich, D. T., Spindler, G. J., Taylor, A. A., and Bartter, F. C., Aldosterone receptors and the evaluation of plasma mineralocorticoid activity in normal and hypertensive states. J. Clin. Invest. 58, 579-589 (1976).

6.   Scatchard, G., The attraction of proteins for small molecules and ions. Ann. N. Y. Acad. Sci. 51, 660-672 (1949).

ANDROGEN RECEPTORS IN PROSTATIC CANCER

R GHANADIAN, G AUF AND G D CHISHOLM

Prostate Research Laboratory, Royal Postgraduate Medical
School and Institute of Urology, University of London
London, England

INTRODUCTION

There are good grounds for the premise that measurement of
androgen receptor proteins in carcinoma of the prostate may be of
value in the prediction of responsiveness to hormone manipulation.
Although a receptor protein which binds dihydrotestosterone has been
identified and characterised in the human prostate by sucrose density
gradient centrifugation and column chromatography, routine quantitative measurements in human prostatic tissues have been beset by a
number of problems in methodology. In the first place, the high
level of sex hormone binding protein (SHBG) and of endogenous
androgens in prostatic tissues interfere with the receptor assay and
the earlier dextran charcoal technique (Mobbe et al, 1975) has proved
to be unreliable. In the dextran charcoal method cytosol is labelled
with either 3H testosterone or dihydrotestosterone. The free and
loosely bound steroids are then separated from tightly bound steroids
by the addition of dextran coated charcoal. However, due to the high
affinity of androgens to SHBG it proved impossible to separate SHBG
from androgen receptors using this technique. This method was
replaced by the "Agar gel electrophoresis technique" (Wagner, 1972),
which can separate SHBG from androgen receptors by agar gel electrophoresis, but in turn has the disadvantage that only (free) receptors
are measured.

Because of the high levels of endogenous androgens in the human
prostate, most of the receptors are bound to androgens and are not
available to bind the radioligand when short term incubation is
applied. In order to overcome this problem, the androgen, which is
tightly bound to the receptor must be exchanged with the radioligand. This can be achieved by long term incubation under appro-

priate experimental conditions which requires a radioligand to be stable at least at 15°C. Tritiated testosterone and dihydro-testosterone have proved to be unsuitable radioligands as they are rapidly metabolised under these conditions. The application of protamine sulphate precipitation has resolved some of these technical problems. In this procedure receptors are precipitated by protamine sulphate and the receptor protamine complex is subsequently labelled with tritiated androgens. Protamine sulphate inhibits the enzymic activity of 5α-reductase on the prostatic cytosol and thus makes it possible to apply appropriate exchange conditions (Ghanadian et al, 1978; Auf and Ghanadian, 1978). It is important to emphasise, however, that there is some loss of receptor during precipitation.

Another useful technique is separation of the receptor by glycerol gradient centrifugation followed by radioimmunoassay of the hormone bound fraction (Rosen et al, 1975). However, this technique is laborious for routine application and furthermore demonstration of the 8s receptor peak in human prostatic tumours has not always been successful.

Bonne and Raynaud (1975) reported on the use of a synthetic androgen methyltrienolone (R1881) which has a high affinity for di-hydrotestosterone, and neither binds to SHBG nor undergoes metabolism.

In a recent report from this laboratory androgen receptors in human benign hypertrophied prostate were measured by an exchange assay using tritiated methyltrienolone (^{3}H R1881). The specificity of this technique was further investigated, and the method was also applied for the measurement of androgen receptors in carcinoma of the prostate (Ghanadian et al, 1978; Auf and Ghanadian, 1978).

MATERIALS AND METHODS

Prostatic tissue from 18 patients with carcinoma of the prostate was obtained by transurethral resection. The tissue was cleaned and the burned surface was carefully removed. Sections of the tissue adjacent to that used for receptor assay was used for histology. Histological examination revealed carcinoma of the prostate in all 18 cases.

In addition, prostatic tissue was obtained from 27 patients undergoing retropubic prostatectomy for benign prostatic hypertrophy.

The details of the cell fractionation, preparation of the cytosol and the assay of androgen receptors have been described elsewhere (Ghanadian et al, 1978[a]; Ghanadian et al, 1978[b]).

RESULTS

Carcinoma

The results for total, free and bound receptors in 18 patients with carcinoma of the prostate are shown in Table I. There was a wide range of receptor level in both treated and untreated groups. At this stage, no attempt was made to relate these data to the clinical condition of the patient.

TABLE I

CONCENTRATION OF TOTAL, FREE AND BOUND CYTOPLASMIC DHT RECEPTOR

IN CARCINOMA OF THE PROSTATE   (ND - None Detected)

(fmol receptor/mg protein)

	Total	Free	Bound	B/F
Untreated (10)	148.0 ± 51.0	4.3 ± 0.7	142.2 ± 51.2	39.2 ± 13.4
	(52.0 - 525.0)	(1.7 - 9.2)	(32.8 - 520.5)	5.6 - 115.3
Treated (7) oestrogen, orchidectomy & cyproterone acetate	119.1 ± 59.4	9.3 ± 2.8	109.8 ± 60.3	27.0 ± 14.1
	(17.5 - 466.0)	(1.5 - 21.4)	(2.6 - 461.0)	0.17 - 92.8
Treated (1) oestrogen	N.D.	N.D.	N.D.	N.D.

BENIGN PROSTATIC HYPERTROPHY

The mean concentration of total DHT receptor in 27 samples of BPH was 90.61 ± 8.50 (Mean $\pm$ SEM fmol/mg protein) (Range 30.7 - 218 fmol/mg protein).

In 14 of the 27 samples, the mean free receptor concentration was 6.88 ± 0.75 (fmol/mg protein) (Range 3.3 - 11.7 fmol/mg protein).

DISCUSSION

Several problems have been encountered in the development of a reliable technique for the quantitative measurement of androgen receptors. There problems are exacerbated when human prostatic tissues are studied. The human prostate is not a homogenous tissue, but consists of at least two types of cells - "epithelial" and "fibromuscular". Their biochemical characteristics are different. Cowan et al (1977) have assessed the yields and homogeneity of the separated epithelial and stromal tissues in BPH, using arginase and hydroxyproline as biochemical markers and recovered about 30% of epithelial and 95% of stromal tissues. They found that dehydro-epiandrosterone sulphate sulphatase was predominantly present in the epithelium, whereas testosterone 5α-reductase activity was predominant in the stroma. These investigators also found no SHBG cortisol binding globulin (CBG) like proteins in the epithelial tissues, whereas substantial amounts of these proteins, as well as receptor proteins, were associated with the stroma (Cowan et al, 1976; Cowan et al, 1977).

In the present report no attempt was made to separate the epithelial and stromal components. Measurement of androgen receptors was carried out in the supernatant preparation from the whole tissue homogenate.

In the present investigation both bound and free androgen receptors have been measured and the bound:free ratio for each tumour has been evaluated. In benign hypertrophied prostate the concentration of the bound receptors was approximately 10 times higher than the free sites. However, this ratio for the untreated carcinoma tissue was much higher. This illustrates the importance of measuring both total and free binding sites, and clearly shows the inadequacy of techniques unable to measure the total receptor population. The specificity of the radioligand (^{3}H R1881) for androgen receptors has been extensively studied and reported elsewhere (Ghanadian et al, 1978; Auf and Ghanadian, 1978).

Apart from the methodological problems and the heterogeneity of human prostatic tissues, another serious shortcoming in this type of investigation relates to the surgical procedure used to obtain tissue samples.

At the present time most of the surgical samples from patients with carcinoma have been obtained by transurethral electro-resection (TUR). Special care should be given to clean the prostatic chips removing all burned tissues and adjacent sections of tissue should be submitted for histological assessment.

REFERENCES

1.   Auf, G. and Ghanadian, R., A comparative study of the binding of androgen receptors to dihydrotestosterone, progesterone and methyltrienolone. Proceeding of the Pharmacological modulation of steroid action, Turin, July 1978. In Press.

2. Bonne, C. and Raynaud, J. P., Methyltrienolone, a specific
    ligand for cellular androgen receptors. Steroids, 26, 227-230
    (1975).

3. Cowan, R. A., Cowan, S. A., Giles, C. A. and Grant, J. K.,
    Prostatic distribution of sex hormone-binding globulin and
    cortisol-binding globulin in benign hyperplasia. Journal of
    Endocrinology, 71, 121-136 (1976).

4. Cowan, R. A., Cowan, S. A., Grant, J. K. and Elder, H. T.,
    Biochemical investigations of separate epithelium and stroma
    from benign hyperplastic prostate tissue. Journal of
    Endocrinology, 74, 111-120 (1977).

5. Cowan, R. A., Cowan, S. A. and Grant, J. K., Binding of
    methyltrienolone (R1881) to a progesterone receptor-like
    component of human prostatic cytosol. Journal of Endocrinology,
    74, 281-289 (1977).

6. Ghanadian, R., Auf, G., Chaloner, P. J. and Chisholm, G. D.,
    The use of methyltrienolone in the measurement of the free and
    bound cytoplasmic receptor for dihydrotestosterone in benign
    hypertrophied human prostate. Journal of Steroid Biochemistry,
    9, 325-330 (1978a).

7. Ghanadian, R., Auf, G., Chisholm, G. D. and O'Donoghue, E. P. N.
    Receptor proteins for androgens in prostatic disease. Brit. J.
    Urol. (1978) (In Press).

8. Mobbs, B. G., Johson, I. E. and Connolly, J. G., In vitro assay
    of androgen binding by human prostate. Journal of Steroid
    Biochemistry, 6, 453-458 (1975).

9. Rosen, V., Jung, I., Baulieu, E. E. and Robels, P., Androgen-
    binding proteins in human benign prostatic hypertrophy.
    Journal of Clinical Endocrinology and Metabolism, 41, 761-770
    (1975).

10. Wagner, R. K., Characterisation and assay of steroid hormone
    receptors and steroid binding serum proteins by agargel electro-
    phoresis at low temperatures. Hopper Seyler's Z. Physiol. Chem.
    353, 1235-1245 (1972).

TRANSRECTAL ASPIRATION BIOPSY OF THE PROSTATE WITH FRANZÉN'S
INSTRUMENT

P L ESPOSTI

Radiumhemmet
Karolinska sjukhuset
Stockholm, Sweden

INTRODUCTION

At Karolinska sjukhuset, Stockholm, the instrument and technique
proposed by Franzén et al (1960) are routinely used in the diagnosis
of prostatic tumours.

In prostatic carcinoma the aspirates generally are rich in
cells, which only occasionally are mixed with blood. The high
cellularity and absence of blood give a distinctive macroscopic
appearance to dried, unstained smears. At microscopy the main
characteristics of a carcinoma are evident: nuclear atypia with
prominent nucleoli, decreased cytoplasmic/nuclear ratio and reduced
mutual adhesiveness of the cells. According to the degree of
deviation from the normal epithelial structure, prostatic carcinoma
can be grouped in highly, moderately and poorly differentiated types
(Esposti, 1971).

Grade I or highly differentiated cancer. Nuclear polymorphism
is of moderate degree, single cells are infrequent. The most
typical feature of the highly differentiated carcinoma is the
microadenomatous complex. The cytoplasm of the malignant cells is
crowded into a central mass while the enlarged nuclei are arranged
in a peripheral circle.

Grade II or moderately differentiated cancer. The general
pattern is similar to that of grade I, however, the number of free
cells in higher and nuclear polymorphism more pronounced.

Grade III or poorly differentiated cancer. The aspirate
consists predominantly of dissociated cells, with polymorphic, often

bizarre nuclear forms and greatly enlarged nucleoli. A tendency to
form patterns reminiscent of the glandular structures is usually
present. More seldom an anaplastic variant is seen with dissociated
cells resembling immature cells.

COMPARISONS BETWEEN CYTOLOGIC AND HISTOLOGIC GRADING OF DIFFERENTIATION

There is no fundamental difference in the criteria of differentiation of prostatic carcinoma in aspirated cell material and in
histological sections. The histological diagnosis of carcinoma rests
mainly on two criteria: cytological abnormalities of individual
cells and abnormalities in the size, configuration and arrangement of
the acini. When such criteria are adopted in histological diagnosis,
comparisons of differentiation grades of prostatic carcinoma in
aspirated material and in histological sections become possible. The
correlation between cytological and histological grades of differentiation in 36 cases of prostatic carcinoma showed the following
results: the five tumours cytologically classified as highly
differentiated received the same histological diagnosis. In 15 of
the 18 cytologically moderately differentiated tumours the histological grading was likewise moderate and in three was poor. In 12
of 13 cytologically poorly differentiated tumours the histological
classification was the same, and one was reported as moderately
differentiated.

CLINICAL SIGNIFICANCE OF CYTOLOGICAL DIFFERENTIATION GRADING OF PROSTATIC CARCINOMA IN PATIENTS RECEIVING HORMONAL THERAPY

Four hundred and sixty nine patients with prostatic carcinoma
had been cytologically diagnosed and graded following the above
mentioned cytomorphological principles. The minimum follow-up was
five years. All the patients were treated with diethylstilboestrol
or ethinylestradiol orally and/or estradurin parenterally. Highly
differentiated prostatic carcinoma was found in 131 (27.9%),
moderately differentiated in 265 (56.5%) while 73 (15.5%) of the
patients were assigned to the poorly differentiated group.

The significance of such differentiation grading was studied
by examining:-
    a)   the response to hormonal treatment in 148 patients as
judged five to seven months from the start of treatment, and
    b)   the survival curves of the patients of the three
differentiation grades after a five year follow-up.
    The results are shown in Table I and are statistically
significant.

It is possible to conclude that the morphological character-

TABLE I

RESPONSE AND SURVIVAL IN RELATION TO CYTOLOGICAL GRADING

DIFFERENTIATION	% RESPONSE			% 5 yr SURVIVAL (Overall 52%)
	Good	Moderate	Poor	
HIGH	73	13.5	13.5	68
MODERATE	46	22	32	55
POOR	9	17	74	11

istics inherent in the cytological differentiation grading of prostatic carcinomas are the expression of different grades of malignancy of the tumours. Cytological malignancy grading of prostatic carcinoma is important for the prognosis. The very low survival rates of patients with poorly differentiated carcinoma lead to the conclusion that hormone therapy is not effective against these tumours. This underlines the urgent need for new types of treatment such as radiotherapy.

REFERENCES

1. Esposti, P. L., Cytologic malignancy grading of prostatic carcinoma by transrectal aspiration biopsy. Scand. J. Urol. Nephrol. 5, 199-209 (1971).

2. Franzén, S., Giertz, G. and Zajicek, J., Cytological diagnosis of prostatic tumours by transrectal aspiration biopsy : a preliminary report. Brit. J. Urol. 32, 193-196 (1960).

TREATMENT OF PROSTATIC CANCER WITH MEDROXYPROGESTERONE-ACETATE (MPA)

C BOUFFIOUX

Service d'Urologie de l'Université de Liège

Liege, Belgium

INTRODUCTION

In 1949, Gutierrez and later Trunnel and Duffy reported favourable results with progestative compounds in prostatic cancer. However, progestative drugs have never had the wide success of oestrogens due to lack of relevant studies such as those of Huggins and because they are weaker compounds as compared to oestrogens. Recently, synthetic and more active progestogens have been available which have stimulated new clinical studies. Imperfections of oestrogen therapy, its palliative and temporary effect, and its cardio-vascular complications led us since 1974 to test the value of MPA as an alternative to oestrogens.

METHOD

Nearly 70 patients treated at the Urological Department of the University of Liège have received MPA for advanced prostatic cancer- Stage III, (T3-4, Nx,MO) and IV (TO-4, NO, M1), at least for a few months. In many cases, subjective, and in some, objective results were observed and we elected:-

1. to evaluate the response of 40 untreated advanced prostatic cancers which were randomly given MPA (20 patients) or oestrogens (20 patients), and
2. to compare the results of estracyt versus MPA in advanced cases who no longer responded to oestrogens.

The doses of the drugs were as follows:

MPA at a dose of 500 mg I.M. 2-4 times a week for one month, followed by MPA 100 mg orally, daily.

Stilboestrol (DES) 3-5 mg a day.
Estracyt 140 mg six times a day for two weeks followed by 140 mg
four times a day.

RESULTS

1.   <u>In previously untreated cases</u> we observed a 40% objective
response rate with MPA and 55% with DES. The mean duration of
remission with MPA was 13.1 months compared to 16.3 months with DES.
The subjective response was less common and shorter in duration with
MPA than with DES. Survival seemed also slighly worse with MPA than
with DES, although this difference was not statistically significant
(Table 1).

TABLE 1

THREE YEARS SURVIVAL RATE IN PATIENTS

TREATED WITH OESTROGENS (DES) OR MPA

	No. of cases	S U R V I V A L		
		1 yr.	2 yr.	3 yr.
Oestrogens	20	16/20 (80 %)	14/20 (70 %)	11/20 (55 %)
MPA	20	19/20 (95 %)	15/20 (75 %)	6/17 (35 %)

2.   <u>Oestrogen resistant cases</u>.   Twelve cases in relapse on
oestrogens were given MPA. Of these five did not show any response
to MPA and died in the following months. A subjective result was
observed in seven patients of whom two reported also an objective
response for periods of six and 12 months respectively. The mean
duration of remission was six months and, except for one case, we
did not have the impression that survival was increased. In six
cases, MPA was administered not only after oestrogens but also after
failure of or intolerance to estracyt. It is noteworthy that three
of those patients displayed good responses for periods of nine to
18 months.

Ten cases in relapse on DES received estracyt. A good
subjective effect with relief of pain was noticed in seven patients,
four of whom also presented an objective effect. The mean duration
of remission was 11 months. In 13 cases resistant to MPA, estracyt

provided a subjective response with a mean remission of seven months, in nine patients.

DISCUSSION AND CONCLUSIONS

The number of cases treated is too small for statistical evaluation. Nevertheless the following conclusions can be drawn from this preliminary study:-

1. MPA, although not inactive, seems less efficient than DES in the treatment of advanced prostatic cancer: periods of remission are shorter and three year survival seems slightly worse. Our impression is that the effect of the progestogen disappears more quickly, which explains our present limited enthusiasm for this drug.

2. In oestrogen resistant cases, estracyt seems better than MPA but progestogens may sometimes provide good results for many months.

3. The main advantage of MPA is that it is usually well tolerated. Impotence occurs in about 60% of the cases but sexual potency returns, in about half the patients, when treatment is stopped. It does not produce gynaecomastia or atrophy of sexual organs and it does not give rise to the cardio-vascular risks of oestrogens.

4. Considering the above criteria and waiting for the results of larger randomised trials going on at the EORTC, we should presently reserve MPA for patients with advanced prostatic cancer who refuse or cannot tolerate oestrogens or who have an increase of cardio-vascular problems.

REFERENCES

1. Gutierrez, R., New horizons in surgical management of carcinoma of the prostate gland. Amer. J. Surg. 78, 147 (1949).

2. Trunnel, J. and Duffy, B., Influence of certain steroids on behaviour of human prostatic cancer. Trans. N. Y. Acad. Sci. 12, 238 (1950).

EXTERNAL IRRADIATION OF PROSTATIC CANCER AND INDICATORS FOR FAILURE OF TREATMENT

B VAN DER WERF-MESSING

Rotterdam Radiotherapy Institute
Groene Hilledijk 297
Rotterdam, the Netherlands

Eighty-four patients with carcinoma of the prostate category T3-4, Mo have been treated by external irradiation to the prostate and surrounding adjacent lymph nodes, but not including systematically all regional lymph nodes. A dose of 7,000 rads was given: 4,000 rads in four weeks with daily fractions of 200 rads, a split of about two weeks, and an additional dose of 3,000 rads in three weeks, again 200 rads daily. The dose was given via four fields (one posterior, one anterior and two lateral). In category T3 cases with well and moderately differentiated growths, three and five year survival was 80% (40 cases). In undifferentiated growths, three and five year survival were respectively 55% and 0% (15 cases).

In category T4 cases differentiated growths had a three and five year survival of 65% (22 cases), whereas in seven patients with undifferentiated growths only 50% lived three years. Due to small numbers the five year survival could not be assessed.

COMPLICATIONS

Of the 84 patients 76 had no complications, five had proctitis for one, three, four, six and eight months respectively; two complained of cystitis for three and eight months. Serious damage was seen in one patient who developed ileus after a preceding operation.

Distant metastases developed in 25 patients. The first indication that clinical metastases would develop was an elevated prostatic acid phosphatase in 14 patients. In the other instances skeletal scan, malignant cells in the bone marrow aspiration, bone

marrow serum acid phosphatase, x-ray and enlargement of lympho-
graphically visualised lymph nodes were the fist indicators. After
the first evidence of such an indicator 50% of the patients developed
clinical metastases within one year but 5% were still free of
metastases 30 months after the first appearance of an indicator.

Regular transrectal cytology has been performed after
irradiation in order to assess whether tumour cells were still
present.   50% of the patients had a positive transrectal cytology
after two years, decreasing to about 20% after three years. This
positive cytology had no bearing on the development of metastases or
on prognosis in general.

CONCLUSIONS

The advantage of radiation therapy is that at the least it
postpones hormone therapy, whilst in the majority of cases hormone
therapy will not be necessary at all (in 80% of differentiated T3
growths and in about 70% of differentiated T4 growths). In view of
the low complication rate, the price for avoidance or postponement
of hormone therapy is acceptable.

This contribution is a summary; the complete article has been
published in Strahlentherapie, 154, 537-541 (1978).

INTRAURETHRAL IRRADIATION OF PROSTATIC CANCER USING AFTERLOADING TECHNIQUE

G LINGÅRDH, J-E JOHANSSON, K MÜLLER, O ODELBERG-JOHNSON,
L-B SCHNÜRER and K-J VIKTERLOF

Departments of Urology, Oncology, Pathology and
Radiophysics, Örebro, Sweden

Prostatic cancer may be irradiated by means of interstitial
irradiation or external megavolt therapy. Since 1973 we have used
a method consisting of intraurethral irradiation by means of an
afterloading technique using a commercially available apparatus (TEM
Cathetron), in combination with external megavolt therapy.

We place an unloaded tube intraurethrally in the centre of the
diseased gland checking by palpation and by x-ray. The radioactive
Cobalt 60 source is then placed in the predetermined position.
After about five minutes irradiation time the source is automatically
retracted to the storage container. During the whole period of
irradiation the personnel are outside the irradiation room. The
relative dose distribution around the source is determined in advance
with a computer. In most cases we give a total dose of 2,800 rads,
referred to a distance of 1 cm from the tube. The dosages are given
in four weekly treatments, each of 700 rads.

Supplementary external irradiation therapy is given, usually by
means of cobalt arc therapy, up to a dose of about 7,000 rads in
total. Our preliminary study (1), including patients with prostatic
carcinoma stage II, has shown that this patient group can be safely
treated with our technique. From a prospective series including 130
new cases of prostatic carcinoma, diagnosed from March 1977 to
July 1978, 22 patients with a medium or poor degree of differentiation were selected for the combined irradiation technique.
Immediate complications were few. Prolonged postradiotherapy lesions
in the urinary tract occurred in three patients; all however, healed
up spontaneously. Initial oedema of the prostatic gland was followed
by a reduction in its size which often was marked. Fine needle
aspirations disclosed a sharp decline in the number of cancer cells

in most cases. A complete disappearance was usually not observed in representative smears. In conclusion the intraurethral irradiation technique has a relatively high radiobiological effect and is simple for the patient. It is performed as an out-patient procedure. Even when supplemented with external irradiation to give a relatively high total intraprostatic radiation dose the treatment gives a reasonably low rate of complications in the bowel and the bladder.

REFERENCE

1.   Fritjofsson, A., Lingårdh, F., Odelberg-Johnson, O. and Vikterlof, K. J., Intraurethral irradiation of prostatic cancer using afterloading technique. In "Prostatic Disease". Alan R. Liss, Inc., New York, 255-266 (1976).

REVIEW OF THE VETERANS ADMINISTRATION STUDIES OF CANCER OF THE
PROSTATE AND NEW RESULTS CONCERNING TREATMENT OF STAGE I AND II
TUMOURS

D P BYAR

Biometry Branch, National Cancer Institute

Bethesda, Maryland, USA

INTRODUCTION

I have been asked to present a progress report on randomised
clinical trials conducted by the Veterans Administration Cooperative
Urological Research Group (VACURG) concerning treatment of prostatic
cancer. I should like to begin by explaining that this group is no
longer in existence because the review committee of the National
Cancer Institute responsible for funding decisions felt that the
project should be terminated. No new patients have been admitted to
protocols since 1975. During the 15 years this group was in existence
data were collected on over 4,000 patients with prostatic cancer in
all stages of the disease who were studied in four randomised prospective clinical trials. The results of these trials have been
published extensively in medical journals and two book chapters have
been prepared which summarise the contributions of the VACURG (1,2).
For convenience the four studies have been designated as Studies 1,
2, 3 and Focal Study. Table I presents information about the stages
of disease, numbers of patients, and the treatments compared in the
various studies. Although the principal objective of these studies
was to compare treatments for prostatic cancer, the data accumulated
have been studied in considerable detail from other points of view.
In particular Dr. Donald Gleason has developed an excellent system
of histological classification of prostatic cancer based on these
data (3-7) and a series of papers have examined the importance of
prognostic factors (8,9) and biochemical measurements (10-14).

Today I should like to divide my presentation into three parts.
First I will review briefly the main conclusions which have emerged
from the treatment comparisons. Second I shall describe Dr. Gleason's
system of histological classification, and finally I shall present

TABLE I. Number of patients and treatments assigned by stage of disease in the VACURG clinical trials

Stage	Study 1[a] (1960-67) Ne	Treatments[f]	Study 2[b] (1967-69) N	Treatments	Study 3[c] (1969-75) N	Treatments	Focal[d] (1964-69) N	Treatments
I	60	Px+Pcb	18	Pcb	20	Pcb	39	Pcb
	60	Px+DES (5.0)	14	Px+Pcb	23	Px+Pcb	36	DES (5.0)
							38	Orch+Pcb
							35	Orch+DES (5.0)
II	85	Px+Pcb	10	Pcb	20	Pcb		
	94	Px+DES (5.0)	11	Px+Pcb	26	Px+Pcb		
III	216	Pcb	75	Pcb	140	Prem (2.5)		
	264	DES (5.0)	73	DES (0.2)	136	Prov (30)		
	55	Orch	73	DES (1.0)	134	Prov+DES (1.0)		
	266	Orch+Pcb	73	DES (5.0)	135	DES (1.0)		
	258	Orch+DES (5.0)						
IV	223	Pcb	53	Pcb	123	Prem (2.5)		
	211	DES (5.0)	52	DES (0.2)	119	Prov (30)		
	57	Orch	55	DES (1.0)	117	Prov+DES (1.0)		
	203	Orch+Pcb	54	DES (5.0)	119	DES (1.0)		
	216	Orch+DES (5.0)						
All Stages	2313		561		1112		148	

[a] Patients admitted from March 1960 through March 1967.
[b] Patients admitted from April 1967 through May 1969.
[c] Patients admitted from June 1969 through September 1975.
[d] Patients admitted from April 1964 through April 1969.
[e] N = number of patients.
[f] Treatment abbreviations.   Pcb = placebo; Px = radical prostatectomy; DES = diethylstilboestrol; Orch = bilateral orchidectomy; Prem = Premarin; Prov = Provera; daily doses in milligrams are given in parentheses following the treatment abbreviations.

new results concerning the comparison of treatments for stage I and
II patients which have not yet been published in detail.

PRINCIPAL CONCLUSIONS CONCERNING THE TREATMENT OF PROSTATIC CANCER

Since the third part of my talk will deal with stage I and II
disease, in this portion I shall confine my attention mainly to the
results for stages III and IV. The staging system used by the VACURG
is shown in Figure 1. In all studies only newly diagnosed patients
were admitted and all cases were confirmed by a referee pathologist.
For Study 1 and the Focal Study this was Dr. F. K. Mostofi of the
Armed Forces Institute of Pathology, and for Studies 2 and 3,
Dr. Donald Gleason of the Minneapolis Veterans Administration
Hospital served as the referee pathologist. All acid phosphatase
determinations were made at a central reference laboratory in
Minneapolis under the direction of Drs. Richard Doe and Ulysses Seal.

The principal result of the treatment comparisons in Study 1 was
that initial treatment with 5 mg of diethystilboestrol (DES) daily
was associated with an excess risk of cardiovascular death when
compared to treatment with placebo or with orchidectomy alone (15,16).
The data did provide evidence that DES was effective in delaying
progression of cancer and in reducing the number of deaths due to
prostatic cancer. However, this beneficial effect was offset by the
cardiovascular toxicity (17). The effect was confined to patients
in stage III where even in the placebo group less than $\frac{1}{3}$ of the
patients died of prostatic cancer. In all the VACURG studies
statistical comparisons of treatments were performed for all patients

STAGE	RECTAL EXAMINATION	PROSTATIC ACID PHOSPHATASE	EVIDENCE OF METASTASES X-RAY OR BIOPSY
I	NO INDURATION 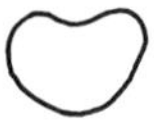	$\leqslant$ 1.0 K.A.U.	0
II	LOCALIZED NODULE 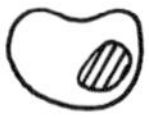	$\leqslant$ 1.0 K.A.U.	0
III	EXTRA-PROSTATIC EXTENSION 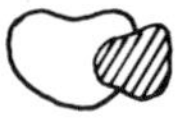	$\leqslant$ 1.0 K.A.U	0
IV	ANY FINDINGS 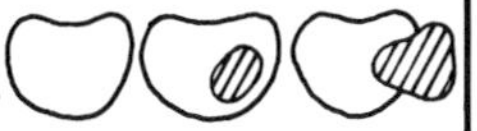	$>$ 1.0 K.A.U. OR	+

FIGURE 1

Staging system for prostatic cancer used by the VACURG.

originally randomised, even though patients showing symptoms of progressive disease often had their treatments changed later, most frequently to oestrogen or orchidectomy. Although some readers have found the results difficult to interpret because of this practice, it is the only correct way to analyse the results of the randomised clinical trial (18). To some extent these studies may be thought of as comparing initial hormone treatment at the time of diagnosis with the possible use of the same treatment later if warranted by the progression of disease. It was justifiably deemed unethical to withhold treatment entirely from patients diagnosed as having prostatic cancer, and principal interests centered on when treatment should be initiated and what that treatment should be. In particular, various initial therapies were compared, but subsequent treatments were left to the discretion of the physician treating the patient. An analysis of the effects of changes from the originally assigned treatment in Study 1 suggested that patients whose initial treatment was placebo were more likely to have the treatment changed later, had their treatments changed when they were in comparatively better health than patients on active therapy, were more likely to benefit from a change of treatment, and survived longer after having their treatment changed (19). In addition, we found no evidence that treatment with oestrogens in the later stages of prostatic cancer was associated with increased risk of death due to cardiovascular causes. It was also of interest to note that a decrease in the acid phosphatase could occur late in the course of disease after a change of therapy, even if the initial therapy included oestrogen, orchidectomy, or both. These results appeared to be consistent with the philosophy that endocrine treatment for prostatic cancer could be withheld until it is required for relief of symptoms.

Study 1 provided no evidence that orchidectomy was superior to 5 mg DES or that a combination of the two was better than either one alone (20). This result sharply contradicted the conclusions of Nesbit and Baum based on a large retrospective study (21). The difference in results can probably be explained by selective factors affecting their data since their study was neither prospective nor randomised. It is interesting to note, however, that there is some hint in the paper by Nesbit and Baum of a relationship between oestrogen and cardiovascular deaths; although not referred to in the text of their paper, the data in their Tables I and II show an increased percentage of deaths not due to prostatic carcinoma among patients treated with DES. The cardiovascular toxicity of oestrogens in a population of men who had already suffered one heart attack was demonstrated in the randomised clinical trial of some 8,000 patients known as the Coronary Drug Project (22). The project had been undertaken because it was believed that oestrogens might actually be beneficial.

Since the practice of treating prostatic cancer patients with oestrogens at time of diagnosis had been practiced widely for at least two decades, it was not surprising that the results of Study 1 excited considerable discussion and criticism. One of the principal criticisms was that the dose of DES was too high. For this reason Study 2 was designed to examine the effects of different doses of DES in treating stage III and IV patients. The doses studied were none (placebo), 0.2 mg, 1.0 mg and 5.0 mg of DES given daily by mouth. The principal result of Study 2 was that 1 mg DES seemed to be as effective as 5 mg in controlling prostatic cancer but was not associated with excess risk of cardiovascular death (23-25).

Study 3 was designed to answer another criticism of the results of Studies 1 and 2, namely that the oestrogen used, DES, was not a natural oestrogen but instead a synthetic compound. There was some speculation that the excess cardiovascular deaths due to DES would not be observed with a natural oestrogen such as Premarin, a preparation of conjugated equine oestrogens often prescribed in the United States. In addition, there was some hope that the anti-androgenic effects of a progestational agent such as Provera (medroxyprogesterone) might be useful in treatment of such patients with stage III and IV prostatic cancer. Although the results of this study have not been presented in detail, they may be summarised briefly by saying that analyses performed to date do not indicate significant differences between the four treatments in either stage III or IV when survival from all causes of death is used as the endpoint. Combining the data from stages II and IV, there was no difference when survival curves constructed for cancer deaths only were examined. It is possible that the dose of Provera used may have been too low, but based on the dose we studied (30 mg per day by mouth), none of the treatments compared were shown to be better than 1 mg daily of DES.

The results of these three studies clearly indicate that prostatic cancer is hormonally responsive and many patients have experienced distinct benefit from the use of oestrogens or orchidectomy, especially with regard to relief of symptoms. A detailed analysis of Study 2 was undertaken to see whether characteristics of the patients could be identified which might allow one to decide whether or not to use oestrogens (26). Although this analysis is rather complex, the results can be summarised fairly simply. Patients who benefited from oestrogens were most often characterised by having primary tumours whose palpable surface area was greater than 30 sq. cm, high grade and advanced stage tumours, and haemoglobin less than 12 grams percent. On the other hand, patients with a history of cardiovascular disease, greater than age 75, confined to bed, or having suffered extreme weight loss were more likely to survive longer if they were treated with placebo rather than 1 or 5 mg of DES. The mathematical models fitted in this analysis allow one to predict the outcome for individual patients based on their characteristics at the time of diagnosis. However, the validity of such analyses would formally depend upon new trials

designed to test them, since the conclusions are based on the retrospective analysis of a study designed for a different purpose.
Nevertheless, it would be reasonable to use results of this analysis
as a rough guide in treating patients and particularly in sharpening
questions to be asked in further clinical trials. In addition to
the indications just mentioned, oestrogen should definitely be
considered when there is progression of disease or pain from
metastases.

Thus far I have described briefly the principal results with
respect to treatment comparisons for stages III and IV. Now I
should like to describe briefly the Focal Study. This study admitted
patients during roughly the same period as Study 1 and was designed
to accommodate those stage I patients who were too old, too ill, or
who refused radical prostatectomy. Treatments compared in this study
were the same as those studied in stages III and IV of Study 1. No
significant differences were detected among the four treatments. A
non-randomised comparison with stage I patients from Study 1 adjusted
for age did not reveal a significant difference in survival, even
though the histologic characteristics of the tumours in both series
were similar (27). This result, although not based on randomised
comparisons, suggested that the role of radical prostatectomy in
treating stage I cancer should be carefully reconsidered. I shall
return to this point in the last part of this paper.

HISTOLOGICAL GRADING FOR PROSTATIC CANCER

One of the most important contributions of the VACURG studies
is the system of histological classification designed by
Dr. Donald Gleason based on review of some 3,000 cases (3-7). Before
his studies were undertaken there was no general agreement about
either the advisability or the possibility of grading prostatic
cancer despite the fact that several authors had shown that a simple
system in which tumours were classified as well differentiated,
moderately differentiated, and poorly differentiated provided useful
prognostic information. One difficulty with all previous studies
was that the authors did not demonstrate that histological grading
added appreciably to the prognostic information provided by tumour
stage. To be useful, any system of grading should work within each
stage.

One of the principal difficulties involved in grading prostatic
carcinoma is the extreme variability of these tumours. It is not
uncommon to find two or more patterns of growth present in the same
histological material. In order to overcome this difficulty
Dr. Gleason decided to record a primary and secondary pattern for
each tumour based simply on the amount present in the specimen.
These patterns were to be chosen from one to five categories designed
to encompass the spectrum of histological appearances encountered

with this disease. A schematic representation of this spectrum of appearances is presented in Figure 2 along with an indication as to the dividing lines along the spectrum which he designated as patterns 1-5 in increasing order of malignancy. This diagram has been extremely useful to a number of pathologists who have tried to learn and use his system. Photomicrographs representing typical appearances of the five patterns are shown in Figures 3-7. A more

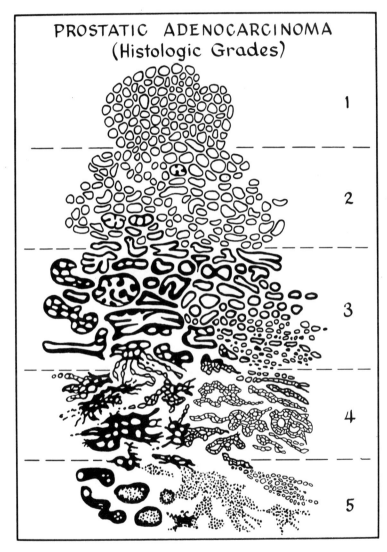

FIGURE 2

Schematic representation of Gleason's five patterns of prostatic carcinoma.

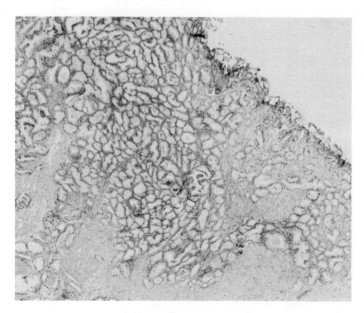

FIGURE 3

Pattern 1, consisting of uniform single separate glands, closely
packed, with definite edges.

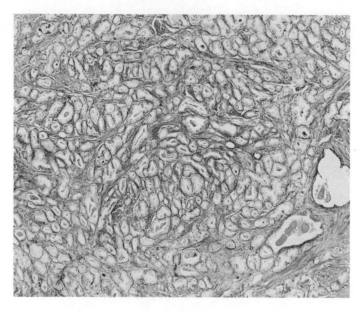

FIGURE 4

Pattern 2, consisting of slightly more variable single separate
glands, loosely packed, with definite but looser edges.

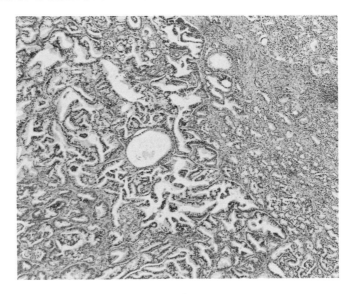

FIGURE 5

Pattern 3, consisting of single separate glands, variable in shape,
ranging from large to very small, and scattered in arrangement.
Pattern 3 also includes smooth round cribriform or papillary masses.

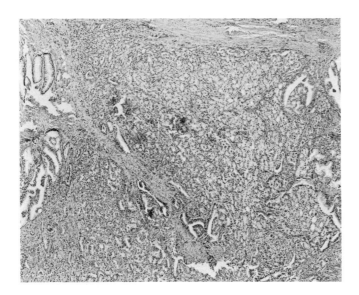

FIGURE 6

Pattern 4, consisting of raggedly infiltrating fused-glandular masses
with dark or light cells.

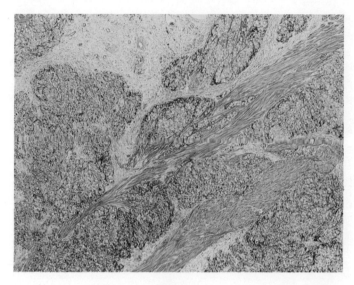

FIGURE 7

Pattern 5, consisting of anaplastic carcinoma.   Pattern 5 also
includes the comedocarcinoma pattern

detailed description can be found in the chapter Dr. Gleason
contributed to the volume Urologic Pathology: The Prostate edited
by Myron Tannenbaum (7) as well as in earlier publications (3-6).
Detailed analysis of his data revealed that the primary and secondary
patterns were about equally important in prognosis. Therefore
Dr. Gleason's system consisted of adding together the numerical
values for the primary and secondary tumour pattern to obtain a
summary score. If the tumour consists of a single type, the number
for the pattern of that type is simply doubled.

     The astonishing thing about this system is that even though
there are nine possible scores, there is a steady progression in the
death rate due to cancer as one progresses from the low scores to the
high scores (Figure 8). This observation has been demonstrated in
each of the three main VACURG studies. In addition, the histological
scores correlate with other prognostic variables at the time of
diagnosis such as metastasis, level of acid phosphatase, dilatation
of the upper urinary tract, and pain (Figure 9). It is also related
to the time until first metastasis for stage II patients (1) and to
the percent with metastases in various major sites at autopsy
(Figure 10).

     Although it is difficult to reproduce the system exactly when
the same pathologist blindly reviews previously graded slides, the

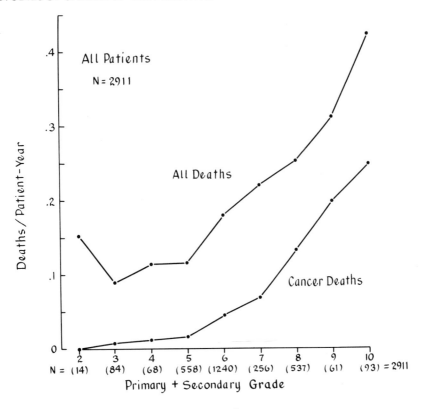

FIGURE 8

Relationship between the histologic score (sum of primary and secondary pattern or grade) and death rates.

degree of reproducibility is quite satisfactory (28). A number of different pathologists in the United States have successfully learned to use this system and it was recently adopted as the standard system to be used in reporting results at a meeting on grading of prostatic carcinoma jointly sponsored by the National Prostatic Working Cadre of the National Cancer Institute and the American Cancer Society (29).

It has become clear through Dr. Gleason's studies that the histological appearance of the tumour at the time of diagnosis is one of the most important prognostic factors for prostatic cancer. This information should be obtained routinely as a guide to therapy in individual patients and is particularly useful in designing and evaluating the results of prospective clinical trials.

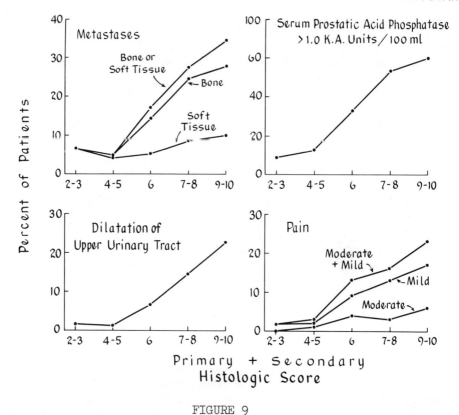

FIGURE 9

Relationship between histologic score and percent metastasis at autopsy in several major sites.

TREATMENT COMPARISON IN STAGE I AND II

Although previous publications of the VACURG have mentioned results of treatment comparisons in stages I and II of Study 1, no analysis has been published for the results of Studies 2 and 3. Since the same treatments were employed in Studies 2 and 3, for simplicity I shall refer to these two studies combined as Study 2.

In Study 1 the goal was to see whether the addition of oestrogen to radical prostatectomy improved survival or delayed progression in stages I and II. The oestrogen used was 5.0 mg of DES daily by mouth. In analysing the results for stage I and II in both Study 1 and Study 2 we found that a number of patients had to be excluded from analysis either because they were mistaged or did not receive the treatment to which they were assigned. Ordinarily it is not a good practice to omit patients from analysis after randomisation

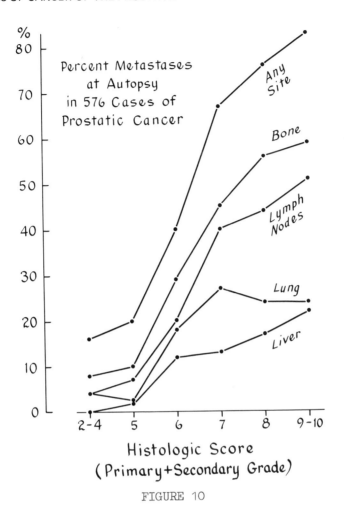

FIGURE 10

Relationship between histological score and percent metastasis at autopsy in several major sites.

since serious biases can arise. However, in this instance, where the number of protocol violations were similar in the various treatment groups and where it was possible to perform careful adjusted analyses based on patient age and the histologic appearance of the tumour, it seemed advisable to restrict attention to those patients who actually received the assigned treatments, particularly since great interest attaches to the natural history of the disease as affected by the treatments. The results of parallel analyses using all patients randomised did not differ appreciably from those to be presented. The numbers of patients omitted can be deduced by

comparing the numbers in these analyses with those in Table I
representing all patients initially randomised.

Comparison of survival curves for stage I patients revealed
that although survival probabilities at 12 years were similar there
was an early separation of the curves in the first two years
favouring the placebo treatment group, significant at p = .02.
Other analyses not presented here indicated that almost all the
excess mortality was confined to patients who had had two operations
within two months, namely the transurethral resection resulting in
diagnosis and the radical prostatectomy. No significant difference
in survival was observed in stage II of Study 1. Here the diagnosis
more often resulted from needle biopsy rather than from transurethral
resection. These data suggest, but do not prove, that major surgical
operations alter the coagulation system in some manner so that it is
more sensitive to the adverse effects of oestrogens.

Progression of disease was defined as occurring at first
evidence of distant metastasis, first rise of the acid phosphatase
above 2.0 King Armstrong Units, or death due to prostatic cancer.
The results for Study 1 by stage and treatment are presented in the
top part of Table II. No significant difference was observed in
progression rates in stage I patients, but in stage II the
progression rate was significantly lower (p = .025) for patients
treated with oestrogen. It will be recalled, however, that no
significant difference was observed in overall survival. This
result is similar to previously published results for stage III
patients (25). Causes of death for patients in Study 1 by stage
and treatment are shown in Table III. In both stages and all
treatment groups cardiovascular causes were the principal causes of
death. Here cardiovascular death includes cerebrovascular accidents,
myocardial infarctions, pulmonary emboli, and congestive heart
failure. In no stage or treatment group did prostatic cancer
account for more than 10% of the total deaths. Although the sample
size is too small to reach statistical significance, we note that
there were a few more deaths from prostatic cancer in the two groups
treated with placebo compared to those treated with oestrogens.

In Study 2 (here taken as the combined results for Studies 2
and 3 for patients in stages I and II) patients were randomised to
placebo or placebo plus prostatectomy. As previously mentioned, the
results of the adjusted comparisons between the Focal Study and
stage I patients in Study 1 suggested that no great benefit was
obtained from radical prostatectomy, so that the treatment
comparisons in Study 2 seemed ethical as well as important. Some
people may feel that failing to treat patients with prostatic cancer
is unethical, while others might feel that performing a possibly
useless operation is unethical. Perhaps the only ethical position
is to study the matter in a randomised clinical trial. At any rate
survival curves for stage I did not reveal a significant difference

TABLE II. Progression rates by study, stage and treatment

	STAGE I			STAGE II		
	Number of Patients	Number Who Progressed[1]	Progression Rate[2]	Number of Patients	Number Who Progressed[1]	Progression Rate[2]
STUDY 1						
Prostatectomy plus Placebo	46	5	1.089	76	11	1.464
			N.S.[4]			p=.025
Prostatectomy plus Oestrogen[3]	43	2	0.617	82	3	0.377
Both Treatments	89	7	0.893	158	14	0.905
STUDY 2						
Placebo	30	2	1.357	20	7	6.029
			N.S.[4]			N.S.[4]
Prostatectomy plus Placebo	31	1	0.532	30	6	3.571
Both Treatments	61	3	0.894	50	13	4.576

[1]Progression was defined as occurring at first metastasis, rise in acid phosphatase above 2.0 King-Armstrong Units, or death due to prostatic cancer.

[2]Expressed as number progressing per 1000 patient-months of observation.

[3]5.0 mgs diethylstilboestrol daily p.o.

[4]N.S. = not significant

TABLE III
CAUSES OF DEATH BY STUDY, STAGE AND TREATMENT

STUDY 1

STATUS	STAGE I		STAGE II	
	Prostatectomy plus Placebo	Prostatectomy plus Oestrogen	Prostatectomy plus Placebo	Prostatectomy plus Oestrogen
Alive	17	13	24	25
Dead	29	30	52	57
Prostate Cancer	4	0	7	2
Cardiovascular	17	19	26	29
Other (Unknown)	8 (1)	11 (1)	19 (5)	26 (2)
	46	43	76	82

STUDY 2

STATUS	STAGE I		STAGE II	
	Placebo	Placebo plus Prostatectomy	Placebo	Placebo plus Prostatectomy
Alive	16	21	14	16
Dead	14	10	6	14
Prostate Cancer	1	1	0	2
Cardiovascular	5	4	0	4
Other (Unknown)	8 (6)	5 (2)	6 (3)	8 (4)
	30	31	20	30

between placebo and placebo plus radical prostatectomy, but the sample sizes were relatively small. Even though the survival curve for the prostatectomy group indicated better survival than that for the placebo group, this difference could easily have arisen by chance. The results in stage II also revealed no significant differences, and in fact the better survival curve was for the group who received only placebo. Again, this result is easily explained by chance when one considers the numbers of patients studied. A comparison of the progression rates in Study 2, defined the same as for Study 1, are shown in the lower part of Table II. Although in both stages the progression rates were somewhat lower for those receiving prostatectomy, in neither case is the difference status statistically significant. In stage II of Study 2 the progression rates for the prostatectomy patients were somewhat higher than those in stage II of Study 1 for patients treated with prostatectomy plus placebo. This difference is in part explained by the fact that there were more high grade tumours in the second study in stage II.

The relationship of the histological grade of the tumour to the progression rates for both Studies 1 and 2 for stage I and II patients is shown in Table IV. For both studies it is clear that the progression rate is strongly related to the histological grade.

The results of Study 2, although based upon relatively small numbers of patients, do not provide evidence supporting the use of radical prostatectomy alone in treating stage I or II patients. These data are consistent with the idea that prostatic cancer is a disease which metastasises early, particularly if the tumour is poorly differentiated. In such instances the operation may be too late to affect the natural history of the disease. In future studies some systemic treatment should be used in addition to or instead of the operation.

A fuller account of the treatment comparisons in stages I and II will appear in Urologia Internationalis (30).

SUMMARY

Although many questions have been answered by 15 years of randomised prospective clinical trials of treatment for prostatic cancer conducted by the VACURG, many more questions remain and the studies themselves have raised further questions. Some of the most important results mentioned in this presentation are summarised below.

1. An excellent system of histological grading for prostatic cancer is now available.

2. Our inability to show any definite benefit from radical

TABLE IV

PROGRESSION RATES BY TUMOUR HISTOLOGY

STUDY	Sum of 1° + 2° Patterns	Number of Patients	Number Progressing	Total Patient Months	Progression Rate[1] per 1000 pt mos.
Study 1	4	50	0	5200	0.00
	5	84	4	7796	0.51
	6	85	7	7977	0.88 p .0001[2]
	7	14	3	1408	2.13
	8-10	11	7	804	8.71
Study 2	4	21	2	1297	1.54
	5	26	1	1631	0.61 p=.007[2]
	6	49	7	2636	2.66
	7-10	11	5	456	10.97

[1]Progression was defined as occurring at first metastasis, rise of acid phosphatase above 2.0 King Armstrong units, or death due to prostatic cancer.

[2]p- values refer to a test for increasing death rate by histological category.

prostatectomy in stages I and II may result from the tendency for higher grade tumours to metastasise early before the operation is performed. In addition, the value of this operation must be weighed against the low probability of death from prostatic cancer in these two stages.

3. Initial treatment with 5 mg of DES carries an excess risk of cardiovascular disease in some groups of patients.

4. Treatment with 1 mg DES daily appears to be as effective as 5 mg in retarding the growth of cancer but is not associated with excess risk of cardiovascular death.

5. Treatment with 2.5 mg of Premarin or with 30 mg of Provera did not appear to confer any benefit over 1 mg of DES in stages III and IV.

6. Our data suggests that not all patients should be treated initially with oestrogen but that the choice of whether or not to treat depends upon the characteristics of the patients.

7. Orchidectomy does not appear to be better than oestrogen in retarding the growth of prostatic cancer and the two treatments together do not appear to be better than either one alone.

REFERENCES

1. Byar, D. P., Contributions of the Veterans Administration Cooperative Urological Research Group studies to our understanding of prostatic cancer and its treatment. Urologic Pathology: The Prostate, ch.13. Ed. M Tannenbaum. New York: Lea and Febiger (1977).

2. Coune, A., Carcinoma of the Prostate. Randomised Trials in Cancer: A Critical Review by Sites. Ed. M. J. Staquet. New York: Raven Press (1978).

3. Gleason, D. F., Classification of prostatic carcinomas. Cancer Chemother. Rep. 50, 125-128 (1966).

4. Bailar, J. C., Mellinger, G. T. and Gleason, D. F., Survival rates of patients with prostatic cancer - Tumour stage and differentiation - Preliminary Report. Cancer Chemother. Rep. 50, 129-136 (1966).

5. Mellinger, G. T., Gleason, D. and Bailar, J. C., III, The histology and prognosis of prostatic cancer. J. Urol. 97, 331-339 (1967).

6.   Gleason, D. F., Mellinger, G. T. and the VACURG. Prediction
      of prognosis for prostatic adenocarcinoma by combined
      histological grading and clinical staging. J. Urol. 111,
      58-64 (1974).

7.   Gleason, D. F., Histologic grading and clinical staging of
      prostatic carcinoma. Urologic Pathology: The Prostate, ch. 9
      Ed. M. Tannenbaum. New York: Lea and Febiger (1977).

8.   Veterans Administration Cooperative Research Group. Factors
      in the prognosis of carcinoma of the prostate: A cooperative
      study. J. Urol. 100, 59-65 (1968).

9.   Byar, D. P., Huse, R., Bailar, J. C., III and the VACURG. An
      exponential model relating censored survival data and
      concomitant information for prostatic cancer patients. JNCI
      52, 321-326 (1974).

10.   Blackard, C. E., Byar, D. P., Seal, U. S., Doe, R. P. and the
      VACURG, Correlation of pre-treatment serum nonprotein-bound
      cortisol and total 17-hydroxycorticosteroid values with
      survival in patients with prostatic cancer. N. Engl. J. Med.
      291, 751-755 (1974).

11.   Blackard, C. E., Byar, D. P., Seal, U. S., Doe, R. P. and
      the VACURG, Correlation of pre-treatment serum 17-hydroxy-
      corticosteroid values with survival in patients with prostatic
      cancer. J. Urol. 113, 517-520 (1975).

12.   Seal, U. S., Doe, R. P., Byar, D. P., Corle, D. K. and the
      VACURG, Response of serum cholesterol and triglycerides to
      hormone treatment and the relation of pre-treatment values to
      mortality in patients with prostatic cancer. Cancer, 38,
      1095-1107 (1976).

13.   Seal, U. S., Doe, R. P., Byar, D. P., Corle, D. K. and the
      VACURG. Response of plasma fibrinogen to hormone treatment
      and the relation of pre-treatment values to mortality in
      prostatic cancer. Cancer, 38, 1108-1117 (1976).

14.   Seal, U. S., Doe, R. P., Byar, D. P. and Corle, D. K. Response
      of serum haptoglobin to hormone treatment and the relation of
      pre-treatment values to mortality in patients with prostatic
      cancer. Cancer, 42, 1720-1729 (1978).

15.   Veterans Administration Cooperative Urological Research Group.
      Treatment comparisons. J. Urol. 98, 516-522 (1967).

16.   Veterans Administration Cooperative Urological Research Group,
      Treatment and survival of patients with cancer of the prostate.
      Surg. Gynaecol. Obstet. 124, 1011-1017 (1967).

17.   Blackard, C. E., Doe, R. P., Mellinger, G. T. and Byar, D. P.,
      Incidence of cardiovascular disease and death in patients
      receiving diethylstilboestrol for carcinoma of the prostate.
      Cancer, 26, 249-256 (1970).

18.   Peto, R., Pike, M. C., Armitage, P., Breslow, N. E., Cox, D. R.
      Howard, S. V., Mantel, N., McPherson, K., Peto, J. and
      Smith, P. G., Design and analysis of randomised clinical trials
      requiring prolonged observation of each patient. Br. J. Cancer
      35, 1-39 (1977).

19.   Hurst, K. S., Byar, D. P. and the VACURG. An analysis of the
      effects of changes from the assigned treatment in a clinical
      trial of treatment for prostatic cancer. J. Chronic Dis.
      26, 311-324 (1973).

20.   Blackard, C. E., Byar, D. P., Jordan, W. P. and the VACURG,
      Orchidectomy for advanced prostatic carcinoma: A re-evaluation.
      Urology, 1, 553-560 (1973).

21.   Nesbit, R. M. and Baum, W. C., Endocrine control of prostatic
      carcinoma. Clinical and statistical survey of 1,818 cases.
      JAMA, 143, 1317-1320 (1950).

22.   The Coronary Drug Project Research Group. The Coronary Drug
      Project - Initial findings leading to modifications of its
      research protocol. JAMA, 214, 1303-1313 (1970).

23.   Bailar, J. C. and Byar, D. P., Oestrogen treatment for cancer
      of the prostate: Early results with three doses of diethyl-
      stilboestrol and placebo. Cancer, 26, 257-261 (1970).

24.   Byar, D. P., Treatment of prostatic cancer: Studies by the
      Veterans Administration Cooperative Urological Research Group.
      Bull NY Acad. Med., 48, 751-766 (1972).

25.   Byar, D. P., The Veterans Administration Cooperative Urological
      Research Group's studies of cancer of the prostate. Cancer,
      32, 1126-1130 (1973).

26.   Byar, D. P. and Corle, D. K., Selecting optimal treatment in
      clinical trials using covariate information. J. Chronic Dis.,
      30, 445-459 (1977).

27.   Byar, D. P. and the VACURG. Survival of patients with
      incidentally found microscopic cancer of the prostate: Results
      of a clinical trial of conservative treatment. J. Urol., 108,
      908-913 (1972).

28.   Harada, M., Mostofi, F. K., Corle, D. K., Byar, D. P. and
      Trump, B. F., Preliminary studies of histologic prognosis in
      cancer of the prostate. Cancer Treat. Rep. 61, 223-225 (1977).

29.   Murphy, G. P. and Whitmore, W. F. Jr., A report of the work-
      shops on the current status of the histologic grading of
      prostate cancer. Cancer, In Press.

30.   Madsen, P. O., Maigaard, S., Corle, D. K. and Byar, D. P.,
      Radical prostatectomy for carcinoma of the prostate, Stages I
      and II. New results of the Veterans Administration Cooperative
      Urological Research Group. Urologia Internationalis. To
      appear.

ESTRACYT

I KÖNYVES

AB LEO, Research Laboratories

Helsinborg, Sweden

ABSTRACT

Estramustine phosphate belongs to a series of compounds where
an alkylating agent is linked to a steroid carrier in the form of a
carbamate. Estracyt is concentrated in the rat ventral prostate, in
DMBA-induced mammary tumours and affects the growth of various
experimental tumours. The drug is used clinically in the treatment
of advanced prostatic carcinoma.

The major advantage of the use of carriers is a higher selectivity of action. The carrier can recognise the target cells and
allow the drug to act either at the surface or intracellularly,
after uptake of the carrier-drug complex (15).

The first paper which mentioned the utilisation of the carbamate
group, containing a cytotoxic agent, was published by Owen and co-
workers in 1956 (12). The carrier group in this case was
cholesterol. Furthermore, Bergel and Wade described in 1959
analogous compounds with amino acids (2) and Nogrady in 1961 with
carbohydrates (11).

In 1961 we started to synthesise compounds where the nor-
nitrogen mustard group is linked to oestrogens in the form of a
carbamate. This activity was initiated by the knowledge that there
is a specific intracellular binding of steroid-hormones in the cells
of neoplasm derived from target tissues for the steroids. This made
it theoretically possible to obtain an intracellular concentration of
the steroid carbamates containing the alkylating agent (6).

TABLE I

STEROID CYTOSTATIC CARBAMATES
SYNTHESISED BY AB LEO RESEARCH LABORATORIES

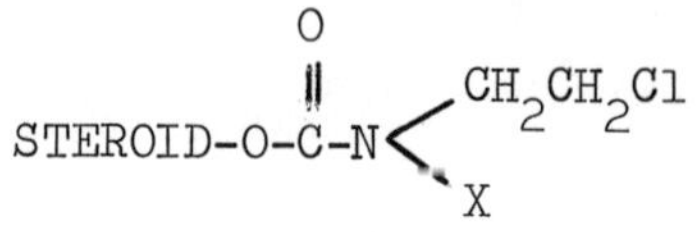

$$STEROID-O-\overset{\overset{O}{\|}}{C}-N\diagdown\overset{CH_2CH_2Cl}{\diagdown X}$$

$$X = CH_2CH_2Cl \text{ or } N = O$$

On the basis of this working hypothesis we have synthesised various oestrogen, androgen, gestogen and corticosteroid carbamates as potential antineoplastic agents.

If the steroid molecule contains two or more hydroxy groups, we could further manipulate the lipophilic properties of these compounds. For instance, increased lipophility could be obtained by esterification with fatty acids. Steroid esters of this kind have prolonged hormonal properties.

On the other hand, water solubility can be achieved by esterification with phosphoric or sulphuric acid. Such esters have a lower hormonal activity and shorter duration.

On the basis of the of the hormonal and cytostatic properties

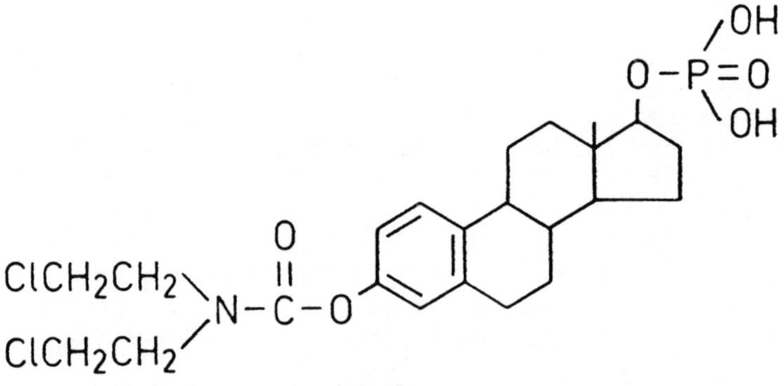

FIGURE 1

STRUCTURAL FORMULA OF ESTRAMUSTINE PHOSPHATE

we selected estramustine phosphate, a phenolic-N-bis-2-chloroethyl
carbamate 17 phosphate of estradiol for further evaluation
(Figure 1).

Estracyt is effective in the following transplantable tumours:

1.   Ehrlich Ascites Tumour in mice (6).
2.   Hepatoma AH 130 in rats (6).
3.   Hormone sensitive R3327 prostatic carcinoma in rats (8).

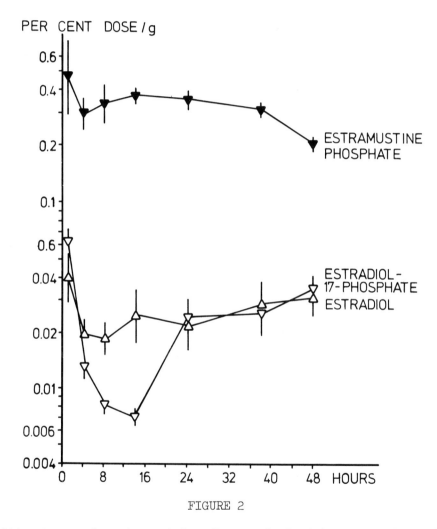

FIGURE 2

Tritium levels in rat prostate after a single intravenous dose of
^{3}H-labelled estradiol-17β (1 mg/kg), estradiol-17β-phosphate
(10 mg/kg) and estramustine phosphate (10 mg/kg). Means of four
animals $\pm$ s.e.

4.   Hormone sensitive R3230 AC mammary carcinoma in rats (16).
5.   Hormone sensitive and resistant DMBA induced mammary tumours
     in rats (9).

     Estramustine phosphate has a high affinity to the rat ventral
prostate. Figure 2, which is in logarithmic scale, shows a
comparison of the uptake in the rat prostate of estradiol, estradiol-
17-phosphate and estramustine phosphate. The in vivo concentration

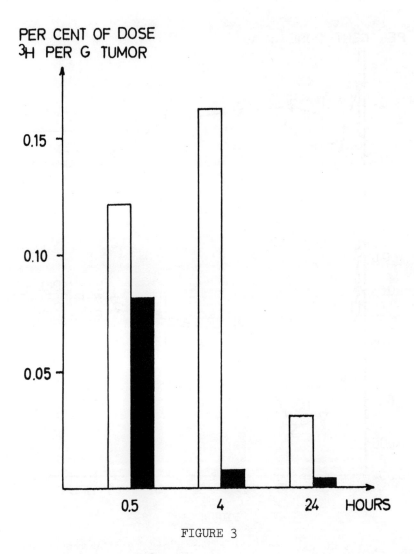

FIGURE 3

Percent of injected dose ^{3}H per gram tumour, 0.5, 4 and 24 hours
after injection of radiolabelled estramustine phosphate (open bars)
or estradiol (solid bars).

of radioactivity in the ventral prostate is about ten times higher
after administration of tritiated estramustine phosphate than after
administration of tritiated estradiol or estradiol 17-phosphate.
Identification studies showed that the radioactivity found after
administration of Estracyt is the dephosphorylated metabolites of
estramustine phosphate (13). The dephosphorylated metabolites were
also found in high levels in plasma from patients treated with
Estracyt (14).

In addition to the prostate two other tissues have been shown
to take up considerably more radioactivity from labelled estramustine
phosphate than after administration of estradiol or estradiol-17-
phosphate. These tissues are the ovary of the rat and the DMBA-
induced rat mammary tumour (9).

Experiments have shown that the uptake of radioactivity by DMBA-
induced mammary tumour tissue is much higher from estramustine
phosphate than from estradiol. Figure 3 shows the percentage of
injected dose of tritium per gram tumour 0.5,4 and 24 hours after
injection of radiolabelled estramustine phosphate or estradiol (9).

In experiments with DMBA-induced mammary tumours made re-
fractory to estradiol treatment, Estracyt had a growth-inhibiting
effect.

Figure 4 shows the progression of tumour growth in the control
rats given daily intraperitoneal injections of 20 mg per kg of
estradiol 17 during four weeks. The animals in the other group were
injected with Estracyt, 20 mg per kg, instead of estradiol. The
tumour growth was reduced significantly by Estracyt in comparison
with estradiol (9).

The cytosol fraction of the rat ventral prostate contains a
specific protein, which is responsible for the concentration of the
dephosphorylated Estracyt (3). Recently, this estramustine binding
protein has been isolated and antibodies against this protein has
been produced (4). By means of this we are searching for the
presence of estramustine binding protein in human prostatic cancer
tissue, in cooperation with the Karolinska Institute, Stockholm.

Estracyt is used today in the treatment of advanced prostatic
carcinoma, above all in oestrogen resistant cases (1,5,7,10).
Randomised trials in Sweden and in the EORTC Urological Group will
indicate the place of Estracyt versus conventional hormone therapy
in patients without previous endocrine therapy.

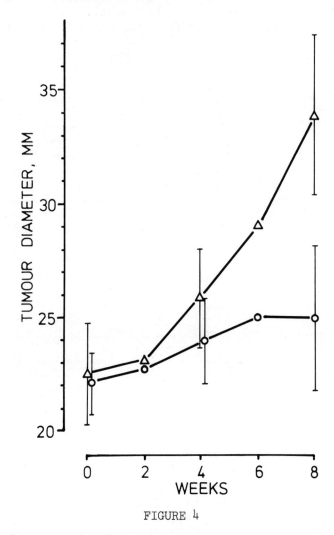

FIGURE 4

Growth of E_2-resistant DMBA-induced mammary tumours in rats injected with Estracyt (o) or Estradiol (-).

REFERENCES

1. Andersson, L., Edsmyr, F., Jonsson, G. and Konyves, I. Recent Results in Cancer Research, 60, 73-77 (1977).

2. Bergel, F. and Wade, R. J. Chem. Soc. 941-947 (1959).

3. Forsgren, B. and Högberg, B. Acta Pharmaceutica Suecica, 15, 23-32 (1978).

4. Forsgren, B., Björk, P., Carlström, K., Gustafsson, J. -Å., Pousette, Å. and Hogberg, B. Proc. Nat. Acad. Sci. In Press.

5. Jönsson, G., Högberg, B. and Nilsson, T. Scand. J. Urol. Nephrol. 11, 231-238 (1977).

6. Könyves, I. and Liljekvist, J. Excerpta Medica International Congress Series No. 375, 98-105 (1976).

7. Mittelman, A., Shukla, S. K. and Murphy, G. P. J. Urol. 115, 4-9-412 (1976).

8. Müntzing, J., Kirdani, R. Y., Saroff, J., Murphy, G. P. and Sandberg, A. A. Urology, 10 439-445 (1977).

9. Müntzing, J., Jensen, G. and Högberg, B. Acta Pharmacol. Toxicol. 44, 1-6 (1979).

10. Nagel, R., and Kölln, C. -P. Brit. J. Urol. 49, 73-79 (1977).

11. Nogrady, T. F. J. Org. Chem. 26, 4177-9 (1961).

12. Owen, L. N., Benn and Creighton, A. M. British Empire Cancer Campaign, 34, 448-9 (1956).

13. Plym-Forshell, G. and Nilsson, H. Acta Pharmacol. Toxicol. 35, Suppl. 1, 28 (1974).

14. Plym-Forshell, G., Müntzing, J., Ek, A., Lindstedt, E. and Dencker, H. Invest. Urol. 14, 128-131 (1976).

15. Trouet, A. Eur. J. Cancer, 14, 105-111 (1978).

16. Wittliff, J., Weidner, N., Park, D. C., Everson, R. B. and Hall, T. C. Cancer Treat. Rep. 62, 1260-1262 (1978).

Editorial Note (F Lund). There can be no doubt that the differentiation of the localised prostatic lesion significantly influences the prognosis and it may be that the higher survival rates in the well differentiated lesions are related more to the nature of the disease than to the treatment given! This does not mean that the attitude of "noli me tangere" towards Veterans Stage I and II lesions is necessarily valid for the poorly differentiated lesions in such stages.

The size of the lesion at diagnosis also exerts an influence on survival as does the presence of an elevated acid phosphatase which seems to carry at least a 50% chance of subsequent progression.

Although oestrogens reduce the growth rate of the local lesion the evidence on the importance of receptor studies in prognosis is still conflicting.

The many well controlled trials now in progress promise well for the future understanding of this capricious disease.

Part 4
Tumors of the Male Genitalia

COMBINED TREATMENT WITH BLEOMYCIN IN PENILE CARCINOMA

F EDSMYR, L ANDERSSON and P-L ESPOSTI

The Radiumhemmet and the Department of Urology

Karolinska Hospital, Stockholm, Sweden

INTRODUCTION

The first clinical studies with Bleomycin (BLM) were conducted by Ichikawa in 1965 and revealed effectiveness against squamous cell carcinoma of the penis. In 1970, at the Radiumhemmet, Stockholm, BLM was given as the sole treatment in three patients with advanced penile carcinoma. Local response of the tumours to therapy was good in two patients; one has now been living over seven years with normal sexual function and micturition.

TREATMENT

Combined treatment with BLM and local irradiation of penile tumours was started in 1973. Through 1977 25 patients have received combined therapy with BLM and irradiation at the Radiumhemmet in Stockholm. All the tumours were verified as squamous cell carcinomas localised to the penis and no clinical metastases were found. Circumcision should be carried out before treatment is started.

Bleomycin was administered two hours before irradiation on each of five days during the first, third and fifth week of treatment. The dose given was 15 mg by intramuscular injection. The total cumulative dose administered during therapy was over 200 mg.

Initially a general tumour dose of 4,500 rads was administered. From the end of 1974 the total tumour dose was increased to 5,800 rads, about 10-15% less than the usual full course for malignant tumours in this region. The whole penis including the shaft was

503

irradiated from two opposing beams of a conventional x-ray machine;
some of the patients are now living over five years and are symptom
free. All are currently free of local penile malignancy. Sexual
function is normal in all patients whose function was normal before
therapy. All patients have normal micturition. Chest x-rays were
carried out every week during treatment and at longer intervals
thereafter. In no patient was pulmonary fibrosis found.

CONCLUSIONS

Amputation of the penis, the conventional method of treatment
of carcinoma of the penis, is associated with psychological trauma
and loss of sexual function. It is also a mutilating procedure.
This combined drug and radiation therapy without amputation will be
more suitable, provided the long term results are acceptable and
complications are few. On the basis of these investigations it
appears advisable to try the combined therapy with subsequent
careful follow-up of the patients. If there is a local recurrence,
amputation is still possible.

REFERENCE

1.   Ichikawa, T., Chemotherapy of penile cancer. Extrait du
      Congres 16^e de la Societe Internationale d'Urologie, (1973).

A complete report has already been published in GANN Monograph on
Cancer Research No. 19, 1976, University of Tokyo Press. Full
information will be given during 1979 in European Urology.

ASSOCIATION OF SURGERY AND CHEMOTHERAPY IN METASTATIC TESTICULAR

CANCER

G PIZZOCARO and S MONFARDINI

Departments of Surgical Oncology and Medical Oncology.

National Tumour Institute, Milan, Italy

Remarkable progress has recently been achieved in the multi-drug therapy of non seminomatous testicular cancer (1,2,5,9) and the association of surgery and chemotherapy has proved useful in improving the prognosis of patients with widespread disease (4,6,11). On the other hand, the role of adjunctive chemotherapy has not yet been clearly defined although it has been suggested it should be able to destroy residual micrometastases (10).

In 1971 we began to investigate the usefulness of combining surgery and chemotherapy in patients with metastatic testicular carcinoma other than pure seminoma. Since January 1976 adjunctive chemotherapy has been systematically given to every N+Mo patient and surgery performed whenever possible in advanced cases.

This report concerns our whole experience of combined surgery and chemotherapy in metastatic non seminomatous testicular cancer from August 1971 up to December 1977. Different chemotherapeutic regimens were employed but the results of chemotherapy itself are not analysed as this paper is an appraisal of the combined treatment modality. Patients who did not receive surgery are not considered.

PATIENTS AND METHODS

From August 1971 to December 1977 54 patients with metastatic testicular carcinomas other than pure seminoma received surgery in combination with chemotherapy: 25 were category N+Mo and 29 had advanced disease. Their age ranged from three to 53 years - median of 28 years. The distribution of cases according to histology of the primary and the N and M categories is listed in Table I.

TABLE I

DISTRIBUTION OF CASES ACCORDING TO HISTOLOGY (W.H.O.)
AND TNM SYSTEM (GENEVA, 1974)

N and M categories	No. Cases	Embryonalca ($\pm$ seminoma)	Embryonalca and teratoma	Immature teratoma
N+ Mo	25	13	7	5
N3 Mo	12	9	1	2
N- M1b	2	2	-	-
N+ M1b	1	1	-	-
N3 M1b	6	3	-	3
N4 M1b	1	-	1	-
N+ M1c	3	3	-	-
N3 M1c	4	3	-	1
TOTAL	54	34	9	11

T category is not taken into consideration because 43 patients (81%) had orchidectomy performed elsewhere from 1 to 18 months before their admission to the Institute (median two months).

The slides of patients who had orchidectomy performed elsewhere were reviewed by members of our Department of Pathology. Clinical stage was determined by clinical examination, bipedal lymphangiography, urography and chest x-rays in all cases. Since January 1976 the beta subunit chorinonic gonadotrophin has been determined in the sera of all cases. Inferior cavography and upper gastrointestinal tract series were performed when deemed necessary. The clinical evaluation failed to demonstrate retroperitoneal involvement in eight cases of Mo category; false positive findings were found in two patients with distant metastases.

All patients had radical orchidectomy and bilateral retroperitoneal lymph node dissection (RPLND). Patients who had had simple orchidectomy performed elsewhere had excision of the spermatic cord and of the cutaneous scar at the time of RPLND. The nodal dissection was usually accomplished through a midline xifopubic incision. The thoracoabdominal approach was used only in three patients: twice to allow the simultaneous removal of lung disease and once to remove pathological nodes in the posterior mediastinum. It was necessary to remove the left kidney in four patients and the inferior vena cava was resected in two. Lung metastases were removed in eight patients and left supraclavicular

nodes in three. Surgery was staged in only one patient who underwent a total pneumonectomy.

Adjuvant Therapy in N+ Mo Patients

Nine cases received both postoperative irradiation and
chemotherapy. Three patients could not have a radical dissection
and another had retroperitoneal metastases of pure seminoma
(histology of his primary was embryonal carcinoma and seminoma).
Radiotherapy was given before or during a split of chemotherapy as
it was impossible to give the two treatments at the same time.
Retroperitoneal irradiation to the lymph node bearing areas ranged
from 4,200 to 5,400 rad in five to eight weeks, but the one patient
with metastases of pure seminoma received 3,200 rad to the abdomen
and 2,600 rad to mediastinum and neck. Four different chemotherapeutic regimens were used in these nine patients: four were
treated with a seven drug schedule (Adriamycin, Mithramycin,
Bleomycin and Vinblastine plus Actinomycin D, Methotrexate and
Chlorambucil); three patients received Vinblastine plus Bleomycin;
one patient was treated with Adriamycin, Vincristine and Methotrexate
(AVM) and another with Adriamycin, Bleomycin and Vinblastine.
Treatment ranged from two to 12 months with a median of six. None
of these patients had previously been treated with radiotherapy or
chemotherapy.

Sixteen patients received only adjunctive chemotherapy: 14
were treated with two to five courses (usually three) of Vinblastine
plus continuous intravenous infusion of Bleomycin (VLB + c.i.v. BLM),
one had three cycles of AVM and the last one received five courses
of Vinblastine, Bleomycin and Cisplatinum (VBP). Beta subunit
chorionic gonadotropin was elevated in the sera of five patients
and in every case returned to normal after RPLND. One patient had
been previously treated elsewhere with a short course of radiotherapy
and chemotherapy and he was the one in the adjuvant therapy group
who required nephrectomy because of neoplastic invasion of the left
renal hilum. Another patient presented with a scrotal recurrence
eighteen months after simple orchidectomy.

Combined Treatment of Advanced Cases

Five patients with operable retroperitoneal nodes and pulmonary
metastases received surgery before chemotherapy. After the
operation, three patients were treated with three courses of VLB +
c.i.v. BLM, one received six cycles of AVM and the last had five
courses of VBP followed by Adriamycin, Vincristine, Actinomycin D
and Methotrexate for consolidation.

The remaining 24 patients were treated with chemotherapy before

surgery, mainly to induce operability of bulky or primarily unresectable retroperitoneal nodes (Table I): 21 received two to four
courses of VLB + c.i.v. BLM, two patients had six cycles of AVM and
one the combination Vinblastine plus Bleomycin. Surgery consisted
of RPLND in all cases and resection of residual pulmonary,
mediastinal or supraclavicular disease in seven. Surgery did not
allow the complete removal of retroperitoneal metastases in five
patients: they received post operative irradiation to the area of
residual tumour. After the operation, a maintenance chemotherapy
was instituted with AVM or Adriamycin and Vinblastine for six
cycles.

Follow-up

Patients were followed every two months after completion of
therapy for the first two years and every four months thereafter.
Chest x-rays and assays of chorionic gonadotropin were regularly
repeated. Other investigations were done when deemed necessary.
Only two patients were lost to follow-up - four and 18 months after
surgery. Follow-up ranged from one to seven years (median 27 months)
for patients receiving adjunctive therapy and from one to five years
(median 21 months) for advanced disease.

RESULTS

Results are recorded as recurrence rate, because relapsing
patients received further therapy which enhanced survival. The
length of the free interval as well as of the survival is considered
from the time of surgery. 31st December 1978 is the date of the
last follow-up.

Adjuvant Therapy in N+ Mo Patients

Relapses were seen in eight of the 25 cases (32%) and 17
patients are living disease free from one to five years (Table II).
Of the three patients receiving radiotherapy and chemotherapy for an
incomplete RPLND one achieved a complete remission (C.R.) and is
alive disease free five years after surgery; one died of sepsis after
the first course of chemotherapy and the third one developed lung
metastases four months after surgery and died of widespread disease
within three months.

The patient with retroperitoneal metastases of pure seminoma is
alive disease free 27 months after surgery.

Only one of the five patients who received post operative
irradiation plus chemotherapy after a radical RPLND developed

TABLE II

RESULTS ACCORDING TO ADJUNCTIVE THERAPY IN

CATEGORY N+ Mo PATIENTS

Adjunctive Therapy	No. Cases	Relapsed		Died of Complications		Alive Disease Free	
		No.	(%)	No.	(%)	No.	(%)
Chemo + RT	9	2	(22)	2	(22)	5	(56)
Chemotherapy	16	6*	(37)	-	-	12	(75)
TOTAL	25	8	(32)	2	(8)	17	(68)

* Two patients in this group got a C.R. by further therapy and are alive disease free.

recurrent disease, six months after surgery. He continued with chemotherapy for slowly progressive lung metastases and died of acute myocardial failure one year later. Three patients are alive disease free from 38 to 41 months and the last one died of intestinal obstruction 20 months after surgery without any evidence of recurrent disease.

Six of the 16 patients (37.5%) receiving post operative chemotherapy alone developed recurrent disease from two to 12 months after surgery: five patients had lung metastases and one a retroperitoneal recurrence above the renal vessels which was disclosed by inferior cavography. However, only one of the relapsing patients died and another one was lost to follow-up with progressive disease. Two patients are living in partial remission and the other two achieved a C.R. by further therapy, so that 12 patients in this group (75%) are alive disease free from 12 to 57 months after surgery.

Relapses were seen in two of five patients with elevated HCG titers before surgery and in five of 13 patients with embryonal carcinoma. Also recurrences were more frequent in patients with more advanced retroperitoneal disease, and the highest incidence was seen in those with neoplastic invasion of spermatic vessels (Table III).

Advanced Cases

Twenty four of 29 patients achieved a complete remission (C.R.) and 14 are alive disease free from one to five years (Table IV).

TABLE III

RELATIONSHIP BETWEEN THE EXTENSION OF RETROPERITONEAL DISEASE
AND RECURRENCE RATE IN 25 N+ Mo PATIENTS UNDERGOING ADJUVANT
THERAPY AFTER RPLND

Extension of retro-peritoneal disease	No. cases	Relapses	
		No.	(%)
Intranodal metastases	8	2	(25)
Extranodal spread or invasion of r.p. fat	10	3	(30)
Incomplete RPLND	3	1	(33)
Neoplastic invasion of spermatic vessels	4	2	(50)
TOTAL	25	8	(32)

TABLE IV

RESPONSE RATE AND DISEASE FREE SURVIVAL IN 29 ADVANCED DISEASE
PATIENTS TREATED WITH THE ASSOCIATION OF SURGERY AND CHEMOTHERAPY

Timing of surgery and chemotherapy	No. Cases	C.R.		Disease Free Survivors	
		No.	(%)	No.	(%)
Surgery + Chemotherapy	5	5	(100)	2	(40)
Chemotherapy + Surgery	24	19	(79)	12	(50)
TOTAL	29	24	(83)	14	(48)

All the five patients receiving surgery before chemotherapy
achieved a C.R., but three developed lung recurrences from five to
17 months after surgery. Two patients are alive disease free from
one to five years.

Surgery did not allow the complete removal of retroperitoneal
disease in five of the patients previously treated with chemotherapy:
these five patients never achieved a C.R. and all developed
progressive disease within seven months. Metastases developed only
in five of the remaining 19 patients (26.3%); 12 are alive disease

free from one to three years, one was lost to follow up four months after surgery and one died of unrelated disease at seven months.

It is noteworthy that in the group of 24 patients receiving surgery before chemotherapy, three had complete destruction of all their neoplastic tissue and only foci of mature teratoma or pure seminoma were found in another two cases. All these patients had a good prognosis.

The disease progressed:

(a) in the five cases who did not achieve a C.R. after the combined treatment,

(b) in the three patients who showed only a minimal response to preoperative chemotherapy, and

(c) in the two who did not fulfil the post operative maintenance chemotherapy as well as in the three patients who had the shortest course of chemotherapy after primary surgery.

The HCG assay was positive before treatment in 14 of 25 tested cases. It returned to normal in nine patients of whom six did well; it remained elevated in five and all progressed. As a whole, patients with elevated HCG did worse (8/14 recurrences) than patients with negative tests (3/11 recurrences).

Twenty one patients had embryonal carcinoma and 11 (52.4%) recurred. Recurrences were seen in only two of eight immature teratomas or mixed tumours (25%).

Bulky or primarily unresectable retroperitoneal nodes were present in 22 patients and eight progressed (36.4%). The prognosis was worse in the seven patients with distant metastases and primarily resectable retroperitoneal nodes (five of them progressed : 71.4%)

The disease recurred locally in three patients and presented as distant metastases in 10. The free interval ranged from one to 17 months, with a median of six.

Complications of Treatment

There were no post operative deaths but seven major complications occurred: two intraoperative haemorrhages, two post operative chyle leakages requiring total parenteral alimentation for four to five days, one intestinal obstruction which needed second look surgery, a severe wound infection which was drained and one instance of viral hepatitis.

Chemotherapy produced toxicity in all patients, but only five required platelet or white cell transfusions. Death can be related to chemotoxicity in two patients: one died of sepsis secondary to severe leukopenia and another one of acute myocardial failure after i.v. injection of Adriamycin.

Post operative radiotherapy was of major concern: late severe bowel damage developed in two patients and one died of this complication. The other one did well after a by-pass procedure. In addition, it was very difficult to combine radiotherapy with chemotherapy in these patients.

                                DISCUSSION

The association of surgery and chemotherapy is nowadays the treatment of choice of advanced non seminomatous testis cancer in many Institutions: this combined treatment modality guarantees about 50% long standing complete remissions (4,6,11) and partial responders to chemotherapy may be made disease free by surgery (2).

On a theoretical basis, surgery should precede chemotherapy in order to reduce the tumour burden and, henceforth, increase drug effectiveness (10). Both our experience and Merrin's (7) suggest that it is preferable to give chemotherapy first: responsive patients are selected and surgery becomes less extensive. RPLND remains the main surgical procedure: it allows one to confirm a C.R. or to transform a partial remission into a complete one, as retroperitoneal disease is often difficult to evaluate and it is usually less responsive to chemotherapy than lung metastases. Some degree of retroperitoneal fibrosis may be found in performing RPLND after chemotherapy, but only on rare occasions does this present any problems.

Relapses in complete responders occur if the disease is poorly responsive to chemotherapy or if a too short post operative treatment is given. It is very difficult to assess how long a patient should be treated after a C.R. has been achieved. Six months is the average length of free interval before relapse, and six months might be the optimal period for maintenance chemotherapy. Treatment should be given in full dosage, however, as minimal residual tumour may be relatively chemoresistant (8).

The role of adjuvant chemotherapy is not yet clearly stated. It was assumed it might destroy residual micrometastases and prevent relapses (10), but the 32% and 42% recurrence rate reported by us and by Hoeffken (3) makes this assumption questionable. If more intensive chemotherapy is needed to prevent recurrences it cannot be lightly given to all patients with nodal metastases. Nowadays, nearly 70% of cases with minor retroperitoneal involvement may be

cured by surgery or radiotherapy alone (12,13) and a significant
number of relapsing patients may be saved by further therapy.
Intensive adjunctive chemotherapy should be therefore restricted to
very high risk patients, and old and new series should be carefully
examined in order to determine the factors of bad prognostic
significance eg. neoplastic invasion of spermatic vessels which
was very ominous in our experience as relapses were seen in all
three patients not receiving adjunctive treatment and in two of
four cases treated with post operative chemotherapy. Such patients
should be regarded as having advanced disease and treated
accordingly.

SUMMARY

The results of combined surgery and chemotherapy in 54 cases
of metastatic non seminomatous testis cancer are presented. The
intensive treatment was generally well tolerated and results were
gratifying in patients with advanced disease: 14 of 29 are alive
disease free from one to five years (48.3%). On the other hand, the
usefulness of post operative adjunctive chemotherapy in N+ Mo
patients is questionable: eight of 25 recurred within one year (32%).
A proper selection of patients and intensive chemotherapy are
believed to be necessary to obtain further improvement.

REFERENCES

1. Cheng, E., Cvitkovic, E., Wittes R. E. and Golbey, R. B., Germ
   cell tumours. VAB II in metastatic testicular cancer. Cancer,
   42, 2162-2168 (1978).

2. Einhorn, L. H. and Donohue, J. P., Cis-diamminedichloroplatinum,
   Vinblastine and Bleomycin combination chemotherapy in
   disseminated testicular cancer. Ann. Int. Med., 87, 293-298
   (1977).

3. Hoeffken, K. and Schmidt, C. G., Chemotherapy for localised
   testicular teratomas. Brit. J. Cancer, 37, 479-480 (1978).

4. Johnson, D. E., Bracken, R. B., Ayala, A. G. and Samuels, M. L.,
   Retroperitoneal lymphadenectomy as adjunctive therapy in
   selected cases of advanced testicular carcinoma. J. Urol., 116,
   66-68 (1976).

5. Klepp, O., Klepp, R., Høst, H., Asbjørnsengg, Talle, K. and
   Stenwig, A. E., Combination chemotherapy of germ cell tumours
   of the testis with Vincristine, Adriamycin, Cyclophosphamide,
   Actinomycin D and Medroxyprogesterone Acetate. Cancer, 40,
   638-646 (1977).

6. Merrin, C., Takita, H., Beckley, S. and Kassis, J., Treatment
    of recurrent and widespread testicular tumour by radical
    reductive surgery and multiple sequential chemotherapy. J. Urol.
    117, 291-295 (1977).

7. Merrin, C. E. and Takita, H., Cancer reductive surgery. Report
    of the simultaneous excision of abdominal and thoracic
    metastases from widespread testicular tumours. Cancer, 42,
    495-501 (1978).

8. Norton, L. and Simon, R., Tumour size, sensitivity to therapy
    and design of treatment schedules. Cancer Treat. Rep. 61,
    1307-1317 (1977).

9. Samuels, M. L., Johnson, D. E. and Holoye, P. Y., Continuous
    intravenous Bleomycin therapy with Vinblastine in stage III
    testicular neoplasia. Cancer Chemo. Rep., 59, 563-570 (1975).

10. Shabel, F. M. Jr., Concepts for systemic treatment of micro-
    metastases. Cancer, 35, 15-24 (1975).

11. Skinner, D. G., Non seminomatous testis tumours: a plan of
    management based on 96 patients to improve survival in all
    stages by combined therapeutic modalities. J. Urol., 115,
    65-69 (1976).

12. Staubitz, W. J., Early, K. S., Magoss, I. V. and Murphy, G. P.,
    Surgical management of testis tumour. J. Urol., 65, 113-117
    (1973).

13. Tyrrell, C. J. and Peckham, M. J., The response of lymphnode
    metastases of testicular teratoma to radiation therapy. Brit.
    J. Urol., 48, 363-370 (1976).

INDEX

515

SPEAKERS

L Andersson, Stockholm, Sweden
J Auvert, Paris, France
G S Barlas, Istanbul, Turkey
E Bercovich, Bologna, Italy
T Berlin, Stockholm, Sweden
M C Bishop, Cambridge, England
J P Blandy, London, England
C Bouffioux, Leige, Belgium
D P Byar, Bethesda, USA
M Camey, Suresnes, France
S Casanova, Bologna, Italy
L Castagnetta, Palermo, Italy
G D Chisholm, Edinburgh, Scotland
L Collste, Stockholm, Sweden
F Corrado, Bologna, Italy
H J de Voogt, Leiden,
  The Netherlands
L Denis, Antwerp, Belgium
M Duchek, Umea, Sweden
F Edsmyr, Stockholm, Sweden
A Ek, Lund, Sweden
H R England, London, England
J O Esho, Lagos, Nigeria
P L Esposti, Stockholm, Sweden
P A Gammelgaard, Copenhagen,
  Denmark
G Grechi, Florence, Italy
R R Hall, Newcastle-upon-Tyne,
  England
M Horňak, Bratislava,
  Czechoslovakia
G Jakse, Innsbruck, Austria
I Könyves, Helsinborg, Sweden
G Kunit, Salzburg, Austria
C E Lindholm, Malmo, Sweden

G Lingardh, Orebro, Sweden
F Lund, Copenhagen, Denmark
J A Martiñez-Pineiro, Madrid,
  Spain
D Melloni, Palermo, Italy
J H Mulder, Rotterdam, The
  Netherlands
R T D Oliver, London, England
S Pauli, Stockholm, Sweden
M Pavone-Macaluso, Palermo, Italy
G Pizzocaro, Milan, Italy
F Putti, Rome, Italy
J Renaud, Amsterdam, The Netherlands
C Rimondi, Bologna, Italy
B Richards, York, England
M R G Robinson, Pontefract, England
S Rocca Rossetti, Trieste, Italy
A Rost, Berlin, Germany
H Rübben, Aachen, West Germany
G Rutishauser, Basel, Switzerland
C C Schulman, Brussels, Belgium
P H Smith, Leeds, England
M Soli, Bologna, Italy
G Stoter, Utrecht, The Netherlands
G Studler, Vienna, Austria
D Tjabbes, Gravenhage, The
  Netherlands
B van der Werf-Messing, Rotterdam,
  The Netherlands
L Wahlqvist, Umeå, Sweden
H Wijkstrom, Stockholm, Sweden
R E Williams, Leeds, England
E J Zingg, Bern, Switzerland